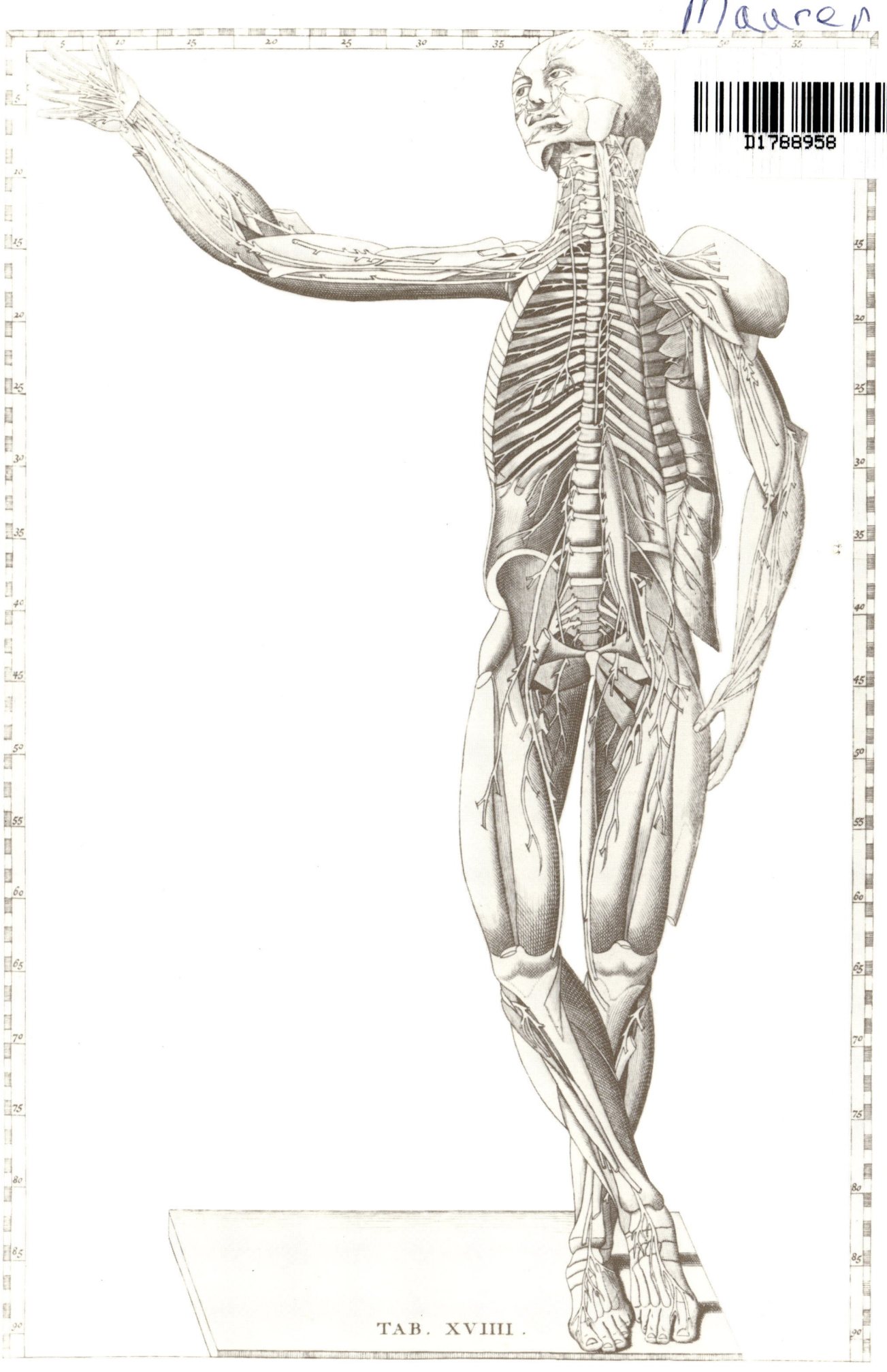

TAB. XVIIII.

Atlas of Orthopaedic Exposures

Detlef von Torklus · Toufick Nicola

Atlas of Orthopaedic Exposures

Second English Edition

Translated by Harry Monsen, Ph. D.
Professor of Anatomy
University of Illinois College of Medicine
Chicago

Urban & Schwarzenberg
Baltimore–Munich 1986

Urban & Schwarzenberg, Inc.
7 E. Redwood Street
Baltimore, Maryland 21202
USA

Urban & Schwarzenberg
Pettenkoferstraße 18
D-8000 München 2
West Germany

© Urban & Schwarzenberg 1986

Detlef von Torklus, Prof. Dr. med., Orthopädische Universitätsklinik, Eppendorf
Martinistraße 52, D-2000 Hamburg 20

A translation of Atlas orthopädisch-chirurgischer Operationsschnitte und Zugangswege;
3. Auflage, Urban & Schwarzenberg, München–Wien–Baltimore 1985

This work first appeared in English as Atlas of Orthopaedic Exposures by Toufick Nicola;
The Williams & Wilkins Company, Baltimore 1966

All rights including that of translation, reserved. No part of this publication may be reproduced, stored in a retrieval system, or transmitted in any other form or by any means, electronic, mechanical, recording, or otherwise without the prior written permission of the publisher.

Library of Congress Cataloging in Publication Data

Torklus, Detlef von:
 Atlas of orthopaedic exposures.
 Includes index.
 1. Orthopaedic surgery--Atlases. I. Nicola, Toufick.
 II. Title.
 RD733.2.T67 1986   617.3   85-31515
 ISBN 0-8067-2061-1

Printed by Kastner & Callwey, Munich.
Printed in Germany.

ISBN 0-8067-2061-1 Baltimore
ISBN 3-541-72061-1 Munich

Preface

The great demand for this Atlas and its popularity are attested to by the need for publishing two German editions and several reprints since 1971. These circumstances and subsequent developments in the field of surgery prompted the undertaking of the sisyphean task of reworking and expanding the Atlas with the inclusion of illustrations in color. The number of illustrations has nearly doubled, which is also reflected in the text.

It should be mentioned that this Atlas has gone through many stages in its development. The *Atlas of Surgical Approaches to Bones and Joints* by Nicola was first published in 1945. It was followed by a new *Atlas of Orthopaedic Exposures* in 1966. The first German edition in 1971 and the expanded edition of 1977 were written in cooperation with Dr. G. Turk, of Hamburg.

The concept of systematic organization, brevity, and simple language as well as a broad scope in regard to text and the creation of illustrative material have also been adhered to in this edition.

In particular, an attempt has consistently been made to tread the narrow path between schematic simplicity and detailed complexity and to include significant and purposeful information.

This Atlas is not meant to be a textbook of surgery. It is more valuable as a quick overview of the available exposures in the field of orthopedic surgery and, ideally, as a guide for "a la carte" procedures.

The exposures are usually presented as anatomical sequences. The method of stepwise progression was chosen to provide the busy surgeon with a good working basis and a quick overview. If one is too tired to read on the evening before the operation, the experienced surgeon can get oriented by studying the illustrations which dovetail with the text. The positioning of the patient is dealt with separately when it is deemed essential.

The presentation of a variety of alternative incisions and approaches is considered to have advantages. The exposures have been evaluated for their effectiveness throughout years of practical experience and they have consistently been supplemented and improved with pertinent details. The exposures are, as so much else in Medicine, applied science and in that respect undergo constant modifications. It is also left up to the user of this Atlas to test the validity of these approaches, which in spite of the careful attention paid to their practicability, may in special cases require deviation from the detailed procedures and sometimes result in failure. For these reasons, suggestions and corrections are welcome.

In the day-to-day surgical practice, the medical-historical basis, which has an eminent anatomical aspect, is easily lost. As a visual reminder of this relationship, the Atlas is "framed" in two old illustrations prepared in the 16th century.

I wish to thank the publishing firm of Urban & Schwarzenberg, and in particular, Mr. Urban, Dr. Müller, and Dr. Dabelstein, for their helpfulness during the preparation of this edition, for their patience, and their much appreciated willingness to consider my demands associated with the expansion of the Atlas.

Mrs. Ingrid von Marchtaler of Hamburg has demonstrated a clear insight into the goals and objectives of the Atlas in her creation of the illustrations. My heartfelt thanks to her for the harmonious cooperation during the many years of reviewing rough drafts and the careful completion of the large number of illustrations, a task that now seems to have been so effortless. I also wish to thank Mrs. Andrea Mesdag of Hannover for the excellent graphics associated with the illustrations in part II of the Atlas. I thank Mrs. Czaplik and Mrs. Strey, our secretaries, for their conscientious participation in the formal layout of the present edition.

Hamburg, Summer 1984   DETLEF VON TORKLUS

Contents

Part I: Upper Limb

Contents 2
Introductory Remarks 4
A. Shoulder Girdle 5
B. Shoulder 16
C. Upper Arm 40
D. Elbow 46
E. Forearm 61
F. Wrist Region 73
G. Hand 83
H. Finger 99

Part II: Neck and Trunk

Contents 111
A. Introduction 112
B. Neck – Cervical Spine 114
C. Thoracic Spine 126
D. Lumbar Region 130
E. Pelvis 141

Part III: Lower Limb

Contents 150
A. Hip Region 152
B. Thigh 170
C. Knee Region 179
D. Leg 199
E. Malleolar Region 210
F. Foot 224
G. Toes 233

Part I
Upper Limb

Contents Part I

Upper Limb

Introductory Remarks 4

A. Shoulder Girdle 5

Clavicle 5
Acromioclavicular Joint 7
   Supraclavicular Exposure 7
   Infraclavicular Exposure 8
Scapula – Medial Margin 9
   Medial Exposure 9
Posterior Surface of Scapula 10
Scapular Notch 14
Sternoclavicular Joint 15

B. Shoulder 16

Applied Anatomy 16
Patient Positions 20
Shoulder Joint 21
   Short Anterior Exposure 21
   Anterosuperior Extension 22
   Long Anterior Exposure 24
   Anteromedial Exposure 26
   Lateral Exposure 28
   Transacromial Exposure of *Kessel* 29
   Transverse Lateral Exposure 30
   Anteroinferior Exposure 31
   Anterior Axillary Exposure 32
   Anterolateral Exposure 33
   Anteroposterior Exposure 34
   Posterior Aspect of Shoulder Joint 37
   Applied Anatomy 37
   Posterior Exposure 38
   Posterior Exposure of *Kocher* 39

C. Upper Arm 40

Shaft of the Humerus 40
   Anterolateral Exposure 40
   Anteromedial Exposure 42
   Musculocutaneous Nerve 43
   Posterior Exposure 44

D. Elbow 46

Elbow Joint (1) 46
   Anterior Exposure 46
   Lateral Exposure 48
Radial Nerve 50
   Applied Anatomy 50
Head of Radius 51
   Posterolateral Exposure 51
Elbow Joint (2) 52
   Medial Exposure 52
   Posterolateral Exposure 54
   Posteromedial Exposure 56
   Posterior Exposure 58
   Posterior Curved Incision 60

E. Forearm 61

Proximal Radius and Upper Fourth
of Ulna 61
Elbow Joint – Posterior Exposure 61
Radial Nerve – Supinator Arch 63
   Lateral Exposure 63
Shaft of the Ulna 65
   Posterior Exposure 65
Shaft of the Radius 67
   Posterior Exposure 67
Shafts of the Radius and Ulna 68
   Posterior Exposure 68
Median Nerve 69
   Volar Exposure 69
Distal Radius 70
   Dorsal Exposure 70
   Volar Exposure 71
Palmar Tendon 72
   Volar Exposure 72

Upper Limb

F. Wrist Region 73

Wrist Joint 73
- Applied Anatomy 73
- Dorsal Exposure 74

Wrist Joint – Palm 76
- Applied Anatomy 76

Carpal Tunnel – Wrist Joint 77
- Volar Exposure 77
- Flexor Retinaculum 79
- Palmar Branch of Median Nerve 79

Distal Ulnar Nerve – Guyon's Tunnel 80
- Volar Exposure 80

Radial Wrist Region – Anatomical Snuff Box 81
- Applied Anatomy 81

Anatomical Snuff Box – Extensor Tendons of Thumb 82

G. Hand 83

Carpus 83
- Applied Anatomy 83

Scaphoid Bone 84
- Medial Exposure 84
- Volar Exposure 85
- Transverse Exposure 85

Lunate Bone 86
- Dorsal Exposure 86
- Volar Exposure 86

Trapezium Bone – Saddle Joint of Thumb 87
- Dorsal Exposure 87

Metacarpal I – Saddle Joint of Thumb 88
- Volar Exposure 88

Long Flexor Tendons of Thumb 89
- Volar Exposure 89
- Tension Lines of the Palm 89

Palmar Aponeurosis 90
- Applied Anatomy 90

Palm – Palmar Aponeurosis 91
- Digitopalmar Zig-Zag Incision of *Bruner* 91
- Y-Incision of *Millesi* 92
- Additional Volar Exposures 93

Palm 94
- Wide Volar Exposure of *Kanavel* 94

Distal Palm 95
- Transverse Exposure 95

Dorsum of Hand – Tension Lines of the Skin 96

Metacarpals II–V 97
- Dorsal Exposure 97

Dorsum of Hand 98
- Dorsal Exposures 98

H. Finger 99

- Volar Exposure 99
- Digitopalmar Z-Incision of *Iselin* 99
- Volar Digital Exposures 100
- Dorsal Exposures 102
- Dorsolateral Exposure 103
- Terminal Phalanx and Nail Bed-Exposures 104
- Finger Tip-Exposures 104

Finger 105
- Midaxial Exposure 105
- Midaxial Hinged Flap 107

Syndactyly of the Fingers – Zig-Zag Incision of *Blauth* 108

Amniotic Syndactyly – Z-Incision of *Iselin* 108

Introductory Remarks

1. Operations on the elbow, forearm, and hand are usually performed on a bloodless limb by the use of a pneumatic tourniquet, in order to gain a detailed overview of structures. The extremity is elevated and exsanguinated by means of a soft rubber bandage, which is wrapped progressively from the distal to the proximal area until it reaches the pneumatic tourniquet.
2. Often a totally bloodless limb is not desirable because some blood affords better visualization of the different structures. This can be achieved by elevating the extended limb for 3–6 minutes. Then apply a pneumatic tourniquet.
3. Pressure in the pneumatic cuff should exceed systolic pressure by 60–100 mm Hg.
4. The cuff should not be pressurized beyond 250–300 mm Hg.
5. Bipolar cautery is preferred for hemostasis.

A. Shoulder Girdle

Clavicle

Indications

1. Irreducible fractures
2. Ununited fractures (pseudoarthroses)
3. Malunited healed fractures exerting pressure on underlying brachial plexus and blood vessels
4. Bone tumors
5. Inflammatory processes

Operative Steps

1. Make the skin incision in the supraclavicular fossa parallel with the portion of the clavicle to be exposed (Figs. I-1 and I-2).
2. Identify the platysma and incise it and the underlying periosteum along the anterior clavicular border.
3. Strip off the periosteum with the attached trapezius muscle and the clavicular portion of the sternocleidomastoid muscle.
4. Elevate the periosteum with the attached deltoid and pectoralis major muscles.
5. Expose the clavicle by retracting the mobilized muscles (Fig. I-3). If necessary, pass a Hohmann retractor under the clavicle.

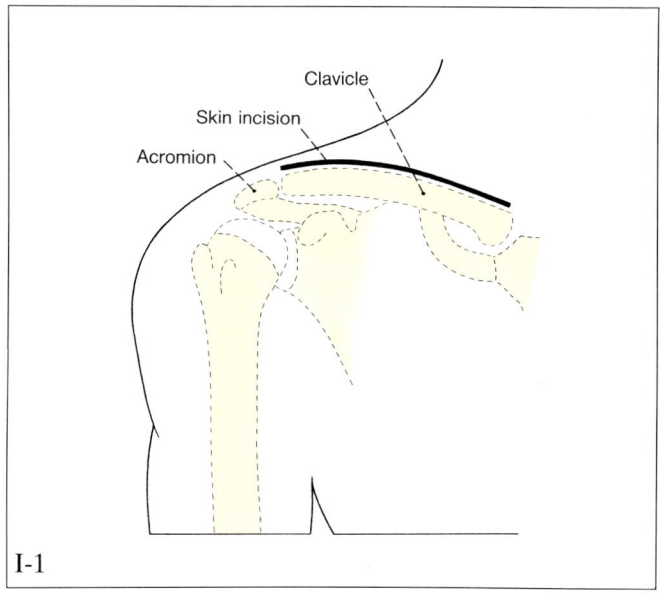

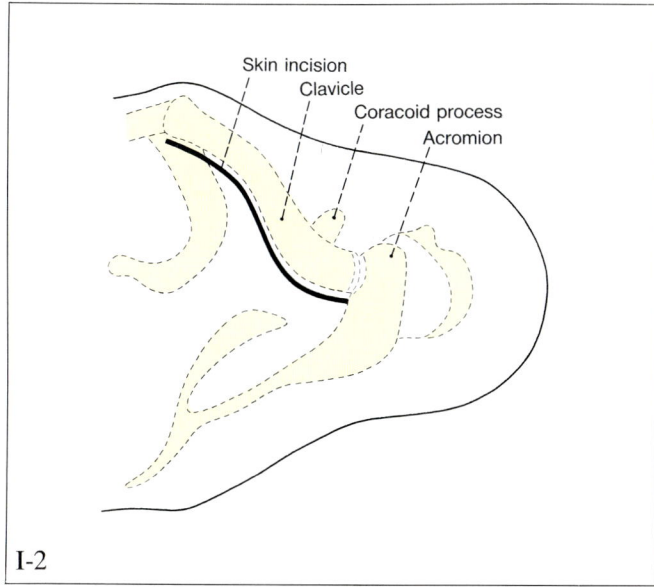

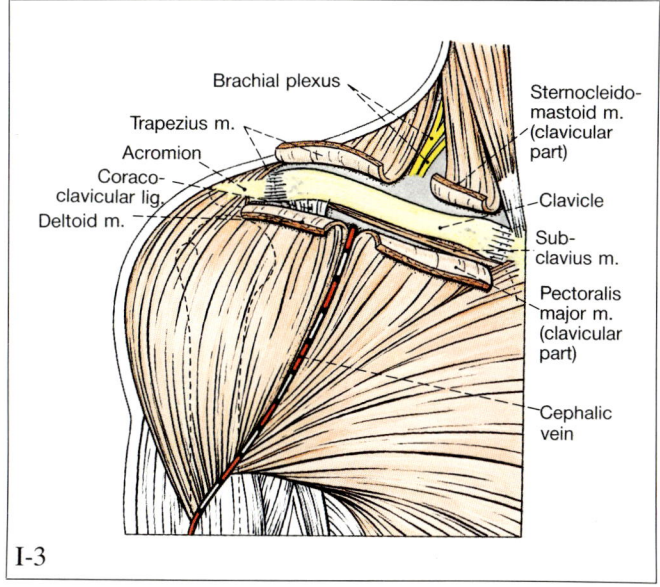

Clavicle

Notes

Placing the skin incision in the supraclavicular fossa leaves a less obvious scar later. Furthermore, the scar is less likely to spread, form keloids, or adhere to the clavicle.

Alternative

Although the approach through the supraclavicular fossa is preferred for cosmetic reasons, a curved incision 1–2 finger breadths below the clavicle may occasionally be selected (Fig. I-4).

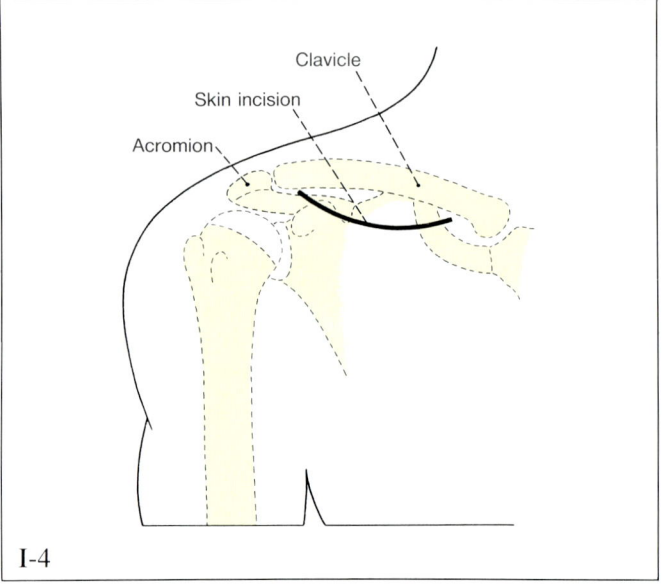

I-4

Acromioclavicular Joint

Supraclavicular Exposure

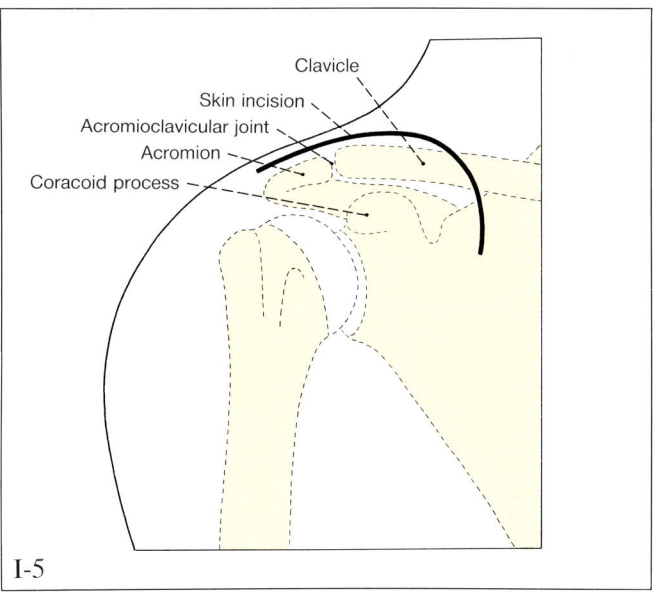

I-5

Indications

1. Acute irreducible dislocation
2. Chronic dislocation
3. Resection of the distal part of the clavicle (excision arthroplasty)
4. Repair of the coracoclavicular ligaments
5. Excision of tumors
6. Inflammatory processes

Operative Steps

1. Make a supraclavicular skin incision along the acromion and the distal clavicle. Continue it across the clavicle at the level of the deltopectoral groove and then downward as a curved extension (Fig. I-5).
2. Frequently a supraclavicular skin incision is adequate without the curved extension (Fig. I-6).
3. The cephalic vein must be avoided.
4. Elevate the deltoid muscle subperiosteally from the anterior border of the clavicle and the acromion.
5. Detach the trapezius muscle subperiosteally from the upper part of the clavicle and the acromion.
6. Reflect the muscles to expose the acromioclavicular joint and the coracoid process with the conoid and trapezoid ligaments (Fig. I-7).
7. Make a longitudinal incision through the middle of the capsule (Fig. I-7). Detach the capsule from the acromion and the clavicle. The joint can now be entered by reflecting the cut edges of the capsule ventrally and dorsally.

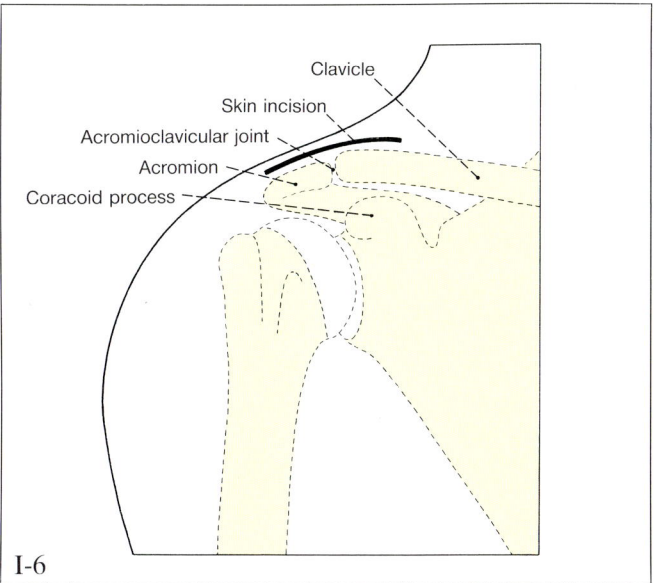

I-6

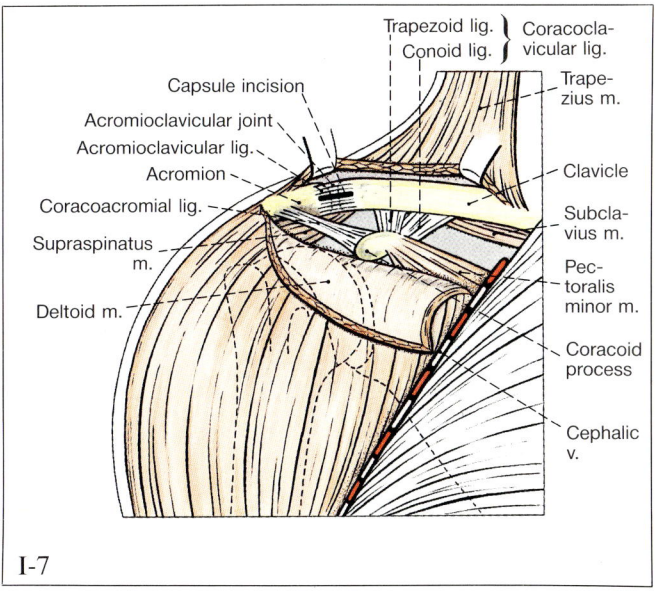

I-7

Alternative Infraclavicular Exposure

Operative Steps

The infraclavicular incision begins at the lateral edge of the acromion and continues beneath the acromion and the clavicle to the level of the deltopectoral sulcus. From this point it curves downward (Fig. I-8).

Notes

1. The articular surfaces of the acromioclavicular joint incline medially and downward, thus favoring an upward displacement of the clavicle.
2. The superior and inferior acromioclavicular ligaments are really thickened portions of the capsule that unite the bony components of the joint. The coracoclavicular ligament with its two parts, the trapezoid and conoid ligaments, represents the main fixation of the clavicle. It extends between the lower surface of the clavicle and the base of the coracoid process and must be avoided.

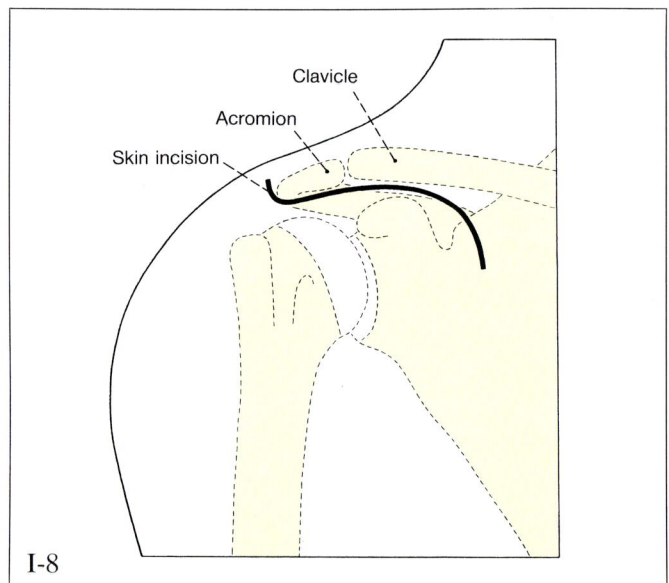

I-8

Scapula – Medial Margin

Medial Exposure

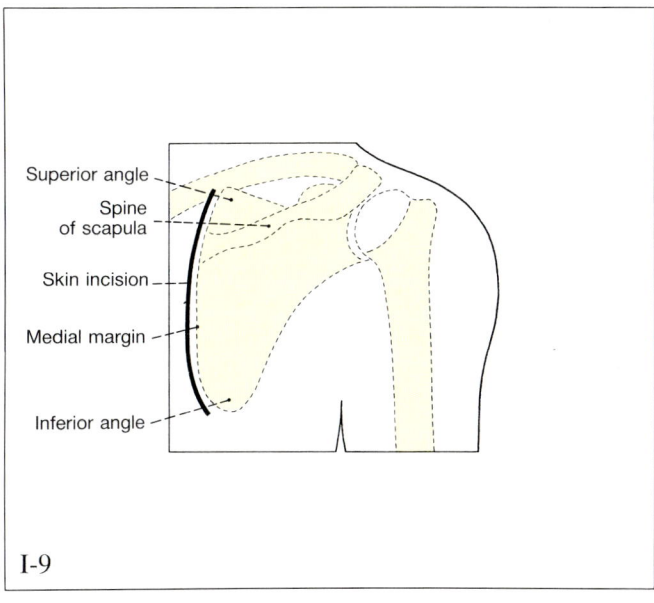

I-9

Indications

1. Inflammatory processes
2. Tumors
3. Irreducible complicated fractures

Operative Steps

To expose the medial margin of the scapula:
1. Make a slightly curved skin incision from the superior angle of the scapula along the inner scapular edge to the inferior angle (Fig. I-9).
2. Expose the muscles attaching to the medial border.
3. Detach the trapezius muscle along line A indicated in Fig. I-10.
4. Retract this part of the trapezius muscle so that the underlying muscle attachments can be seen.
5. Detach these muscles subperiosteally – levator scapulae, major rhomboid, minor rhomboid, supraspinatus, infraspinatus, teres minor, and teres major – close to the medial scapular border along line B (Fig. I-11) so that the bony scapular edge is visible.
6. With subperiosteal elevation of the musculature, hemorrhage is reduced to a minimum.

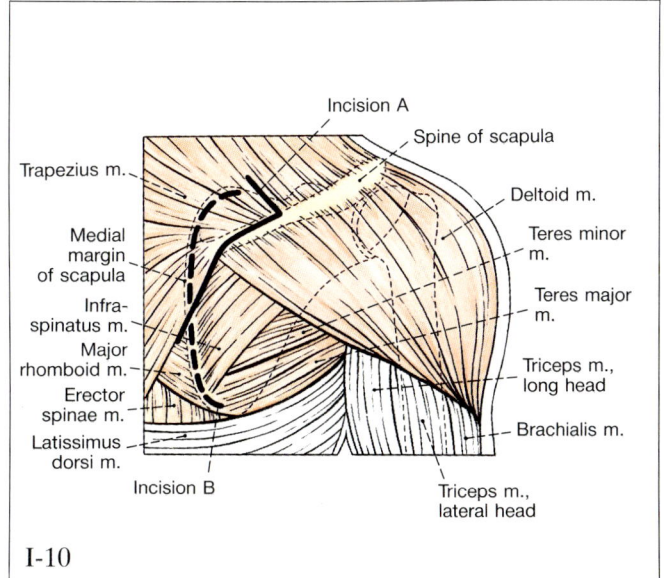

I-10

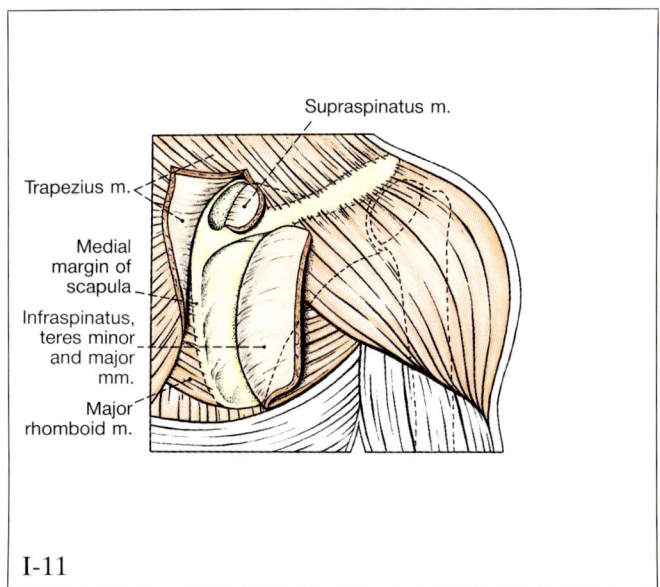

I-11

Posterior Surface of Scapula

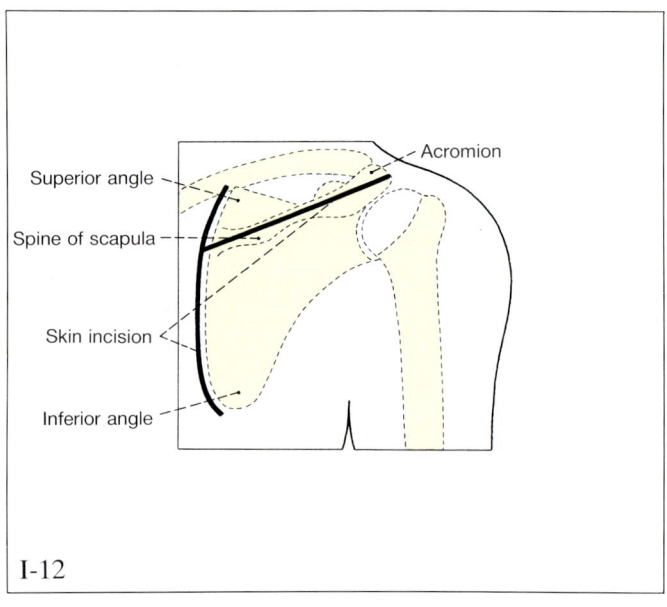

I-12

Operative Steps

1. Make a T-shaped skin incision. Begin the first incision at the superior angle of the scapula and continue along the inner lip of the scapular border to the inferior angle.
2. Begin the second incision at the intersection of the first with the spine of the scapula, and extend it to the tip of the acromion (Fig. I-12).
3. The muscle incisions correspond to the skin incisions. The first cut is made into the periosteum over the spine of the scapula, following line A in Fig. I-13. Continue it medially through the trapezius muscle for about 2 cm.
4. Then strip the trapezius muscle subperiosteally off the spine and reflect it upward.
5. Likewise, elevate the deltoid muscle subperiosteally from the spine and reflect it downward and laterally.
6. The muscles attaching to the inner scapular border (Fig. I-13, Incision B) are separated from the posterior scapular surface by sharp dissection and reflected laterally (Fig. I-14).
7. Hemorrhage is reduced to a minimum if the dissection is conducted close to the bone.

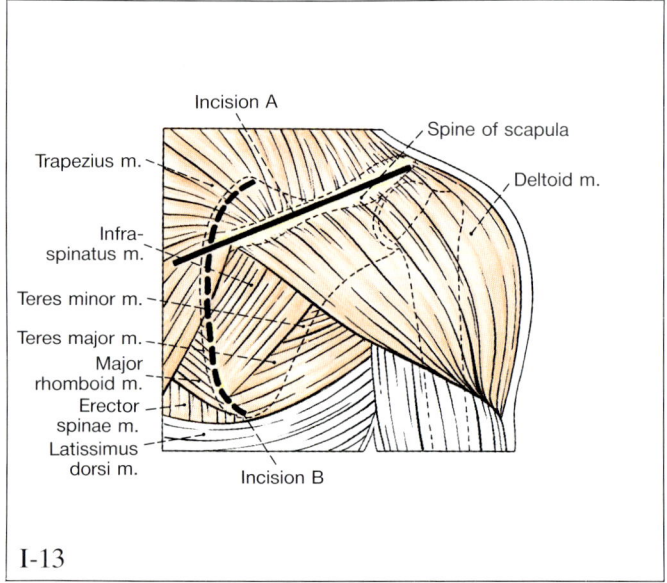

I-13

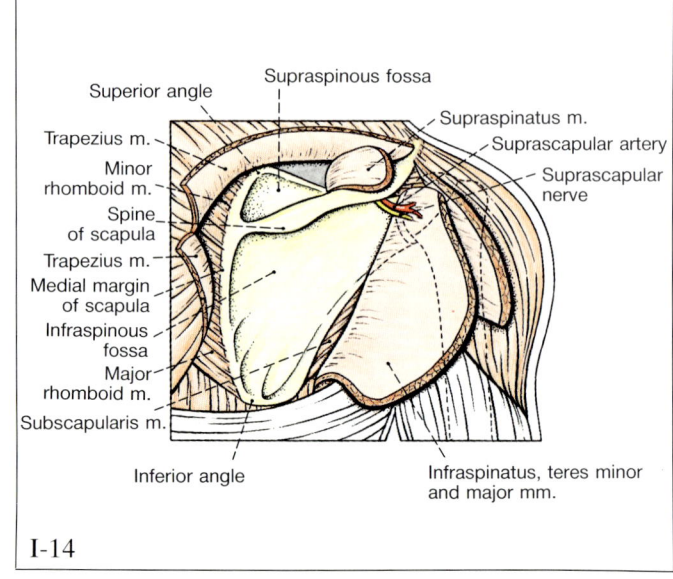

I-14

Posterior Surface of Scapula — Exposures

8. When the supraspinatus muscle is reflected, the suprascapular nerve, which passes through the scapular notch and innervates the supra- and infraspinatus muscles, must be protected (Fig. I-15).
9. When the group of muscles below the scapular spine is reflected, the neurovascular bundle to the infraspinatus muscle must be guarded against injury as it passes under the spine in the upper, outer corner of the field (Fig. I-15).

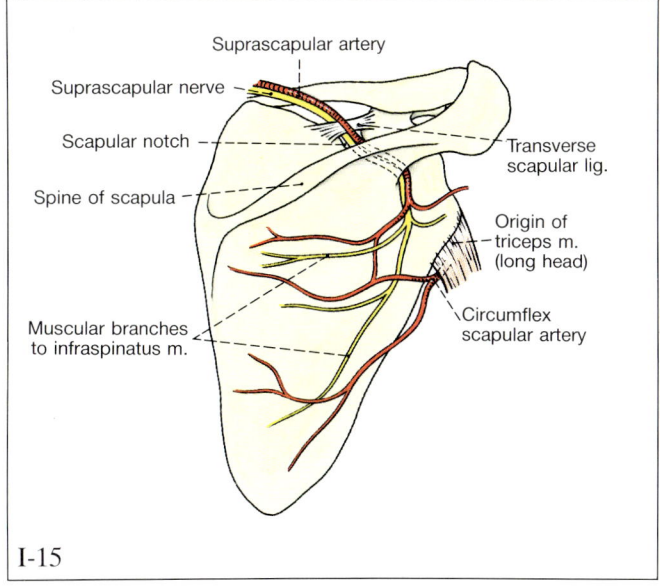

Posterior Surface of Scapula — Alternative A

Alternative A

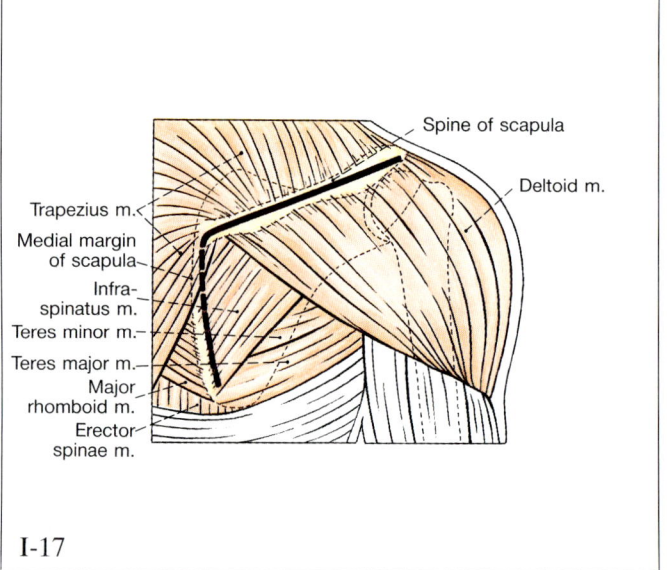

I-16

1. In a limited approach that does not involve the supraspinous fossa, a shorter incision is adequate.
2. In this case an angular skin and muscle incision follows the spine of the scapula and the infraspinous medial scapular border (Figs. I-16 and I-17).
3. Detach the deltoid muscle subperiosteally from the spine and reflect it laterally. The trapezius muscle remains intact.
4. Detach the infraspinatus and teres minor muscles subperiosteally by sharp dissection and reflected them laterally (Fig. I-18).
5. The suprascapular nerve with accompanying vessels is visible in the upper, outer corner of the field and should be protected (Fig. I-18). Compare with Fig. I-15).

I-17

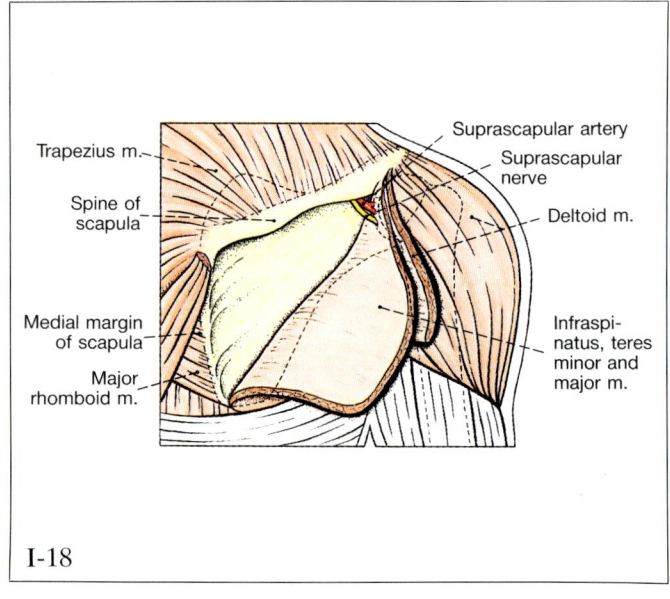

I-18

Posterior Surface of Scapula — Alternative B

Alternative B

1. With minor procedures, such as a biopsy, a less extensive incision may be adequate.
2. Make an oblique, slightly curved incision under the scapular spine (Fig. I-19).
3. Detach the deltoid muscle subperiosteally from the spine of the scapula.
4. Make a blunt entry between the infraspinatus and teres minor and retract the muscles (Fig. I-20).

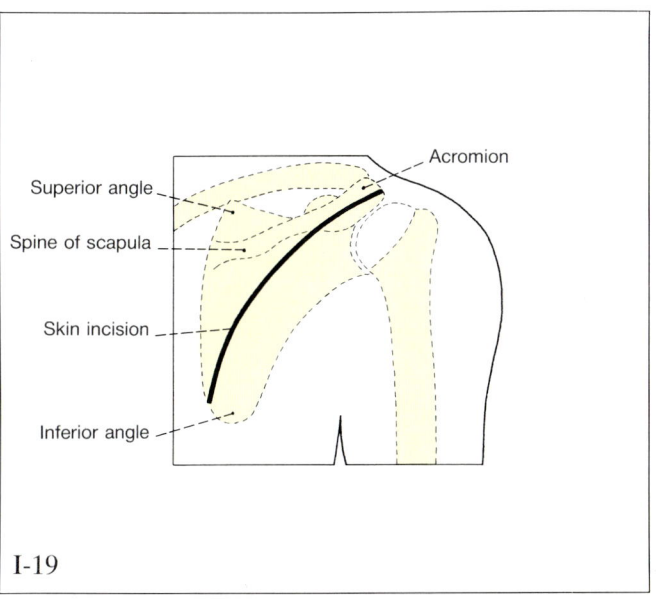

I-19

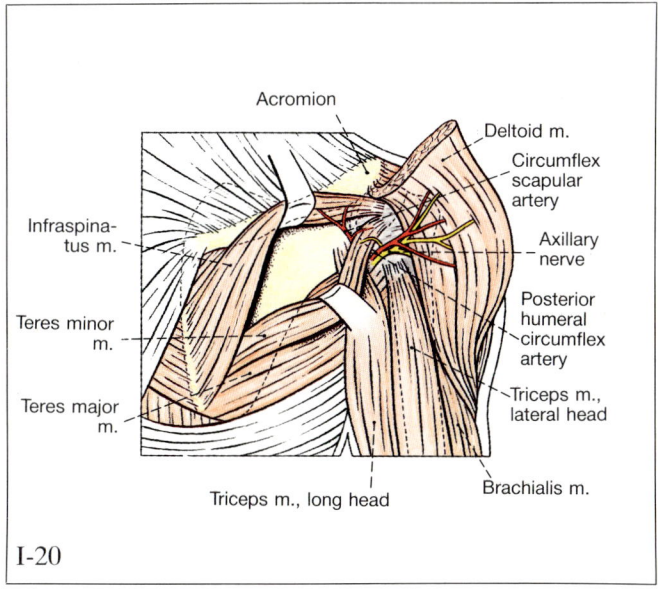

I-20

Scapular Notch

Indication

Suprascapular nerve entrapment syndrome

Operative Steps

1. Make the skin incision over the middle of the scapular spine, with an angular extension along the fiber direction of the trapezius muscle (Fig. I-21).
2. Release the trapezius attachment on the spine subperiosteally. Bluntly separate and bilaterally retract the trapezius muscle fibers near the medial aspect of the incision.
3. The relationship of structures is indicated schematically in Fig. I-22. While the suprascapular nerve runs through the scapular notch under the transverse scapular ligament, the suprascapular artery passes over the ligament into the supraspinous fossa.

Notes

1. The development of the scapular notch is variable.
2. The superior transverse scapular ligament may be ossified.
3. The inferior transverse scapular ligament, which bridges the neurovascular bundle and extends to the posterior glenoid lip, is inconstant (Fig. I-22).

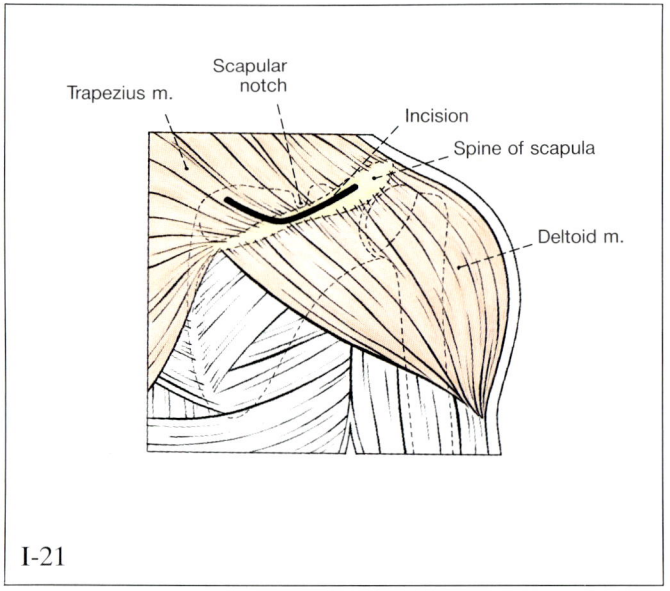

I-21

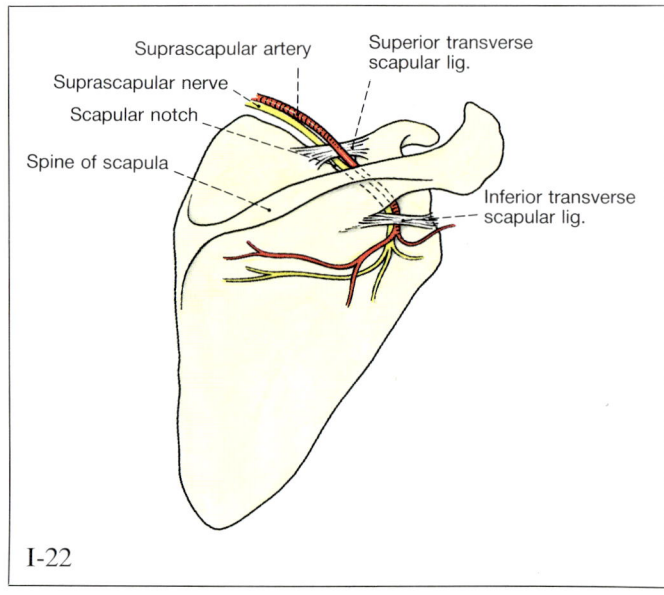

I-22

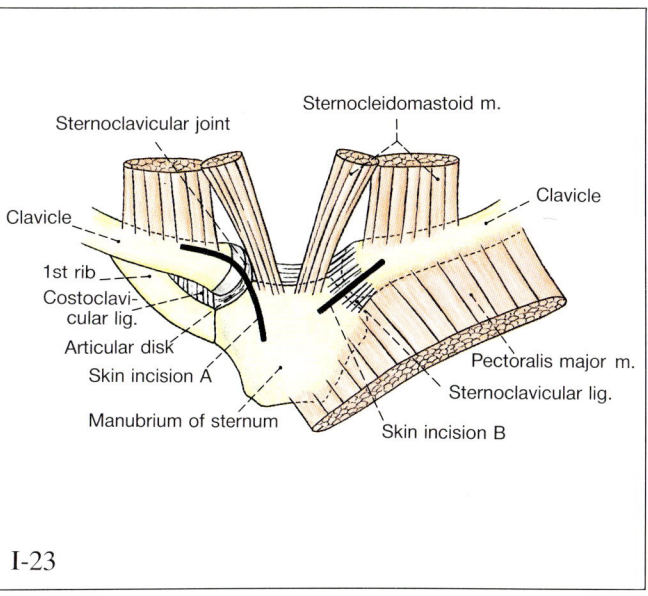

I-23

Sternoclavicular Joint

Indications

1. Acute irreducible dislocation
2. Chronic dislocation
3. Tumors in the medial clavicular region
4. Inflammatory and osteonecrotic processes

Operative Steps

1. Make a curved skin incision over the sternoclavicular joint beginning in the supraclavicular fossa about 2 cm from the medial end of the clavicle. Continue it medially to the lateral border of the sternal head of the sternocleidomastoid muscle and then downward for a distance of 2 cm over the manubrium of the sternum (Fig. I-23, skin incision A).
2. Alternative: for a limited exposure (i.e., biopsy), a straight incision over the sternoclavicular joint may be sufficient (Fig. I-23, skin incision B). The joint is then entered directly.
3. Expose the clavicular and sternal heads of the sternocleidomastoid muscle.
4. After cutting the platysma, incise the periosteum on the anterior surface of the clavicle.
5. Detach the sternocleidomastoid and pectoralis major muscles to expose the articular capsule.
6. Incise the capsule transversely and reflect the ends upward and downward for entry into the joint.
7. A thin articular disk attaching cranially and caudally to the capsule is seen inside the joint (Fig. I-24).

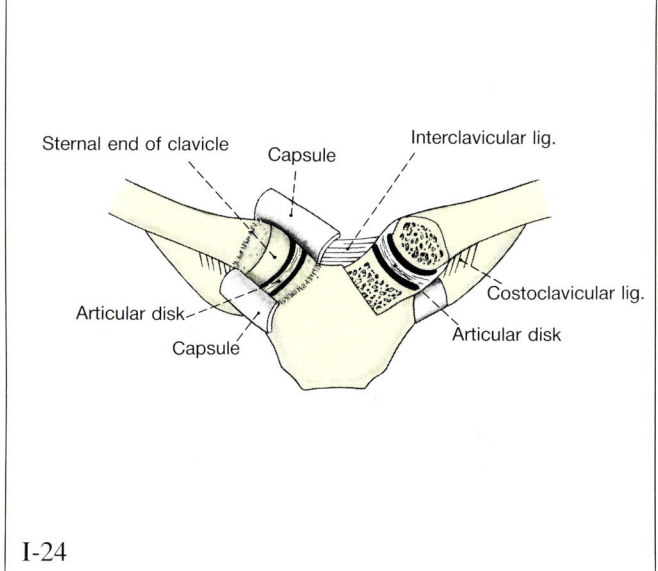

I-24

Notes

1. The clavicle is attached by means of the interclavicular, the anterior and posterior sternoclavicular, and the costoclavicular ligaments (Fig. I-24).
2. When necessary, a part of the sternal end of the clavicle may be resected without fear of disarticulation. The ligaments and the posterior capsular wall must remain intact.

B. Shoulder

Applied Anatomy

Topography of the "Arch" of the Shoulder

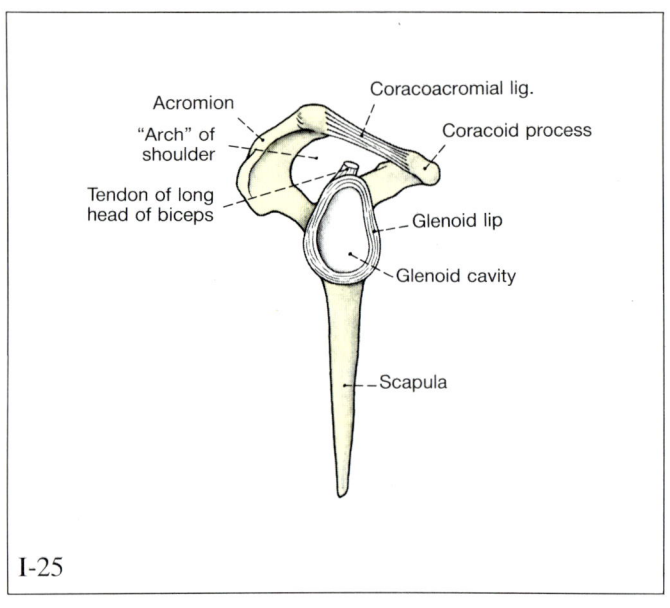

I-25

The "arch" of the shoulder joint (seen in a lateral view in Fig. I-25) is formed by the acromion, the coracoacromial ligament, and the coracoid process.

Topography of the Rotator Cuff

1. In a lateral view, the raised, fan-shaped muscles of the rotator cuff are clearly seen with the tendons radiating from their horseshoe-like area of attachment (Fig. I-26).
2. Side view (Figs. I-27 and I-28).
3. Front view (Fig. I-29).

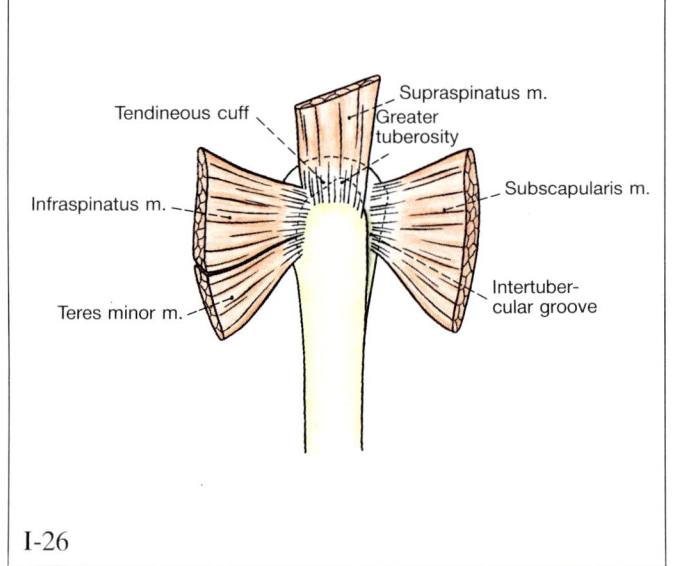

I-26

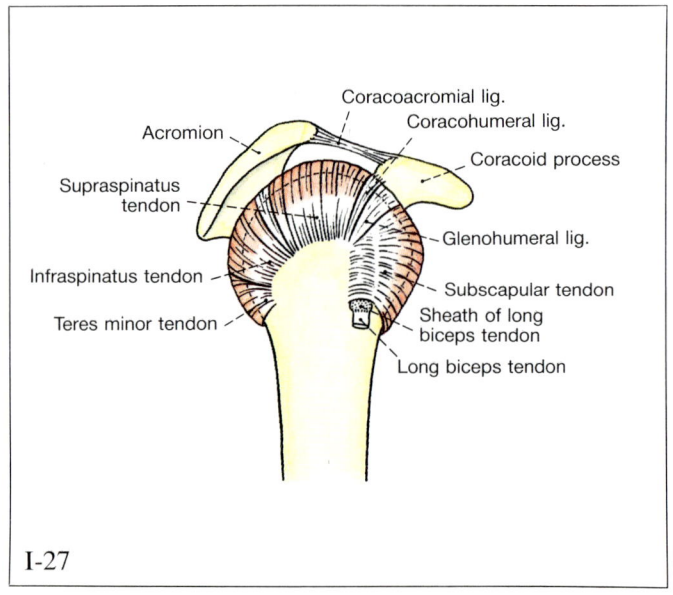

I-27

Shoulder — Applied Anatomy

Topography of the Shoulder Joint

1. The schematic frontal section (Fig. I-30) shows the close relationship between the rotator cuff and the shoulder joint. The acromion, peripheral structures of the articular surface, the coracoacromial ligament, and the coracoid process, in front, take part in the formation of the "arch" of the shoulder.
2. The subacromial bursa lies under the acromion and extends distally, covered by the subdeltoid fascia. An isolated subdeltoid bursa may be present at this point. The tendon of the supraspinatus muscle lies directly underneath the subacromial bursa.

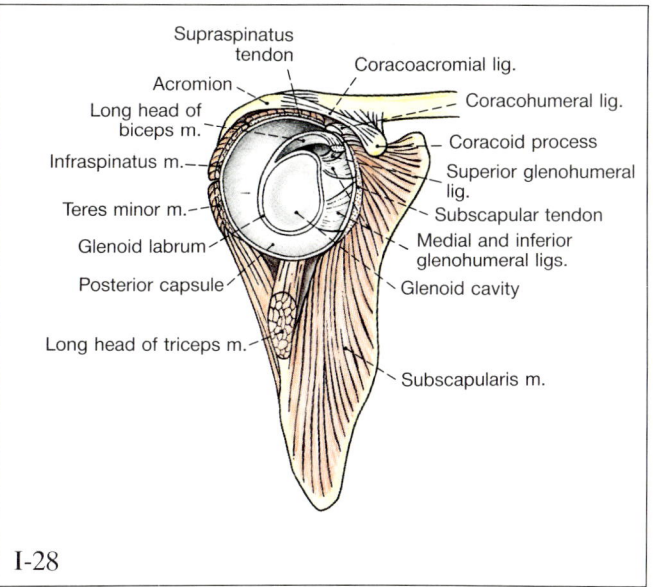

I-28

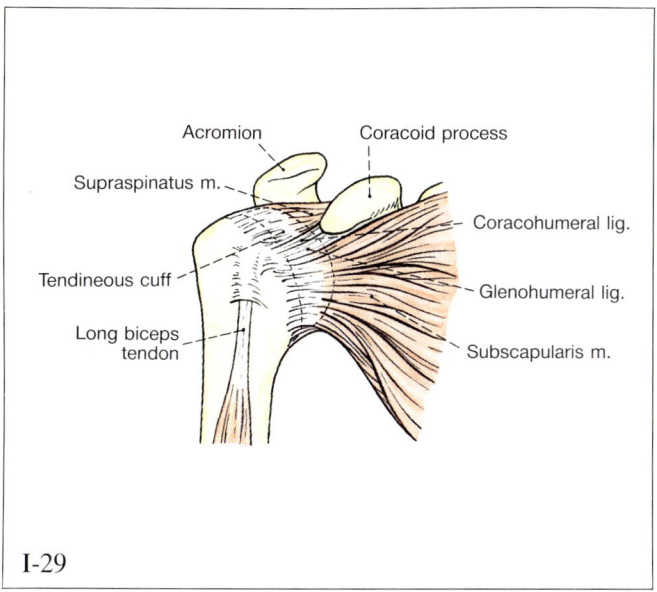

I-29

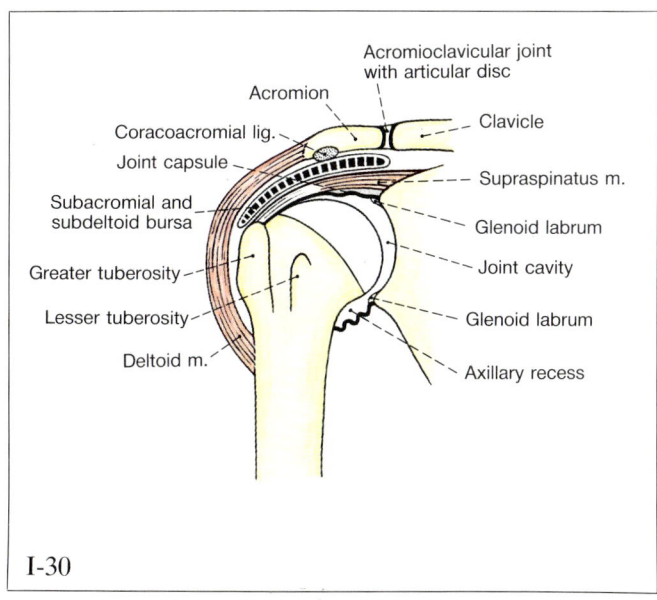

I-30

3. The subcapsular, intraarticular course of the long biceps tendon is shown in Fig. I-31.
4. The synovial component of the shoulder joint is seen frontally in Fig. I-32.
5. The close relationship of the coracoacromial ligament to the joint, the proximity of the synovial sac to the acromioclavicular joint, and the sleeve enveloping the long biceps tendon are important practical considerations.

Notes

1. Preoperative control of the patient's position is extremely important in shoulder operations.
2. A flexible position that permits movements of the shoulder joint in all planes also offers the option of expanding the operative field, as needed.
3. Preoperative failure to correctly position the patient hampers the proper execution of many shoulder operations because of inability to evaluate the overall situation.
4. In a partially frozen shoulder, the mobilization of the joint is bloodless prior to the corrective operative procedure.

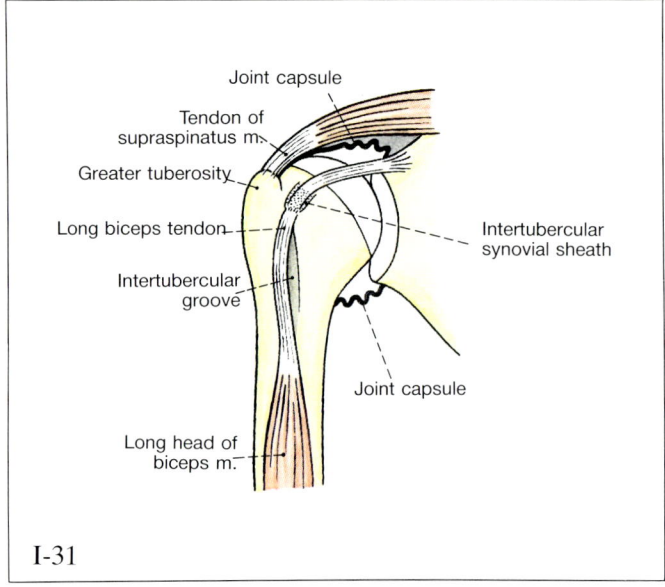

I-31

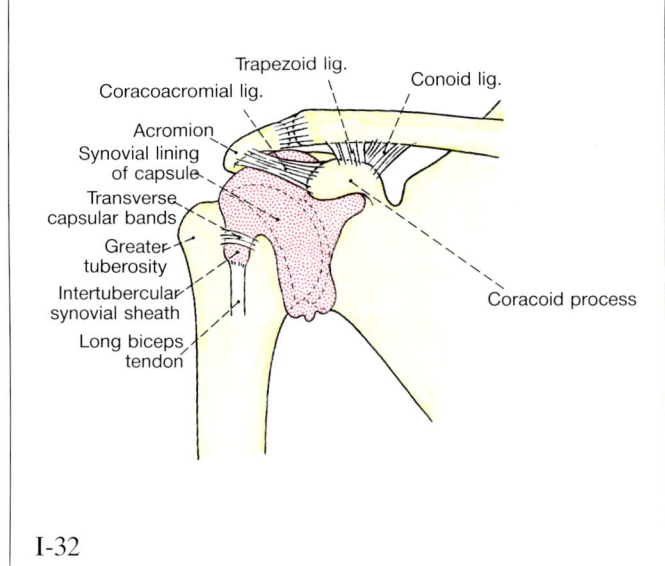

I-32

Collateral Circulation in the Shoulder Region

During the course of operations in the shoulder region, the following arteries may be injured (Fig. I-33):
1. Subclavian
2. Thoracoacromial with its two branches:
   a. Acromial branch
   b. Deltoid branch
3. Posterior humeral circumflex
4. Anterior humeral circumflex
5. Axillary
6. Deep brachial
7. Subscapular
8. Brachial
9. Superior ulnar collateral
10. Suprascapular

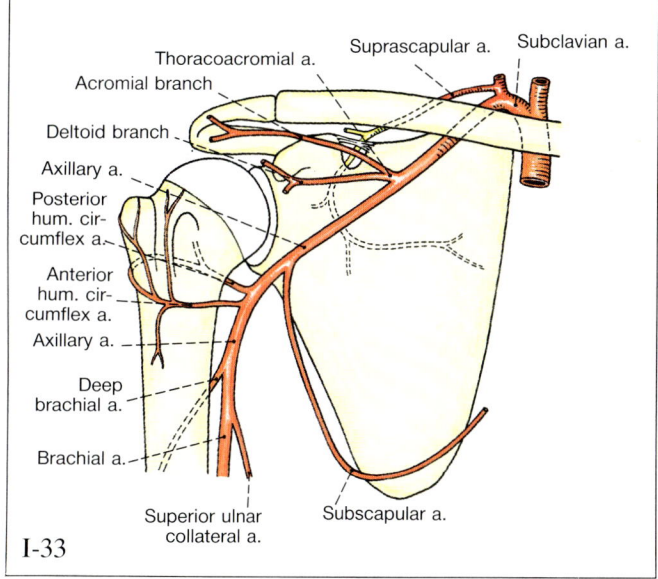

I-33

Shoulder

Patient Positions

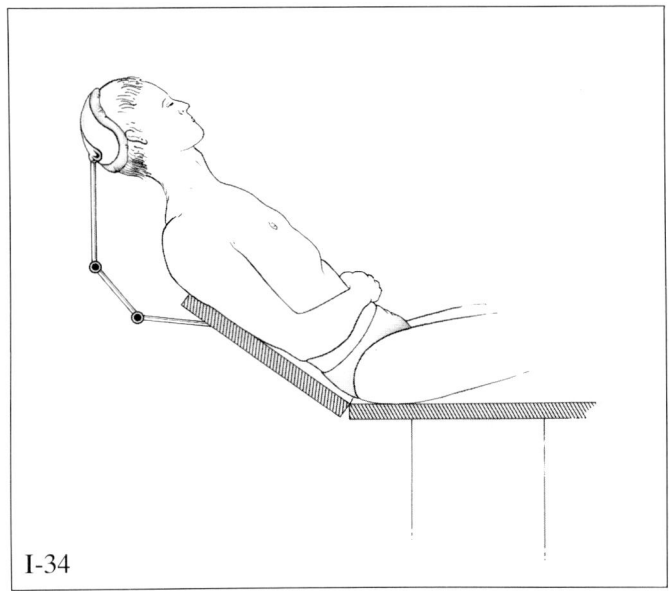

I-34

1. Many shoulder operations may be performed with the patient in a simple supine position. In general, the limb should be movable.
2. Extensive operations on the shoulder demand a generous operative field with full freedom of movement of the corresponding limb. This must be considered when the patient is draped and placed on the table.
3. A great degree of freedom of movement of the limb is achieved when the head support of the operating table is pulled out so that the shoulders are elevated (Fig. I-34).
4. Furthermore, both the head support and the patient should be moved toward the side of the operation so that the shoulder extends slightly beyond the edge of the table.
5. Finally, the head and upper torso are placed in an inclined position by elevating the head end of the table (Fig. I-35). This makes it possible to reach the dorsal aspect of the shoulder, which can become necessary for the exposure of a ruptured rotator cuff.
6. To prevent the patient from sliding down, the foot end of the table is also angled so that the lower limbs are correspondingly elevated. It is helpful to place a pillow under the knee and a padded ring under the heel.
7. The anesthetist sits on the opposite side of the patient so that there is full freedom of movement toward the head. In addition, the head may be tilted somewhat to the contralateral side. A mask over the head would be in the way and therefore is either not used or only placed on the contralateral side.
8. The position offers a full view of the "arch" of the shoulder over the rotator cuff (supraspinatus muscle and also partly the infraspinatus muscle) by pushing the adducted arm backward (Fig. I-36). The arm also may be rotated.
9. The shoulder should be appropriately draped so that it is accessible from all sides and freely movable.

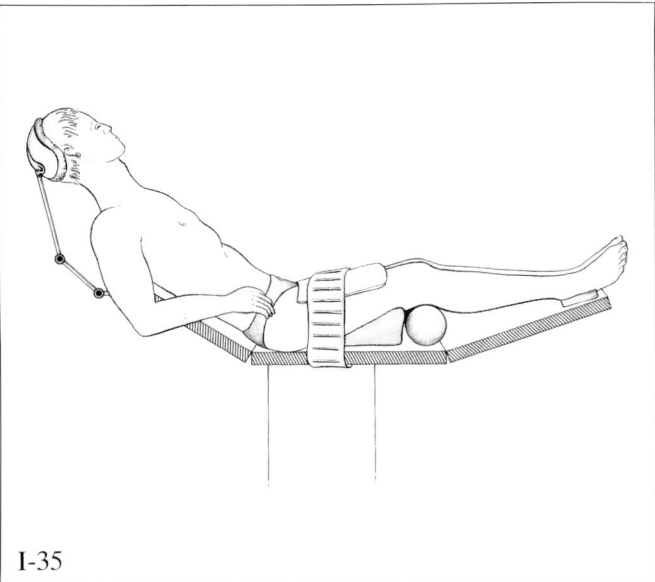

I-35

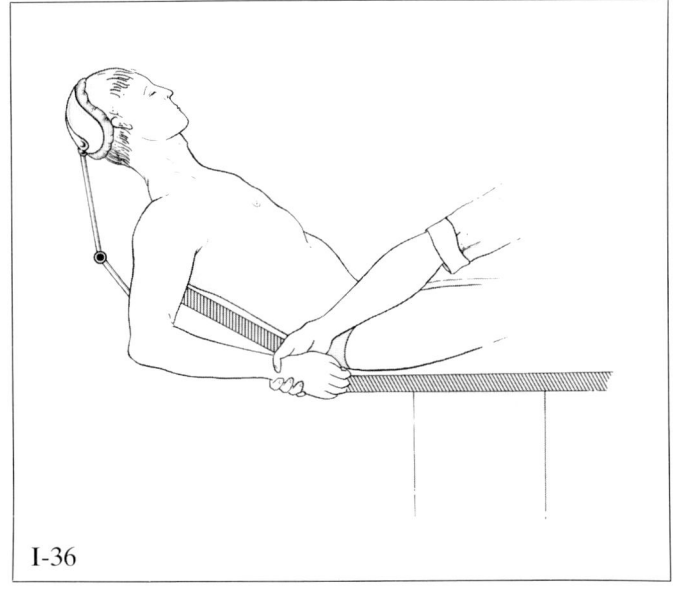

I-36

Shoulder Joint

Short Anterior Exposure

Standard Exposure A

Indications

1. Exploration of the shoulder joint
2. Exploration of the rotator cuff
3. Rupture of the rotator cuff
4. Rupture of the long biceps tendon
5. Calcium deposits in tendons
6. Excision of the coracoacromial ligament in impingement syndrome

Operative Steps

1. Make a 4- to 5-cm longitudinal incision beginning at the acromioclavicular joint and continuing along the fiber direction of the deltoid muscle (Fig. I-37).
2. Bluntly enter the deltoid muscle (Fig. I-38). Retract the edges medially and laterally until the subacromial bursa is visible. The bursa may be retracted medially or incised. The coracoacromial ligament also may be divided or resected.
3. By appropriate rotation of the arm, the anterior or lateral aspects of the joint capsule can be brought into view. The readily palpable intertubercular sulcus is a good landmark.

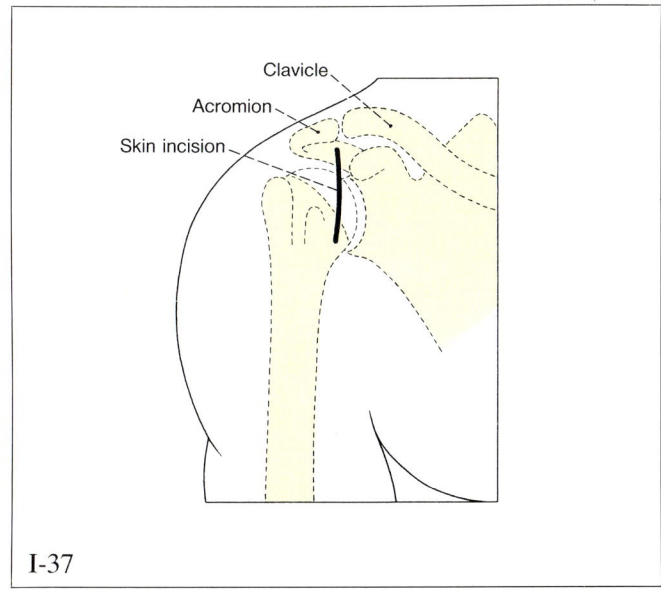

I-37

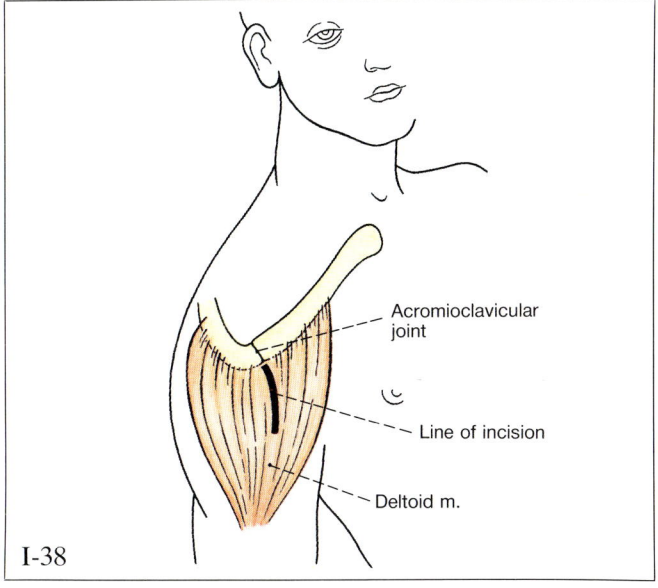

I-38

Shoulder Joint — Anterosuperior Extension

Alternative Anterosuperior Extension "Sabre Cut"

Operative Steps

1. A wider exposure is obtained by continuing the incision about 3–4 cm beyond the acromioclavicular joint (Fig. I-39).
2. In addition, the anteromedial part of the acromion may be resected as far as the acromioclavicular joint (Fig. I-40).

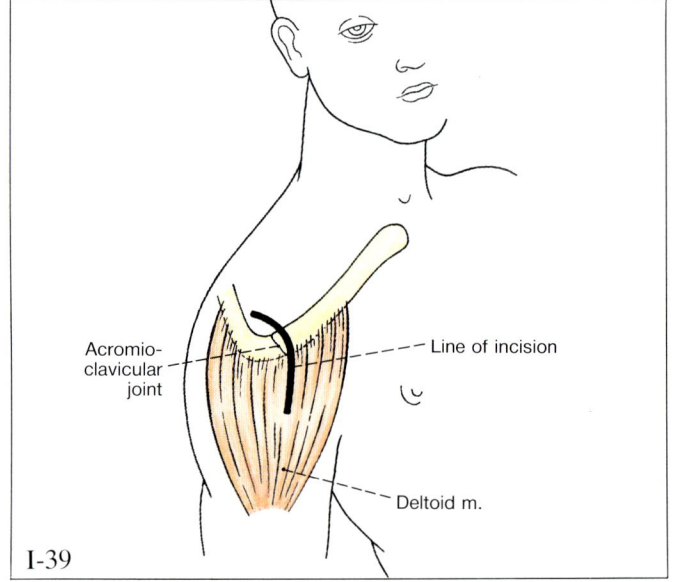

I-39

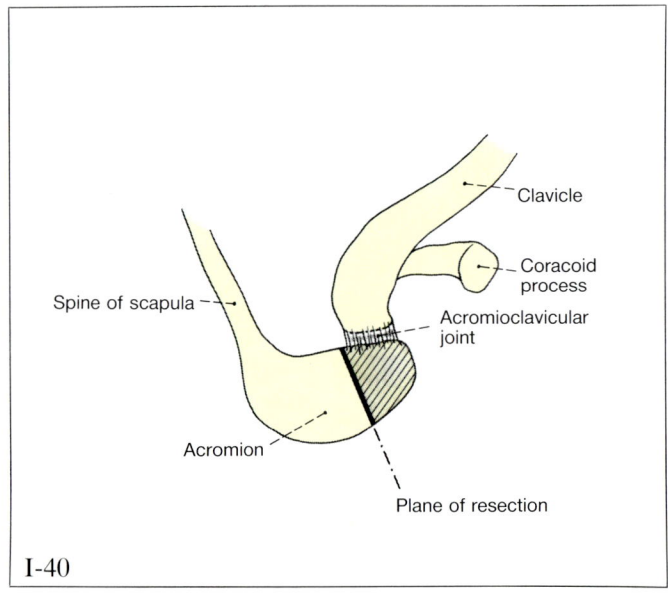

I-40

On occasions, the disc and a 0.5- to 1-cm length of the lateral end of the clavicle may also be resected (Fig. I-41). In this case, the coracoclavicular ligaments must be meticulously guarded.

3. An extensive total or subtotal acromionectomy is usually not desirable. It is especially important to save the lateral portion of the acromion, which serves as attachment for the deltoid muscle. If required, however, a subtotal medial acromionectomy may be performed (Fig. I-42).
4. A partial resection of the anterior lower surface of the acromion and/or removal of bony overgrowth near the edges of the acromioclavicular joint is also possible.

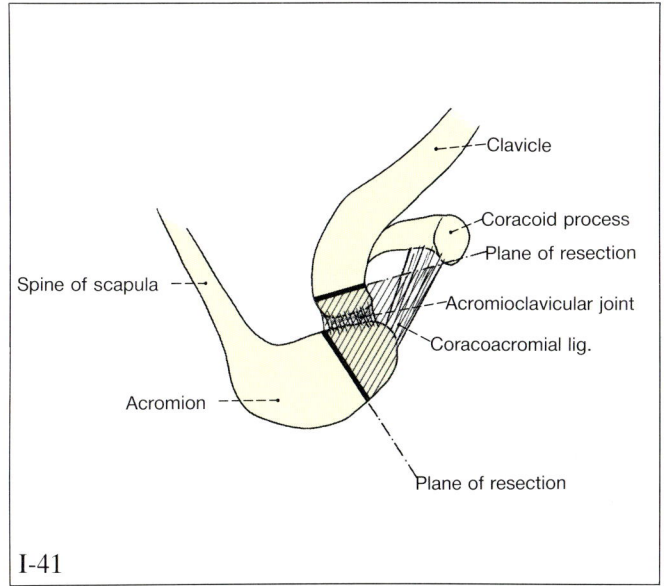

I-41

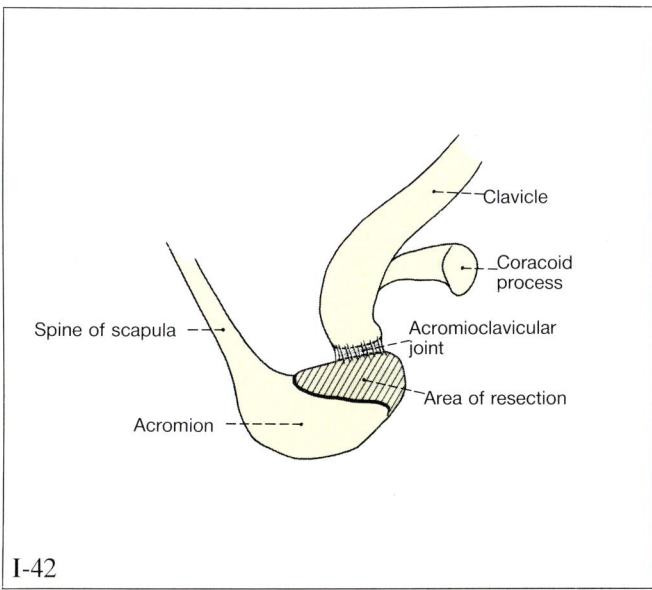

I-42

Long Anterior Exposure
Standard Exposure

Indications

1. Fracture dislocation of the humeral head
2. Anterior (recurrent) shoulder dislocation
3. Rupture of the long biceps tendon
4. Chronic shoulder dislocation
5. Calcium deposits in tendons (with medial rotation of the arm)
6. Rupture of the rotator cuff

Operative Steps

1. Make a slightly curved skin incision beginning below the clavicle at the level of the coracoid process and following the deltopectoral groove caudally (Fig. I-43).
2. Bluntly dissect the deltoid muscle about 1 cm from the sulcus to prevent injury to the cephalic vein and the deltoid branch of the thoracoacromial artery, which may be seen in the upper third of the incision (Fig. I-44).
3. Retract the edges of the deltoid muscle medially and laterally to bring into view the anterior aspect of the shoulder joint. The following structures are now exposed: the coracoid process with the short head of the biceps, the coracobrachialis, the pectoralis minor, the long head of the biceps, and the tendons of the subscapularis and pectoralis major muscles, as well as the anterior humeral circumflex artery (Fig. I-45).

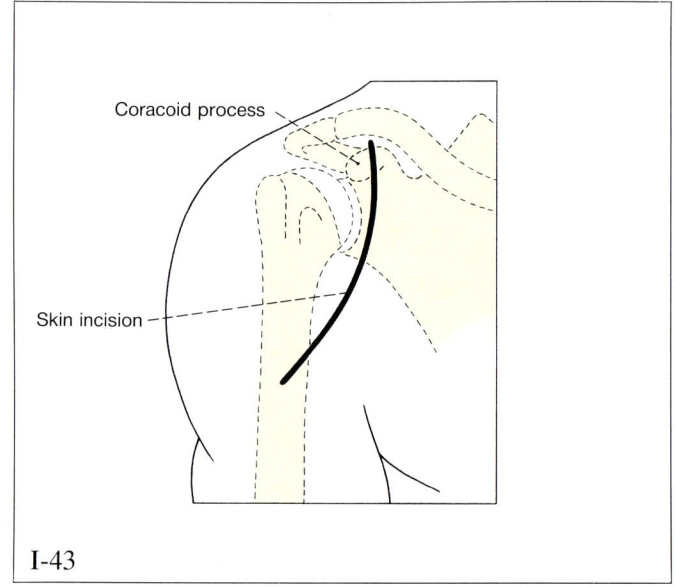

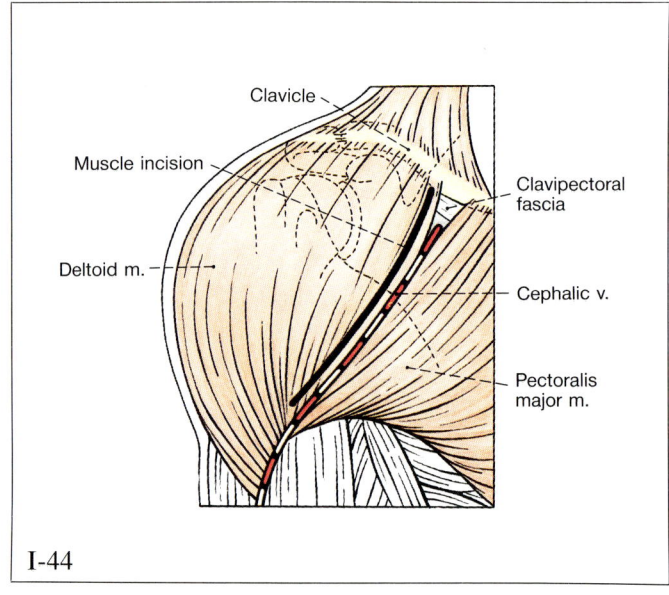

Shoulder Joint — Long Anterior Exposure

4. The readily palpable intertubercular groove with the long biceps tendon is a good landmark.
5. Lateral rotation exposes the subscapularis muscle with its tendinous capsular fibers. Medial rotation brings the greater tuberosity into view.
6. The deltoid muscle may be reflected far enough laterally so that, if needed, a Hohmann retractor can be passed behind the proximal shaft of the humerus.
7. The supraspinatus muscle is seen by extending the arm (see "Positioning of the Patient").
8. In the presence of scar tissue (old rotator cuff rupture), the thickened subacromial bursa may simulate an intact tendinous cuff. In these cases the bursa should be partially or totally removed.
9. By following the steps outlined in 2, the deltoid muscle may later be approximated without injuring the cephalic vein.

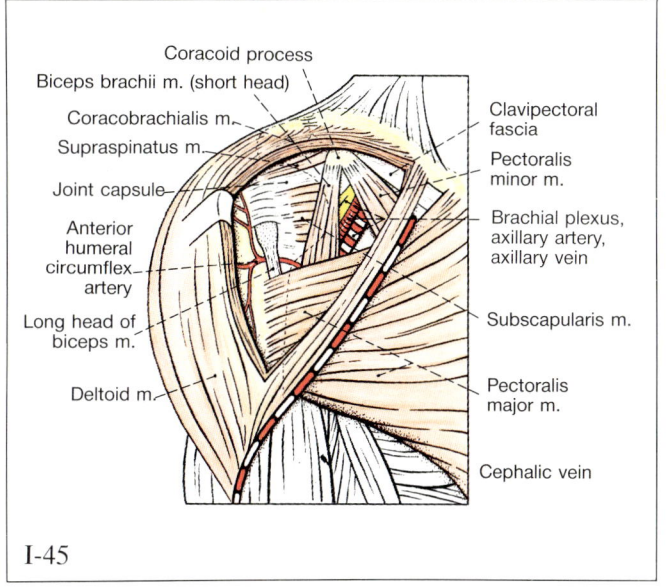

I-45

Notes

1. This is a particularly useful standard approach.
2. An extension of the incision is possible by the anterosuperior approach ("sabre cut") indicated earlier, with anteromedial partial acromionectomy.
3. Proper positioning of the patient is important in approaches to the shoulder joint.
4. If the cephalic vein is injured, it must be doubly ligated and excised.
5. Spread of scar tissue is likely to occur with this incision.

Anteromedial Exposure
Standard Exposure C

Indications

1. Arthrotomy
2. Fracture dislocation of the head of the humerus
3. Open reduction of anterior shoulder dislocation
4. Rupture of the long biceps tendon
5. Open reduction of an old shoulder dislocation
6. Insertion of a humeral head prosthesis
7. Rupture of the rotator cuff
8. Synovectomy

Operative Steps

1. The skin incision begins over the anterior border of the acromioclavicular joint, continues medially along the anterior surface of the lateral third of the clavicle, angles sharply downward, and follows the anterior border of the deltoid muscle to a point two-thirds of the distance between the origin and insertion of the deltoid muscle (Fig. I-46).
2. Identify the cephalic vein in the deltopectoral sulcus. By blunt dissection elevate the medial border of the deltoid muscle and reflect it laterally. To ensure the safety of the cephalic vein, the incision may be 1 cm lateral to the medial border of the deltoid muscle (Fig. I-47).
3. Transect the deltoid muscle approximately 1 cm below the clavicle to facilitate reattachment. During this procedure one must be prepared, in case of hemorrhage, to ligate a large branch of the thoracoacromial artery (Fig. I-47).

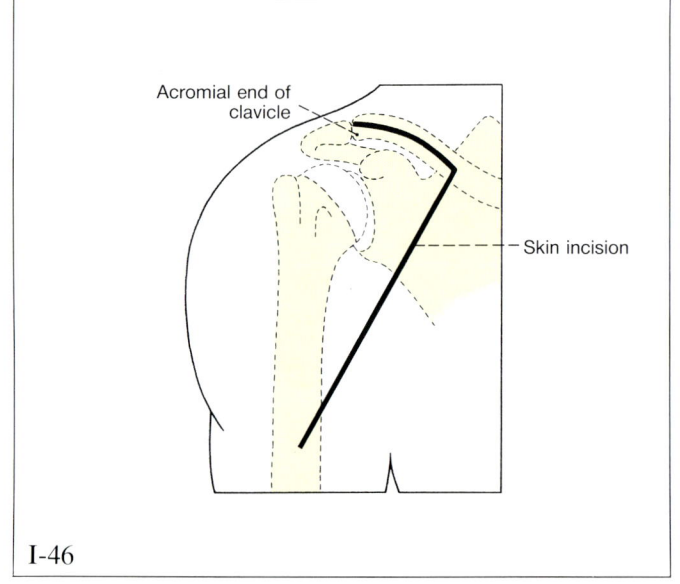

I-46

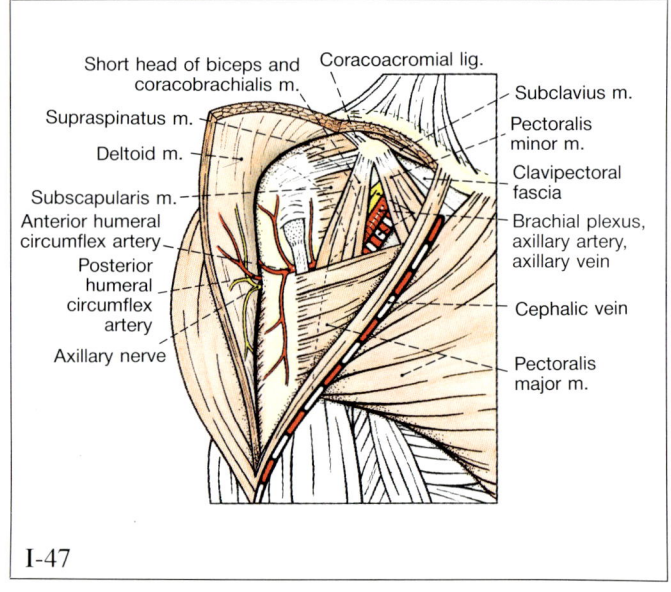

I-47

Shoulder Joint — Anteromedial Exposure

4. Reflect the anterior, detached part of the deltoid muscle laterally to expose the structures at the level of the coracoid process and the anterior aspect of the joint capsule.
5. If a wider exposure of the capsule is needed, the tip of the coracoid process with the attached musculature may be resected (see Notes).
6. Rotate the arm laterally to see the subscapularis muscle. Undermine the subscapularis muscle bluntly with scissors, and after placing a stay suture in the muscle, detach it as close to the insertion as possible. The stay suture (or an appropriately placed clamp) is essential to prevent rapid medial retraction of the muscle.
7. To achieve an extensive exposure of the anterior and inferior aspects of the capsule, mobilize the coracoid process with its muscle attachments and reflect the subscapularis muscle medially. The joint may now be opened by a longitudinal incision (Fig. I-48).
8. During wound closure reattach the coracoid process and approximate the retracted portion of the deltoid muscle to the part still attached to the clavicle. Medially the deltoid muscle will be sutured to the pectoralis major muscle.

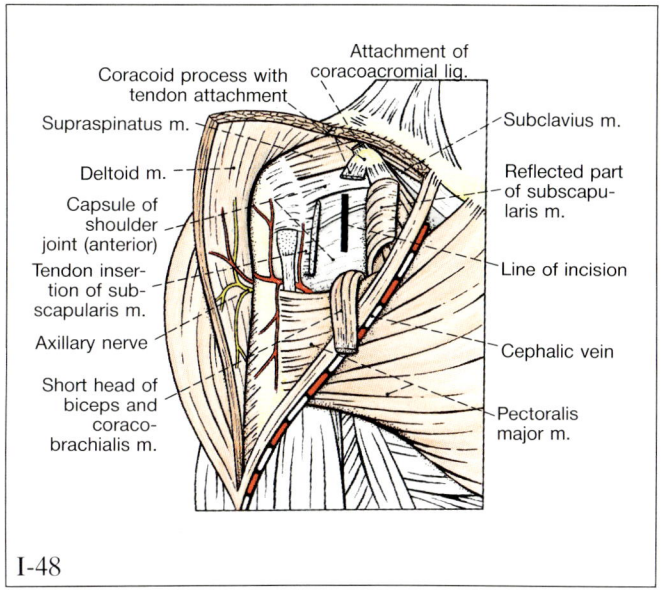

I-48

Notes

1. This approach affords a wide exposure.
2. The proper positioning of the patient is important in approaches to the shoulder joint.
3. As a variation of point 5, the muscles attached to the coracoid process may be reflected by cutting the common tendon of the coracobrachialis and short head of the biceps muscles. In this case, a 1 cm long tendon should remain attached to the bone for easier reattachment (Fig. I-48).
4. The skin incision may be curved rather than angled.
5. To reinforce the joint against future dislocation, the subscapularis muscle may be attached farther laterally on the capsule.

Lateral Exposure

Indications

1. Lesions associated with the supraspinatus tendon
2. Exposure of the subdeltoid or subacromial bursa
3. Calcium deposits in tendons (depending on location)

Operative Steps

1. Make a skin incision from the lower border of the acromion to a point 5 cm distal (Fig. I-49).
2. Separate fibers of the deltoid muscle by blunt dissection.
3. By lateral rotation of the humerus and right-angle flexion of the elbow, the intertubercular groove may be palpated, and the greater tuberosity with the tendinous insertions of the supraspinatus, infraspinatus, and teres minor muscles are seen (the latter by medial rotation).
4. By further lateral rotation of the humerus, the lesser tuberosity with the attachment of the subscapularis muscle is brought into view.
5. For a wider exposure, approximately 2.5 cm of the origin of the deltoid muscle can be stripped from the acromion and the clavicle.

I-49

Notes

1. If the lengthwise incision of the deltoid muscle is longer than 4–5 cm, as measured from the acromial border, there is danger of injury to the anterior humeral circumflex artery and the anterior muscular branch of the axillary nerve. Cutting the nerve branch will cause partial paralysis of the deltoid muscle, with a weakened anterior portion and a subsequent change in the contour of the shoulder.
2. Spread of scar tissue is observed with this incision.
3. This approach is suited only for limited procedures.
4. Extension of the arm affords a better overall view.
5. In cases of calcified deposits, their locations must be ascertained by preoperative roentgenograms with the arm rotated laterally as well as medially.

Transacromial Exposure of *Kessel*
Standard Exposure D

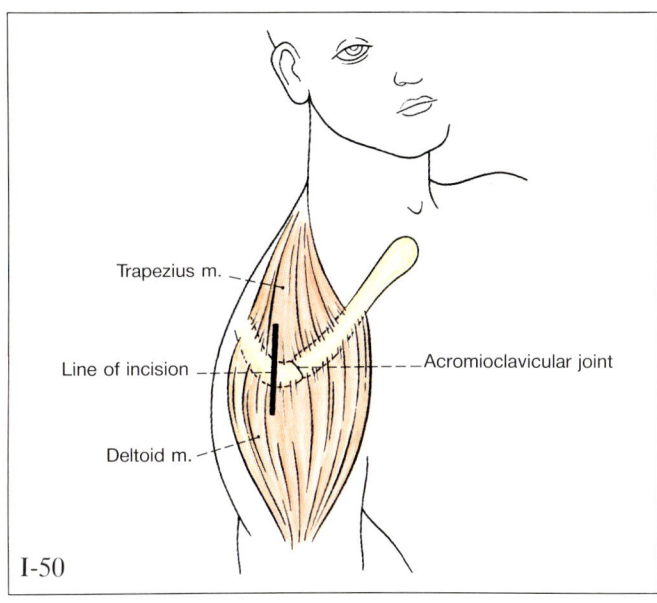

Indication

Ruptures of the rotator cuff

Introduction

With extensive ruptures of the rotator cuff, the standard anterior approach is occasionally inadequate. It can be difficult to obtain satisfactory exposure in this region from the front for mobilization and repair of the deeply placed muscles, tendons, and capsular portions. The transacromial approach is an alternative.

Operative Steps

1. The most lateral point of the supraclavicular fossa is a good landmark and may be palpated with the index finger as a depression between the clavicle and the spine. Make a skin incision at this point and extend it medially and laterally for about 4 cm, respectively (Fig. I-50).
2. Bluntly separate the fibers of the trapezius and deltoid muscles along the line of the skin incision and reflect them ventrally and dorsally. Then detach them from the acromion without severing the connective tissue bridge that connects the trapezius and deltoid muscles.
3. With an oscillating saw or an osteotome, split the acromion in the frontal plane along the line of the skin incision.
4. Hold apart the anterior and posterior portions of the split acromion with a self-retaining retractor. This permits a view of the subacromial bursa and the rotator cuff (Fig. I-51).
5. The subacromial bursa may be cut through or resected.

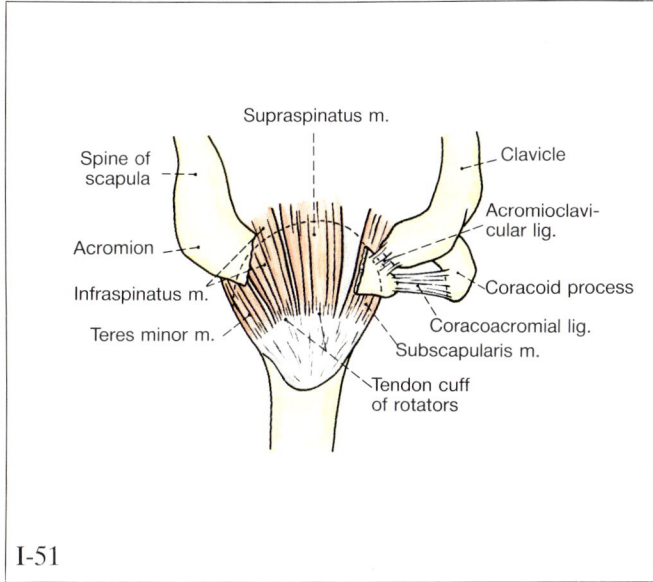

6. Expose the individual parts of the rotator cuff and shoulder joint by rotating the arm.
7. At the end of the operation and after removal of the self-retaining retractor, it is sufficient to approximate the two parts of the acromion and suture the overlying soft tissues across the union.

Note

When making the incision it should be noted that the anterior muscular branch of the axillary nerve runs approximately 5 cm below the acromion.

Transverse Lateral Exposure

Indications

The same as for the lateral exposure

Operative Steps

1. Make an approximately 4 cm long transverse skin incision about 1.5 cm below the tip of the acromion (Fig. I-52).
2. Split the deltoid muscle 5 cm longitudinally (Fig. I-53).
3. By lateral rotation of the humerus and right-angle flexion of the elbow, the intertubercular groove may be palpated, and the greater tuberosity with the tendinous insertions of the supraspinatus, infraspinatus, and teres minor muscles are seen (the latter by medial rotation).
4. For a wider exposure, approximately 2.5 cm of the origin of the deltoid muscle can be stripped from the acromion and the clavicle (Fig. I-53).

Notes

1. This lesion will heal without a later spreading of the scar.
2. It should be noted further that the anterior muscular branch of the axillary nerve runs about 5 cm below the acromion and may be injured.

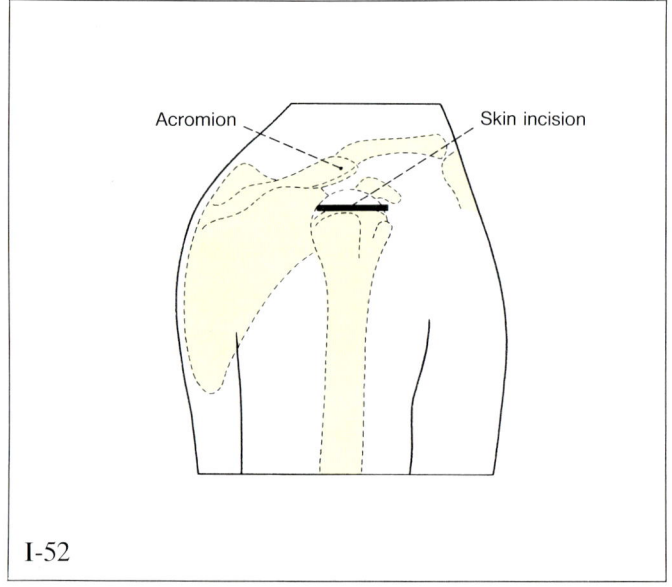

I-52

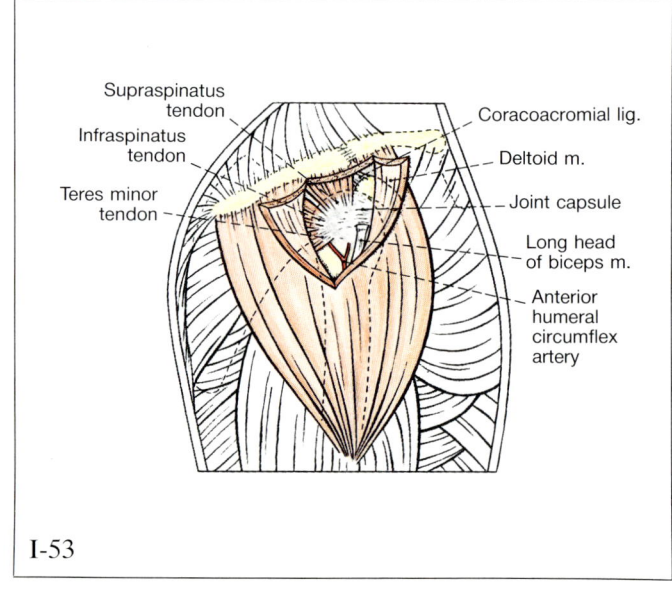

I-53

Anteroinferior Exposure
Low Axillary Exposure

Indications

1. Anterior dislocation of the shoulder
2. Rupture of the long tendon of the biceps
3. Fracture dislocation of the head of the humerus

Operative Steps

1. Make a skin incision over the lower part of the deltopectoral sulcus (Fig. I-54).
2. Bluntly undermine the skin upward to the clavicle.
3. Using strong traction, expose the area up to the coracoid process.
4. Subsequent steps are the same as those depicted in Fig. I-45.

Notes

1. Blunt undermining of the skin prevents injury to the cephalic vein.
2. This incision is cosmetically advantageous, but it is difficult to obtain an adequate view.

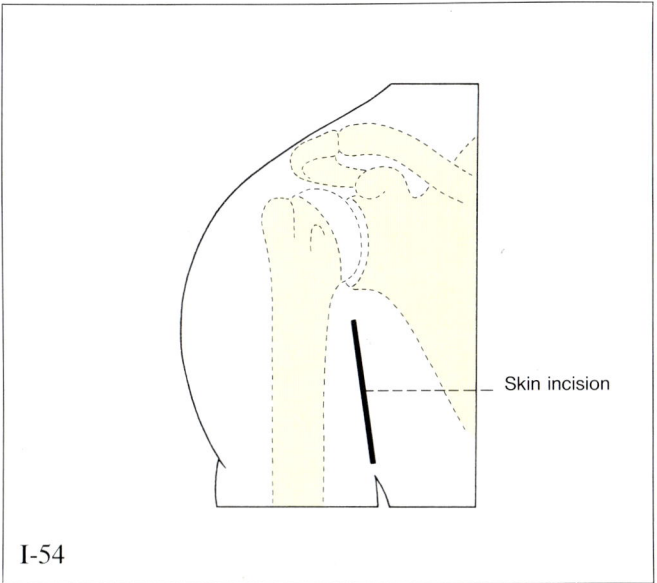

I-54

Shoulder Joint — Anterior Axillary Exposure

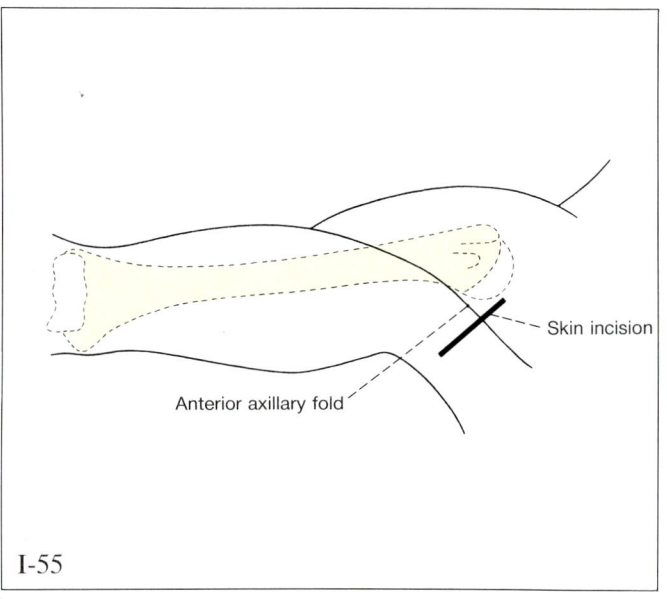

I-55

Anterior Axillary Exposure

Indications

1. Recurrent anterior dislocation of the shoulder
2. Rupture of the long biceps tendon

Operative Steps

1. Position the limb on a side table in lateral rotation and 90 degrees abduction.
2. Begin the incision at about the middle of the anterior axillary fold over the pectoralis major muscle and continue it dorsally for about 5 cm into the axilla (Fig. I-55).
3. Perform wide, blunt undermining of the skin area from the upper end of the incision to the coracoid process (Fig. I-56).
4. Reflect the skin upward and laterally so that the cephalic vein and the deltopectoral sulcus can be seen. When the groove is developed, retract the deltoid muscle laterally and the cephalic vein medially.
5. Detach the tendon of the pectoralis major muscle either partially or totally at its insertion and retract the muscle medially and downward (Fig. I-57).
6. If a better exposure is needed, release the short tendon of the biceps and the coracobrachialis muscle from the coracoid process. Visualize the joint capsule by cleaning and mobilizing the subscapular tendon (Fig. I-57).
7. At the time of wound closure, reattach the mobilized tendons. Subcutaneous sutures are not required because the arm will be rotated medially and held against the chest wall.

Note

By careful approximation of the wound edges, the skin incision will appear as a hairline scar and is therefore particularly well suited for female patients.

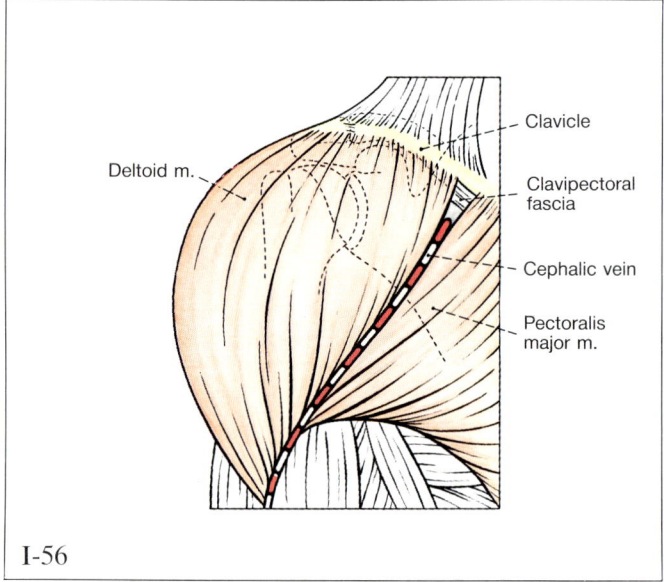

I-56

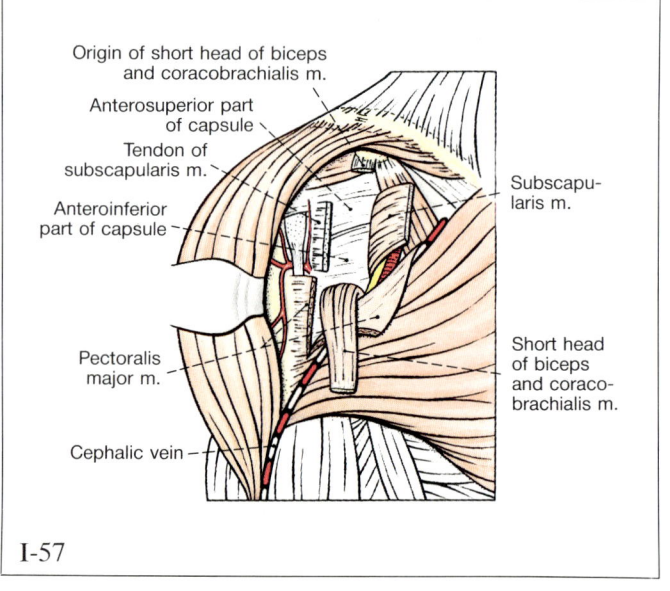

I-57

Anterolateral Exposure

Indications

1. Operative repair of injuries to the rotator cuff
2. Irreducible fractures of the greater tuberosity of the humerus

Operative Steps

1. The anterior part of the incision is similar to that in the anteromedial approach in which the incision was continued around the lateral edge of the acromion. The posterior limb of the incision extends along the lateral half of the scapular spine (Fig. I-58).
2. Detach the deltoid muscle from the clavicle, the acromion, and that part of the scapular spine exposed by the skin incision (Fig. I-59).
3. Obtain access to the joint by corresponding incisions of the capsule in front and behind, or:
4. Expose the articular surfaces of the shoulder joint by a continuous incision of the capsule from the anterior aspect of the joint upward, over the head of the humerus, and then downward behind the head (inverted "U"). Take care to avoid cutting the long biceps tendon.

Note

Any part of this approach can be used for operations that require only limited exposure.

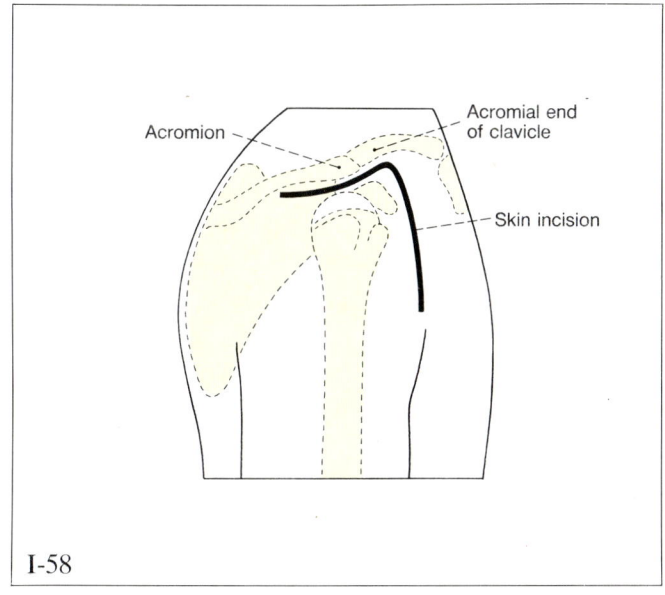

I-58

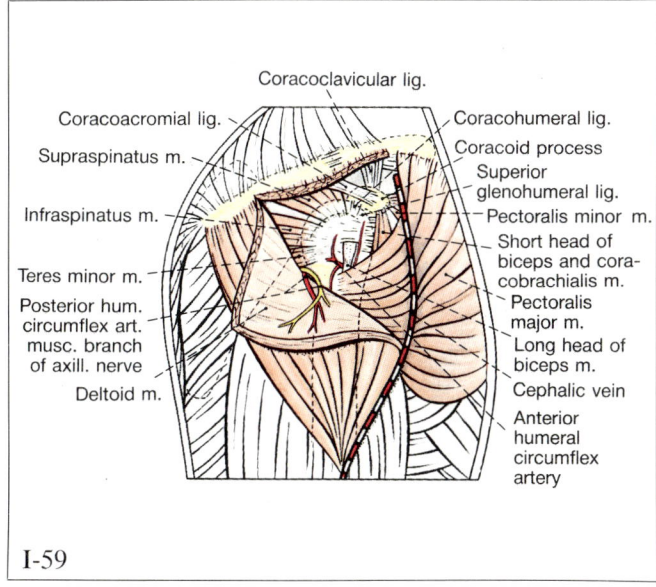

I-59

Anteroposterior Exposure

Arched Incision from Front to Back

Indications

1. Repair of ruptured rotator cuff
2. Irreducible fracture of the greater tuberosity
3. Arthrodesis of shoulder joint

Operative Steps

1. Make a incision in the shape of an inverted "U" (Figs. I-60 and I-61).
2. Begin the incision anteriorly, 7–8 cm below the head of the humerus; then extend it over the medial third of the deltoid muscle, over the acromioclavicular joint, and caudally over the posterior third of the deltoid muscle, terminating it 5 cm below the acromion (Fig. I-61).

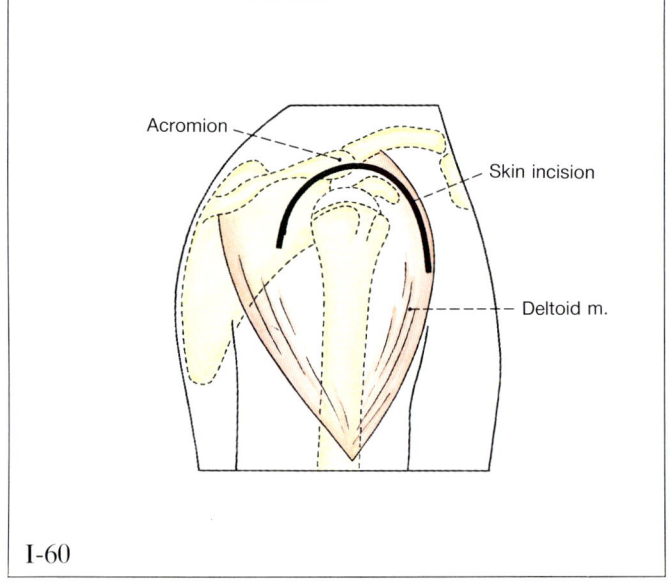

I-60

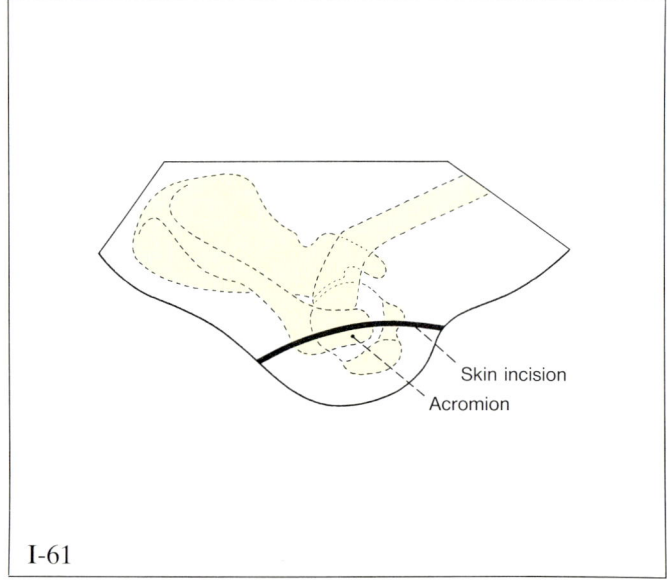

I-61

Shoulder Joint — Anteroposterior Exposure

3. Separate the deltoid fibers craniocaudally in front and in the back (Fig. I-62).
4. Perform an acromial osteotomy somewhat lateral to the acromioclavicular joint (Figs. I-62 and I-63).
5. Reflect the bone with the attached deltoid muscle laterally to avoid injury to the suprascapular nerve and artery. The nerve runs through the scapular notch; the artery passes over the transverse scapular ligament.
6. At this stage of the procedure there is an excellent view of the rotator cuff muscles (Fig. I-63).
7. An alternative to procedure in point 4 in case a wider exposure is needed: open the acromioclavicular joint and sever the acromion from the spine of the scapula (Fig. I-64); then reflect the acromion with the attached deltoid muscle laterally. This procedure affords a full view of the upper and lateral aspects of the joint (Figs. I-65 and I-66).

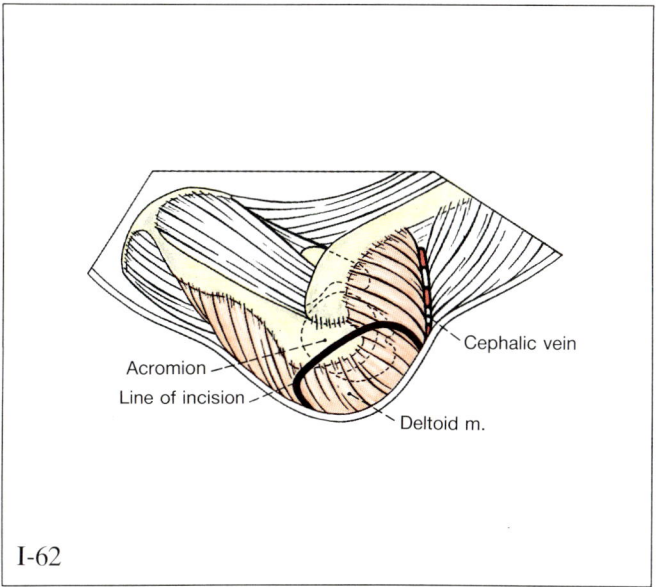

I-62

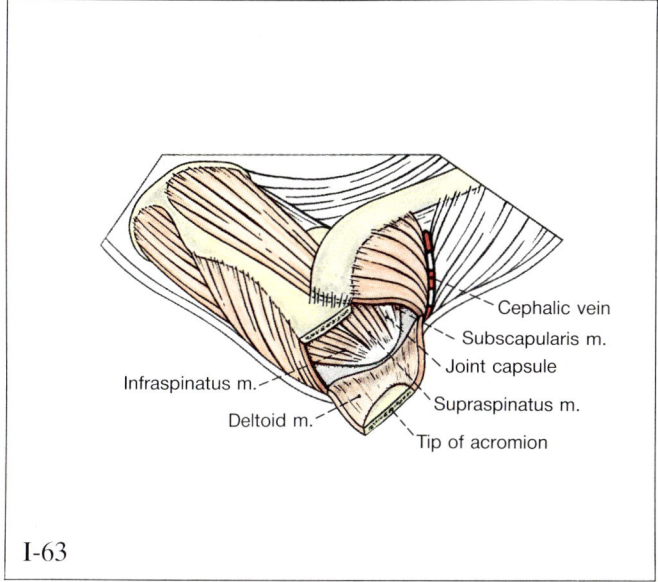

I-63

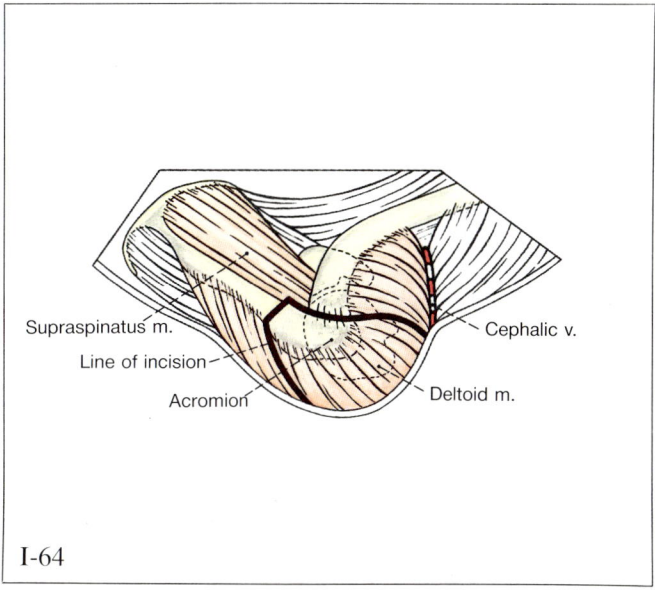

I-64

Shoulder Joint — Anteroposterior Exposure

Notes

1. The axillary nerve enters the posterior margin of the deltoid muscle and runs anteriorly on its deep surface. If the muscle fibers are separated at a distance greater then 5 cm from the acromion, the main trunk of the nerve is in danger of being severed. When splitting the deltoid muscle along its fiber direction, the greatest hazard lies in injury to those branches of the axillary nerve that supply the anterior part of the muscle.
2. A pseudoarthrosis may develop and cause complications following replacement of the detached acromial piece.

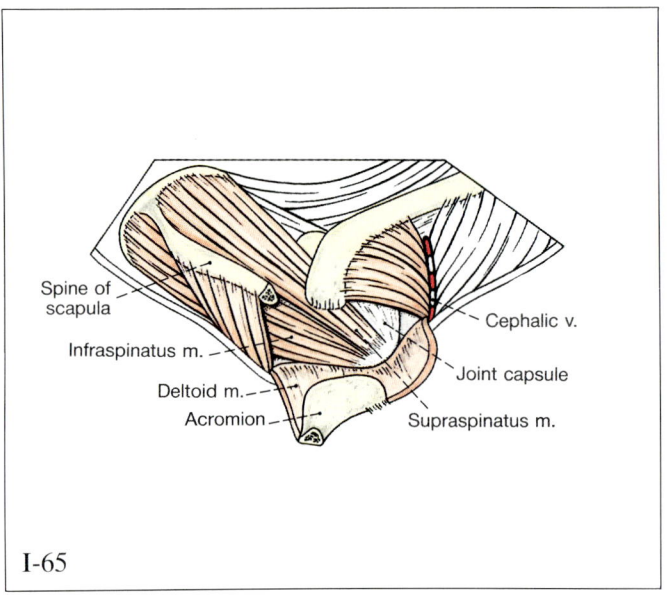

I-65

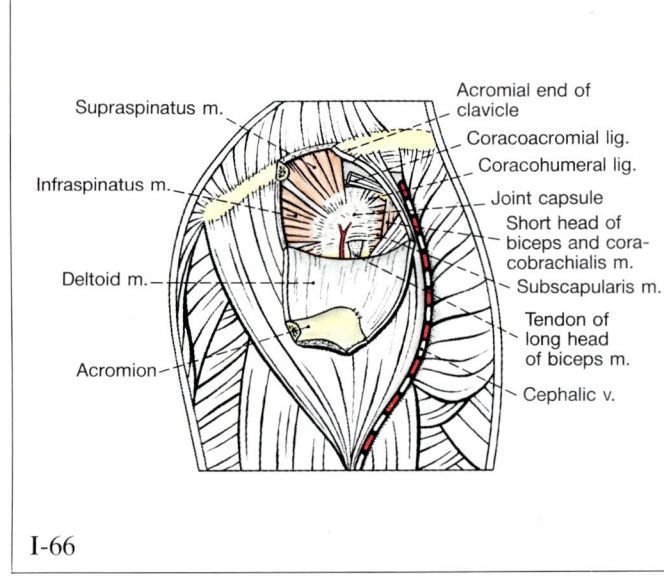

I-66

Posterior Aspect of Shoulder Joint

Applied Anatomy

1. Muscles, seen from behind (Fig. I-67).
2. Nerves on posterior aspect (Fig. I-68).

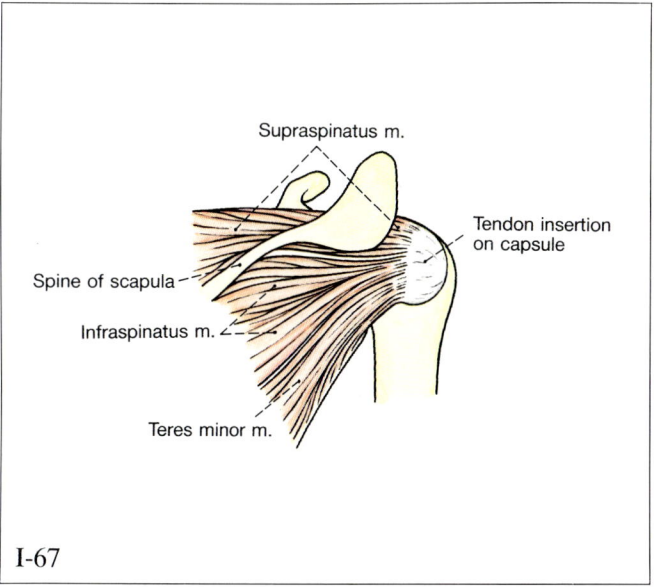

I-67

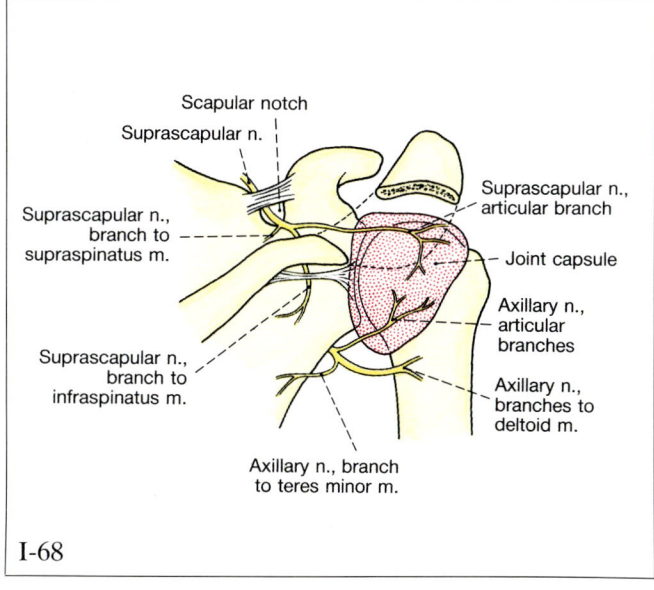

I-68

Shoulder Joint

Posterior Exposure

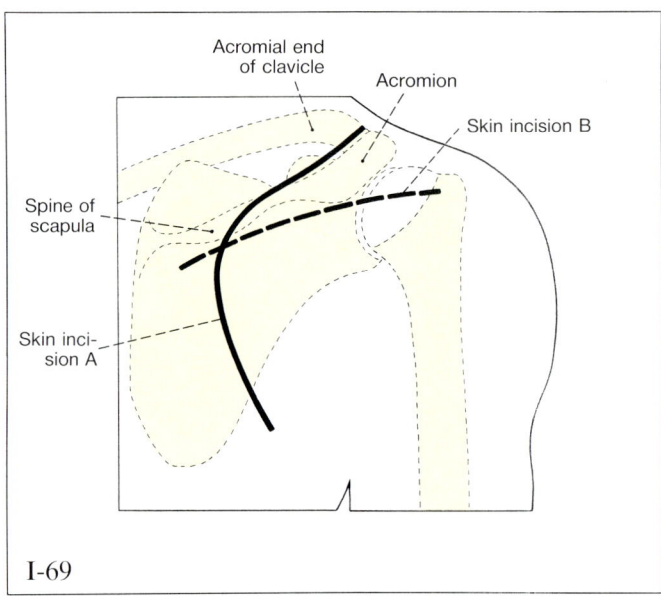

I-69

Posterior Exposure

Indications

1. Recurrent posterior dislocation of the shoulder
2. Loose bodies in the posterior compartment of the shoulder joint
3. Repair of tear in the posterior joint capsule
4. Irreducible fractures of the posterior part of the greater tuberosity
5. Arthrodesis of the shoulder joint

Operative Steps

1. Begin the skin incision at the acromioclavicular joint and carry it along the upper border of the acromion and the spine of the scapula to about the middle of the latter. From here, curve the incision downward to a point approximately 3 cm above the posterior axillary fold (Fig. I-69, skin incision A).
2. Insert a finger at this level under the deltoid muscle and separate it from the deep muscles to which it is bound by loose connective tissue.
3. Cut the deltoid muscle away from the spine of the scapula all the way to the acromioclavicular joint, if necessary, leaving about 1 cm of the muscle on the spine for convenient reattachment later (Fig. I-70).
4. Retract the deltoid muscle. Injury to the axillary nerve and the posterior humeral circumflex artery can be avoided by careful reflection of the muscle (Fig. I-71).
5. At this stage of the operation, the infraspinatus, teres minor, and lateral and long heads of the triceps muscles are seen, as well as the upper, posterior part of the shaft of the humerus.
6. If it becomes necessary to expose more of the posterior aspect of the capsule, divide the supraspinatus, infraspinatus, and teres minor muscles near their insertions and reflect them medially (Figs. I-71 and I-72). These muscles have a broad attachment to the capsule and are intimately bound to it.
7. Before the muscles are released from the capsule, introduce a small hemostat or scissors between capsule and musculature.
8. If the joint cavity must be opened, incise the supraspinatus, infraspinatus, and teres minor muscles at their tendinous junction together with the capsule which lies immediately underneath them.
9. When closing the wound, include muscles and capsule in the same suture.
10. As an alternative, a more medially placed vertical incision of the capsule permits a better overlapping of the individual layers during closure (Fig. I-72).

Notes

1. This approach offers a potentially wider exposure of the posterior parts of the shoulder joint.
2. Reflection of the supraspinatus muscle is not required in posterior exposure of the joint.
3. A posterior reinforcement of the capsule can be achieved by partial overlap of the infraspinatus and teres minor muscles.

Shoulder Joint — Posterior Exposure of Kocher

Alternative Posterior Exposure of *Kocher*

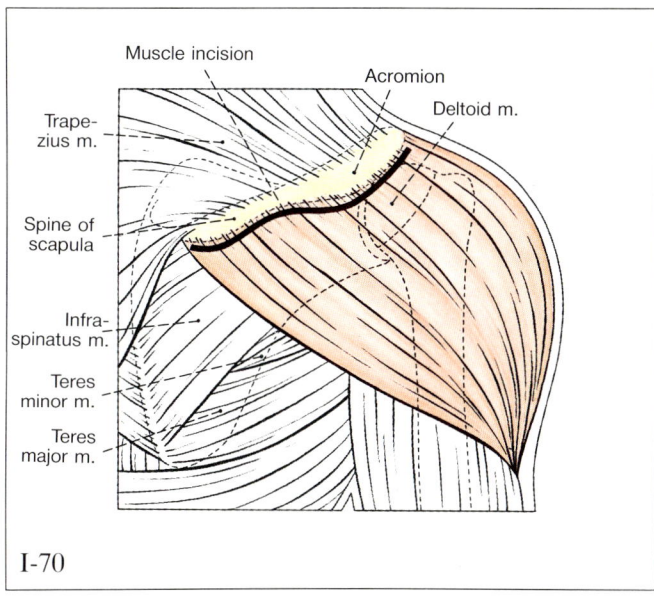

I-70

Operative Steps

1. Begin the incision below and lateral to the acromion. Continue it medially along the posterior border of the acromion and immediately under the spine of the scapula (Fig. I-69, skin incision B).
2. Separate the deltoid muscle from the spine of the scapula, leaving about 1 cm of the muscle attached to the spine (Fig. I-70).
3. Reflect the deltoid muscle only to the level of the teres minor muscle while carefully protecting the axillary nerve (Fig. I-68).
4. The point at which the suprascapular nerve passes under the scapular spine is untouched to prevent damage to the nerve (Fig. I-68).
5. Expose the posterior aspect of the joint capsule by retracting the infraspinatus muscle upward and the teres minor muscle downward.
6. For further exposure of the posterior part of the joint capsule, cut both muscles at their tendinous junction vertically approximately 1 cm from their attachments to the greater tuberosity (Fig. I-71) and reflect them.
7. Incise the capsule parallel with and about 1 cm from the medial edge of the joint (Fig. I-72).
8. When the muscles are later reapproximated, overlap the individual layers to assure a strong closure.

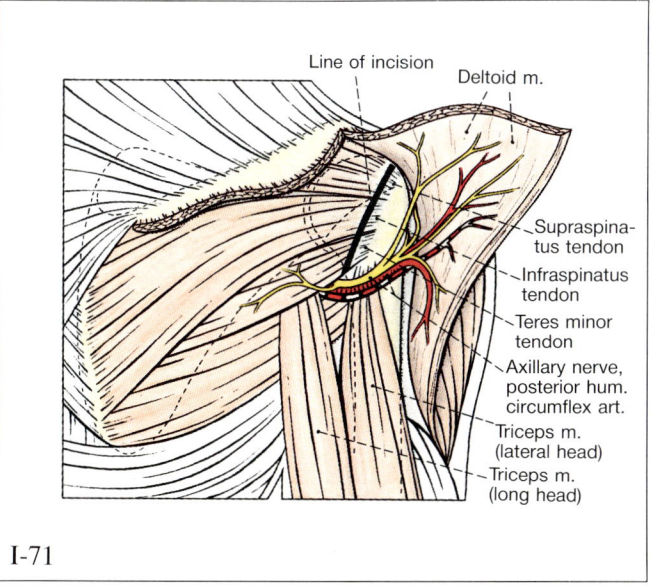

I-71

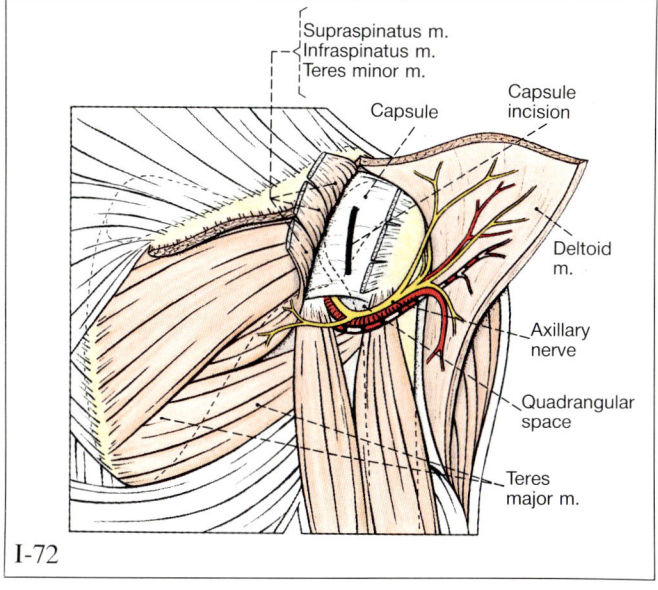

I-72

C. Upper Arm

Shaft of the Humerus

Anterolateral Exposure

Indications

1. Irreducible fractures
2. Inflammatory processes
3. Pseudoarthroses
4. Tumors

Operative Steps

1. The best and safest method of exposure of the upper third of the humerus is achieved through the anterolateral approach between the pectoralis major and the deltoid muscles (Fig. I-73).
2. Adequate exposure frequently requires reflection of the deltoid muscle. In these cases the incision is extended along the anterior axillary fold toward the clavicle to the acromioclavicular joint, about 1 cm lateral to the deltopectoral sulcus (Fig. I-73, incision A or B). This corresponds to the standard anterior approach to the shoulder joint.
3. Expose the middle and lower thirds of the humerus by making an incision from the medial border of the deltoid muscle distally along the lateral edge of the biceps muscle to a point in the middle of the upper third of the forearm (Fig. I-73).
4. Expose the brachialis muscle by reflecting the deltoid muscle laterally and the biceps muscle with the cephalic vein medially. Split the brachialis muscle longitudinally down to the bone and displace it subperiosteally, medially and laterally (Figs. I-74 and I-75). During this procedure flex the elbow to relax the brachialis muscle.

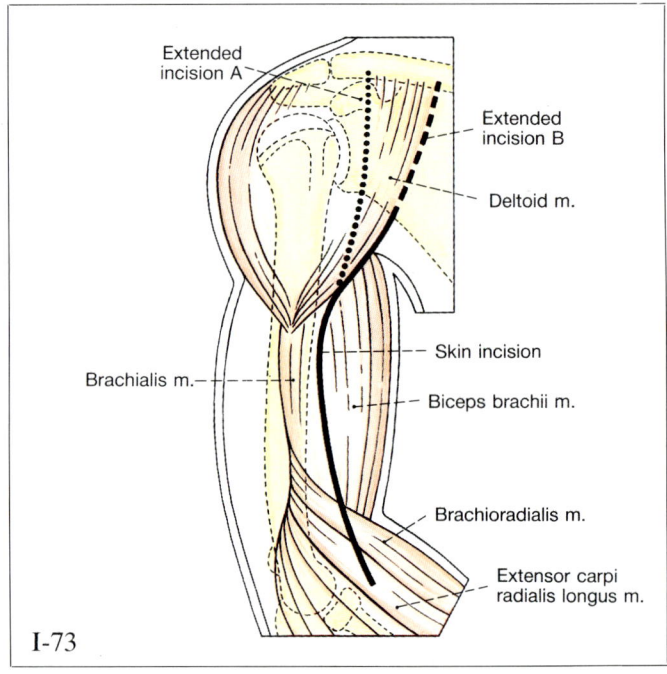

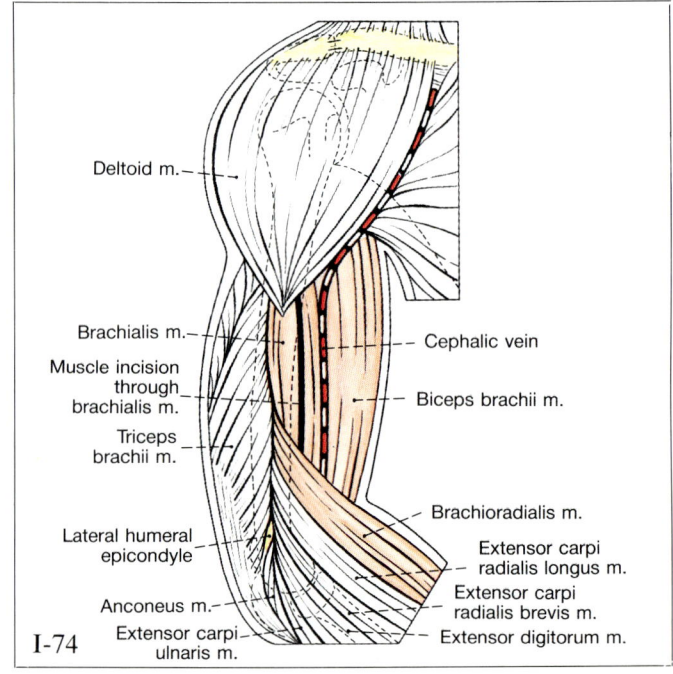

Shaft of the Humerus — Anterolateral Exposure

5. Reflect the radial nerve and the posterior half of the brachialis muscle dorsally by passing a Hohmann retractor under the structures (Fig. I-75). The brachial artery, the musculocutaneous nerve, and the median nerve lie medial to the incision (compare, however, with Fig. I-77).
6. Expose the shaft of the humerus by extending the incision proximally and reflecting the deltoid muscle in the lateral bicipital sulcus.

Notes

1. A temporary radial nerve paresis can be caused by excessive traction on the dorsolateral portion of the brachialis muscle.
2. Frequently, only a part of the incision may be needed.

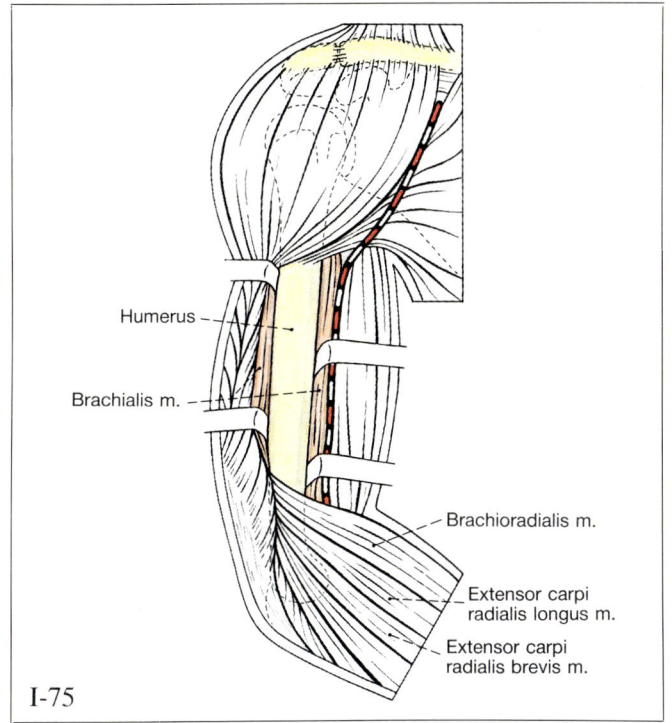

I-75

Anteromedial Exposure

Operative Steps

1. In patients with poorly developed musculature, the incision can be made on the anteromedial aspect (Fig. I-76). This skin incision will give a better cosmetic appearance.
2. Begin the incision lateral to the deltopectoral sulcus and continue it over the medial border of the deltoid muscle in the anterior axillary fold. If necessary, extend it farther distally along the medial edge of the biceps muscle to the medial epicondyle.
3. Incise the fascia medial to the biceps muscle. Expose the shaft of the humerus medial to the inner bicipital sulcus.

Notes

1. Frequently, only a portion of this incision may be needed. It is not without risk.
2. The anteromedial approach to the shaft of the humerus may endanger the musculocutaneous nerves and a careful, blunt dissection is recommended.

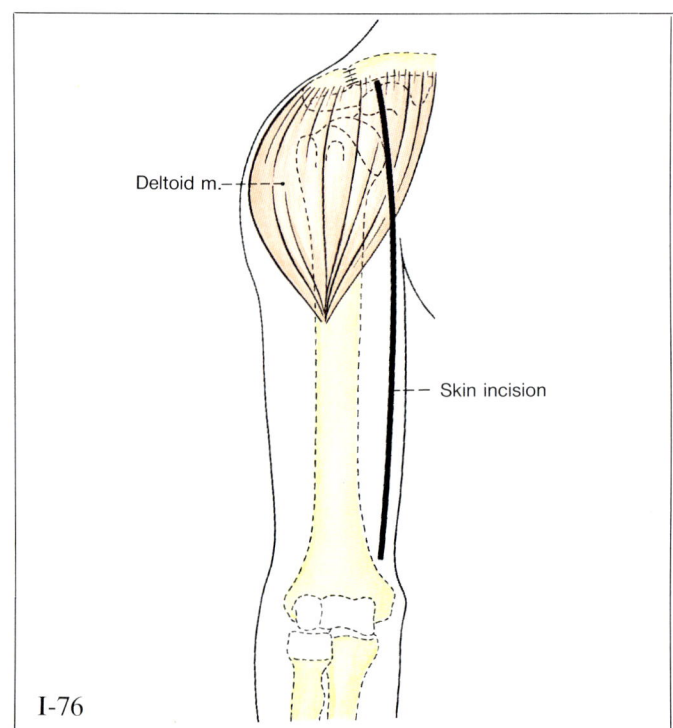

I-76

Musculocutaneous Nerve
Applied Anatomy

1. This nerve is easily injured in shoulder and arm operations.
2. It arises from the lateral cord of the brachial plexus and runs between the coracobrachialis muscle and the axillary nerve. It supplies branches to the coracobrachialis muscle and then penetrates this muscle (Fig. I-77) to lie between the short head of the biceps and the brachialis muscle.
3. When the short head of the biceps and the coracobrachialis muscle are released from their origin and retracted distally, there is danger of paralyzing the biceps and brachialis muscles by excessive traction on the nerve. Its cutaneous branches to the forearm will also be affected.
4. In the anteromedial approach the nerve may also be injured when the brachial fascia is incised medial to the biceps muscle.

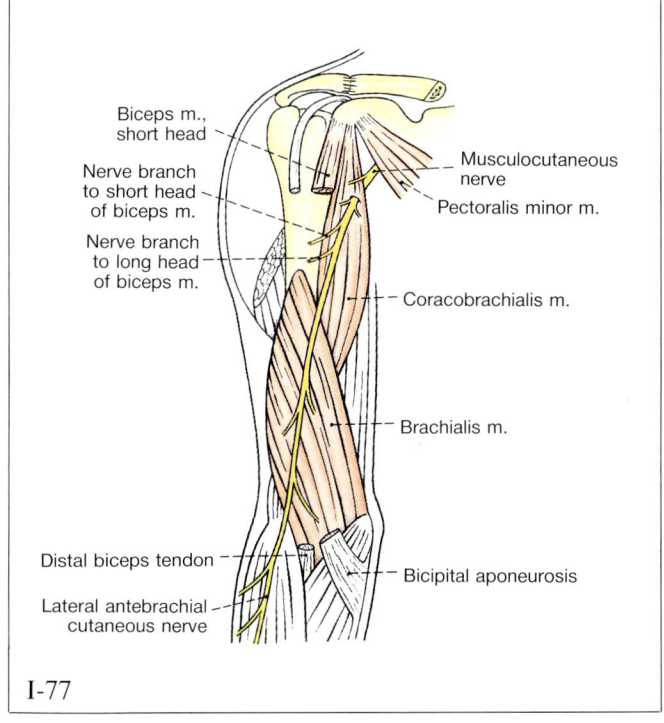

I-77

Shaft of the Humerus — Posterior Exposure

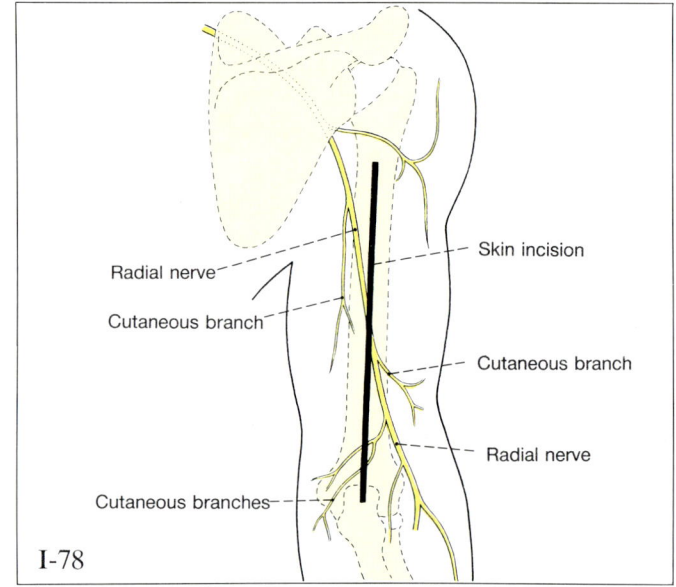

I-78

Posterior Exposure

Indications

1. Tumors
2. Injuries to the radial nerve
3. Complicated fractures of the shaft of the humerus

Operative Steps

1. Position the patient face down, with the arm abducted and resting on a side table.
2. Begin the skin incision about 5 cm below the acromion and continue it to the olecranon (Fig. I-78).
3. Open the deep fascia by blunt dissection close to the outer border of the long head of the triceps muscle.
4. Insert the index finger in the V-shaped niche between the heads of the triceps (Figs. I-79, I-80 and I-81).

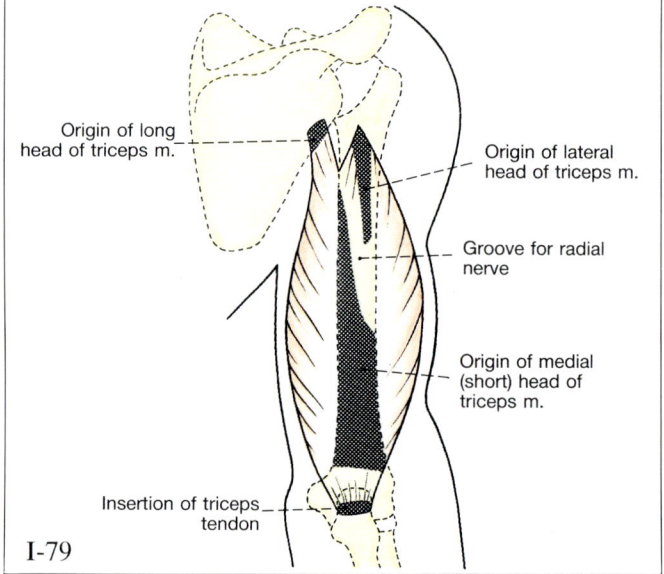

I-79

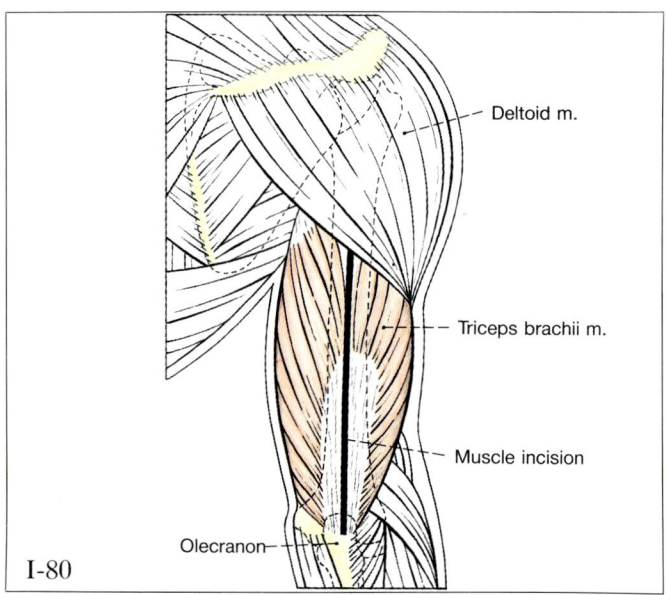

I-80

Shaft of the Humerus — Posterior Exposure

5. Raise the muscle off the underlying structures and split it between the long and lateral heads down to the olecranon.
6. The large neurovascular bundle consisting of the radial nerve and the deep brachial vessels is now brought into view (Fig. I-82).
7. By reflecting these structures, the medial head of the triceps can be split and retracted to expose the shaft of the humerus. While performing these cuts, avoid the branch of the radial nerve to the lateral head of the triceps; compared to the main trunk it runs more transversely (Figs. I-82 and I-83).
8. When the medial head of the triceps is split, also avoid the muscular branch from the radial nerve to the most medial part of this head. The substantial, parallel-running branch to the lateral half of the medial head can be protected by retracting it with the muscle.
9. While splitting the triceps muscle in its distal portion, it is essential to stay close to the lateral head to prevent transection of the ulnar nerve.

Notes

1. In this approach the anatomical dissection must be executed with painstaking precision and care to avoid injury to branches of the radial nerve.
2. The incision can be extended proximally along the posterior border of the deltoid muscle. In doing so, the axillary nerve must be watched.

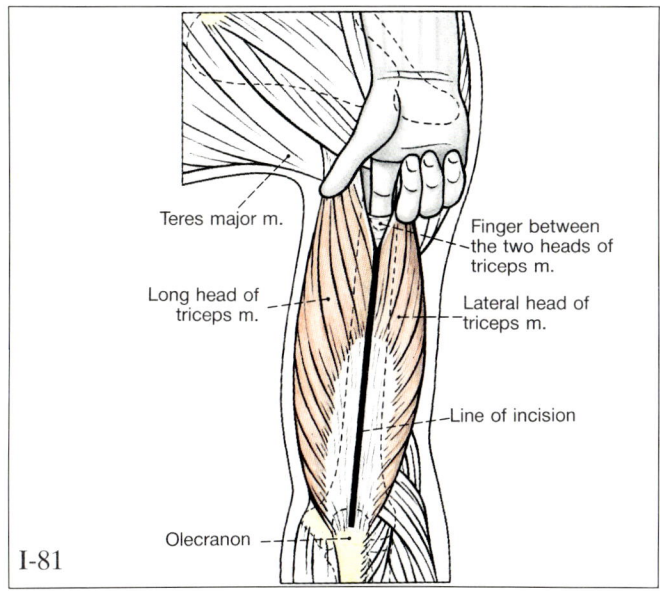

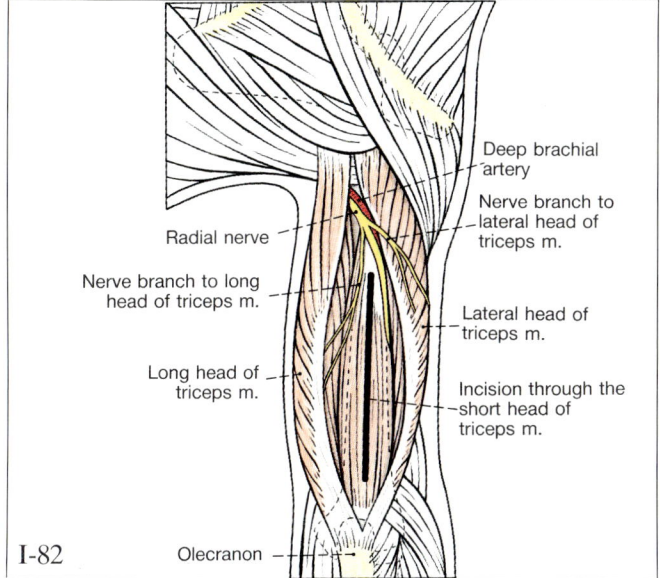

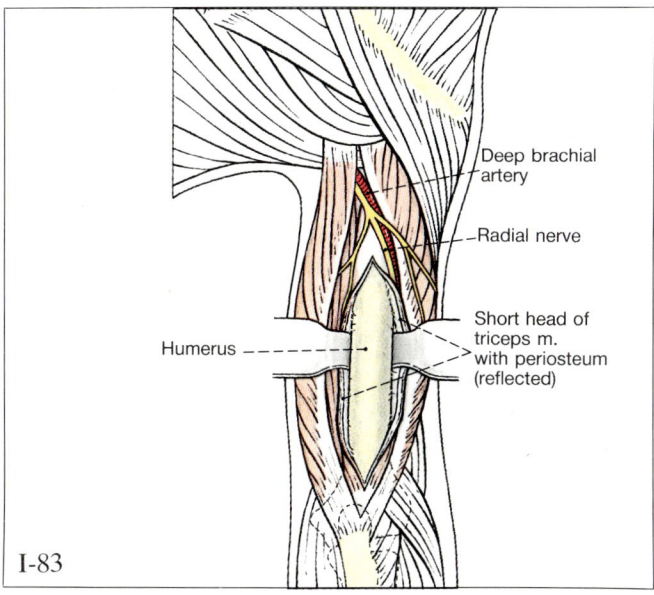

Elbow Joint — Anterior Exposure

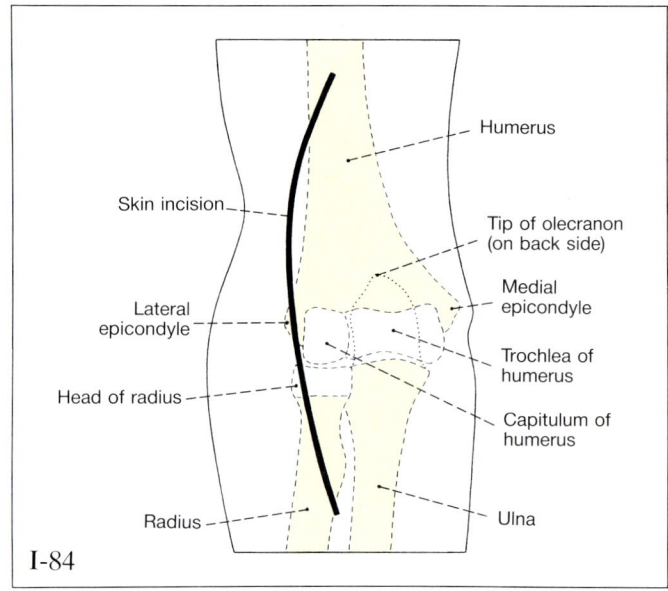

I-84

D. Elbow

Introduction

All operations on the elbow joint should be performed on a bloodless limb with a pneumatic tourniquet. The required pressure depends on the degree of muscular development but must be 250–300 mm Hg or 60–100 mm Hg higher than systolic pressure. Compare also the introductory remarks at the beginning of Part I.

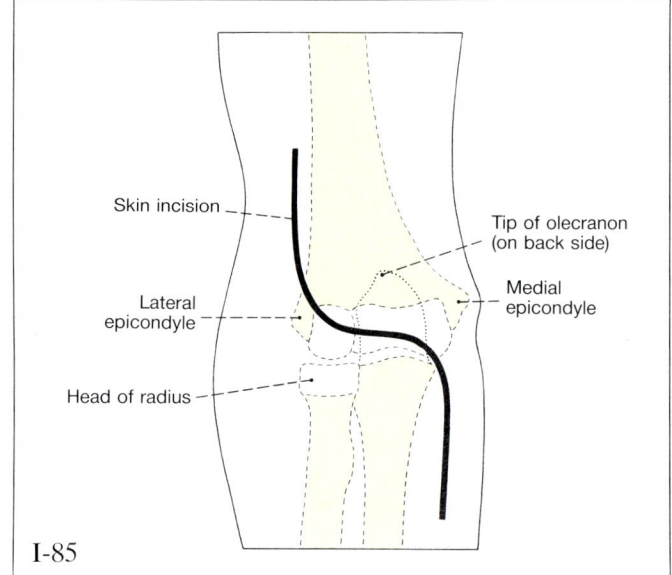

I-85

Elbow joint (1)

Anterior Exposure

Indications

1. Distal rupture of the biceps tendon
2. Loose bodies in the anterior compartment of the joint
3. Tumors near the distal end of the humerus
4. Injuries to the radial nerve

Operative Steps

1. Make a curved anterior skin incision lateral to the midline; extend it about 5–8 cm proximal and 5 cm distal to the elbow joint (Fig. I-84).
2. Alternatives are shown in Figs. I-85, I-86 and I-87.

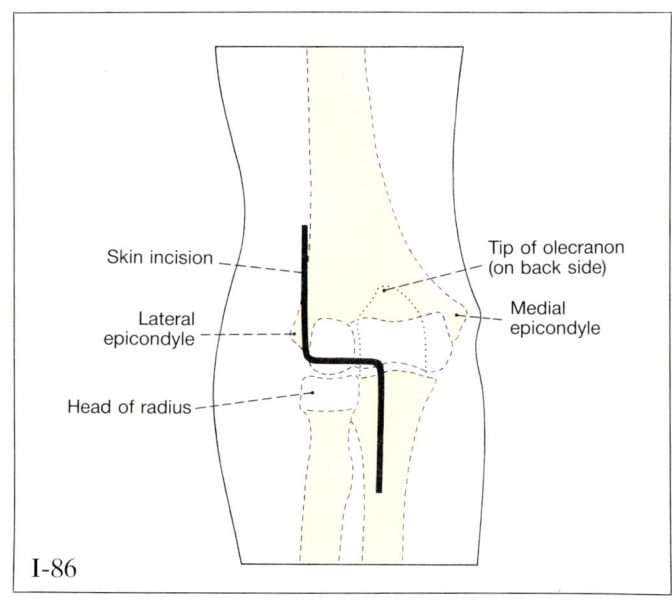

I-86

Elbow Joint — Anterior Exposure

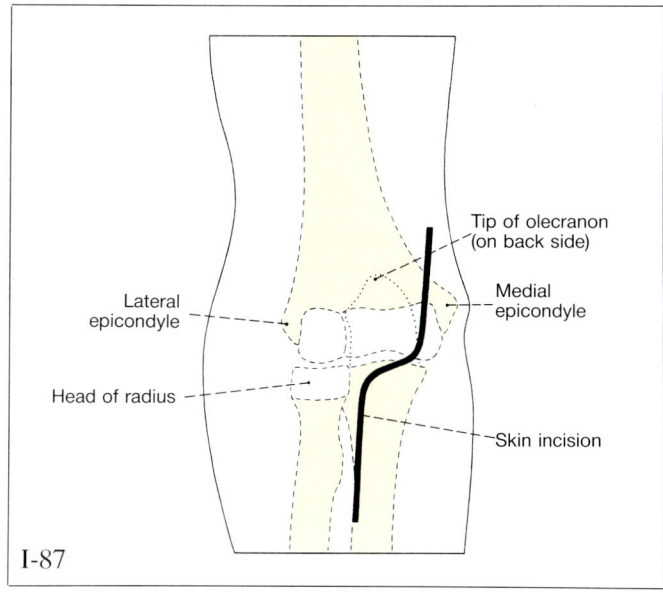

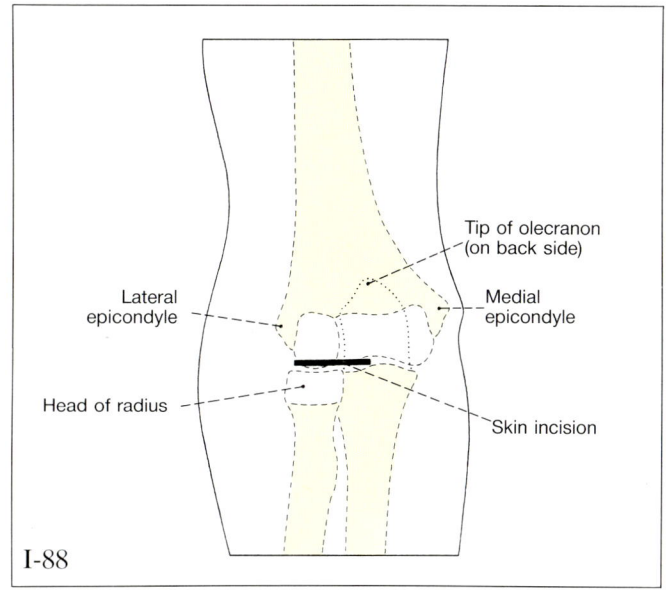

3. The bayonet-shaped medial incision (Fig. I-87) is particularly well suited for exposure of the median nerve and adjacent vessels.
4. Begin the transverse incision inside the lateral margin of the biceps tendon and continue it along the transverse skin crease of the elbow to the lateral epicondyle (Fig. I-88). This incision leaves a good cosmetic appearance, but continuation of this approach demands extra caution.
5. The nerves and vessels may be retracted either medially or laterally, depending on which part of the capsule is to be exposed.
6. Deep anterolateral approach: incision of the deep fascia. Look for the space between the brachialis and brachioradialis muscles immediately above the elbow joint (Fig. I-89).
7. Visualize the radial nerve. Retract the brachioradialis with the radial nerve laterally (Fig. I-90). By this method the muscular branches of the radial nerve will be spared.

Notes

1. With careful dissection this approach is not difficult.
2. The slender lateral cutaneous nerve of the forearm must be protected.

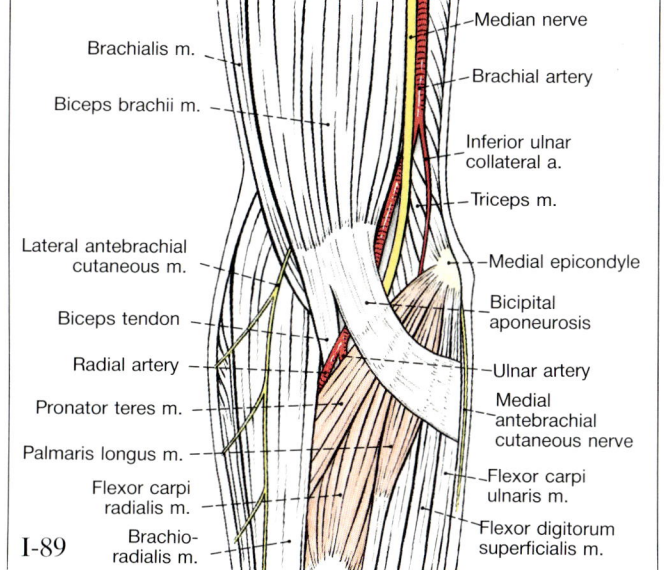

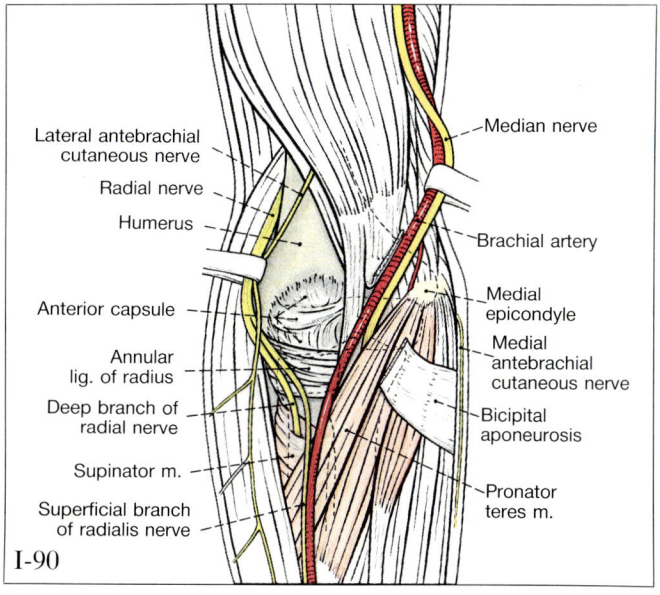

Elbow Joint

Lateral Exposure

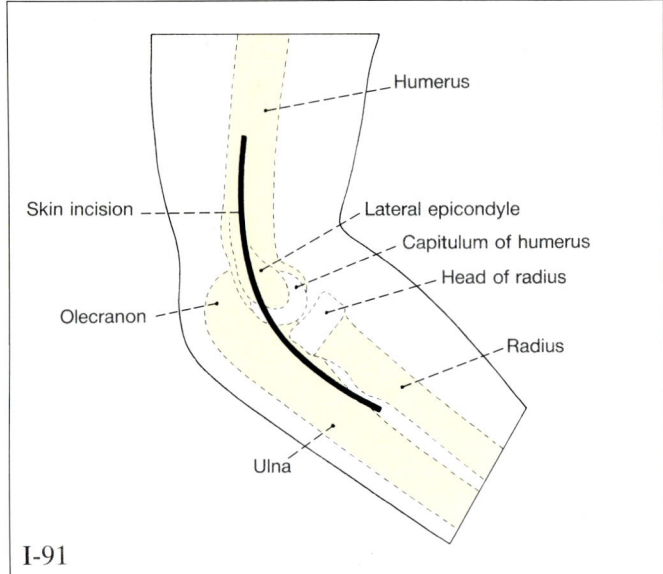

I-91

Lateral Exposure

Indications

1. Fractures of the neck and head of the radius
2. Loose bodies in the anterior or posterior compartment of the joint cavity
3. Comminuted fractures near the elbow joint
4. Lesions of the radial annular ligament
5. Synovectomy
6. Inflammatory processes
7. Bone tumors
8. Arthroplasty

Operative Steps

1. Begin a supracondylar skin incision on the outside of the elbow joint about 4–5 cm above the joint line. Extend it distally over the head of the radius and then over the anconeus muscle of the forearm (Fig. I-91).
2. Alternative: S-shaped incision (Fig. I-92).
3. Incise the muscle between the extensor carpi ulnaris and the anconeus muscles (Fig. I-93).

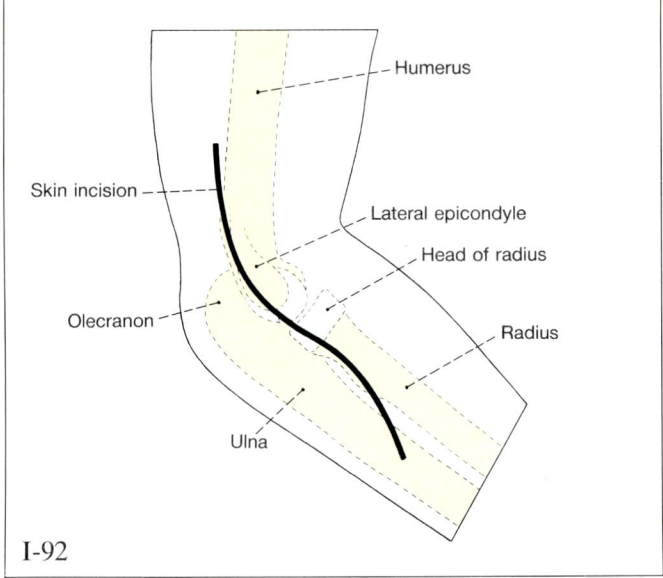

I-92

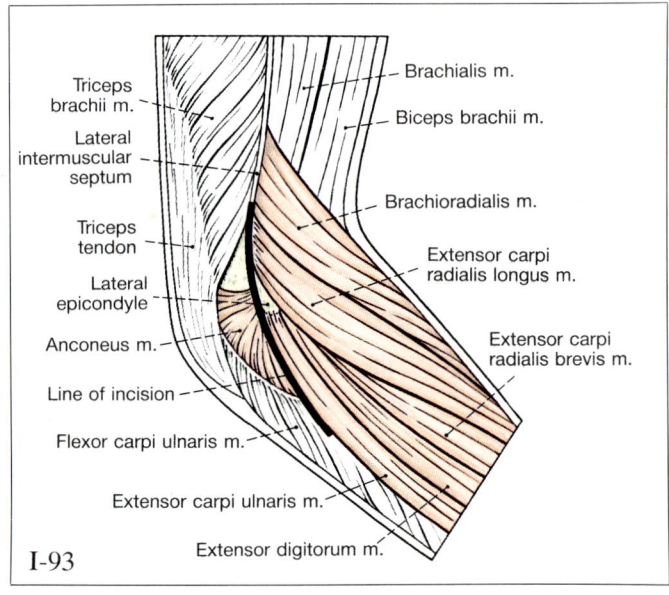

I-93

Elbow joint — Lateral Exposure

4. Alternative: Incise the muscle between the extensor carpi radialis longus and extensor digitorum or extensor carpi radialis brevis (Fig. I-94).
5. Sharply strip the muscles from the distal end of the humerus, both in front and in the back, staying close to the bone. This will prevent injury to the deep branch of the radial nerve (Fig. I-95), which runs in intimate contact with the anterior aspect of the joint capsule and over the head of the radius.
6. Make a deep incision of the capsule over the lateral aspect of the head of the radius. This exposes the articular surfaces of the head of the radius and the distal end of the humerus (Fig. I-95).
7. A better exposure of the joint is obtained by dividing the radial collateral ligament temporarily and retracting the triceps muscle dorsally (Fig. I-95). However, see notes.

Notes

1. After cutting through skin and fascia, the incision may be so chosen that the elbow joint can be opened with a lateral longitudinal cut through the common extensor tendon. This incision should be made immediately in front of and/or behind the radial collateral ligament after the skin is undermined.
2. In this way a wide anterior and/or posterior exposure is obtained while leaving the radial collateral ligament intact.

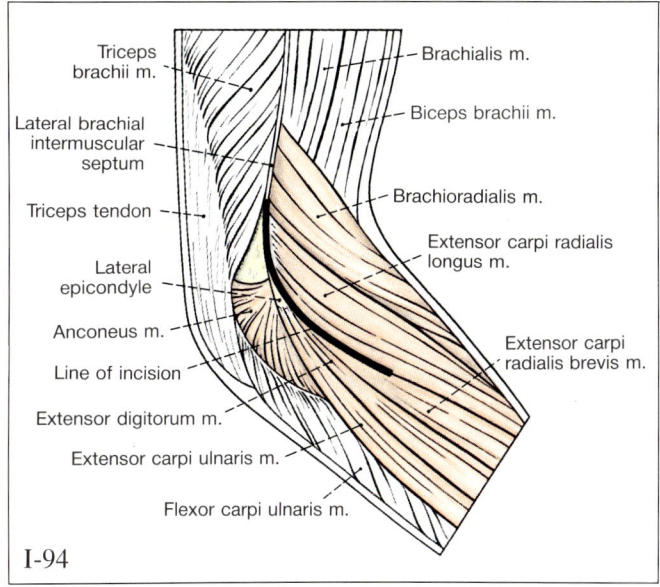

I-94

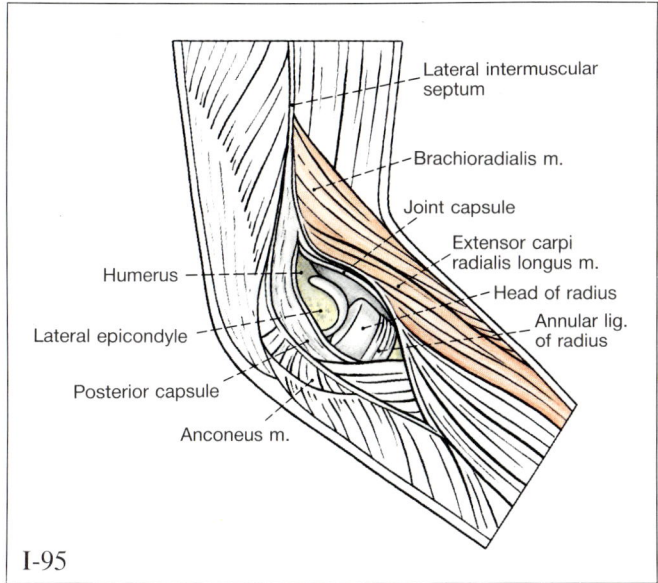

I-95

Radial Nerve

Applied Anatomy

1. Fig. I-96 shows schematically the course of the radial nerve.
2. Important anatomical details include the still undivided radial nerve trunk curving around the distal shaft of the humerus, its intimate relationship to the anterior aspect of the head of the radius, and the bifurcation of the nerve at this level into superficial and deep branches.
3. The deep branch enters the supinator muscle under its superficial tendinous part (the arch of Frohse, under which it may be compressed) to emerge again distal to the muscle.

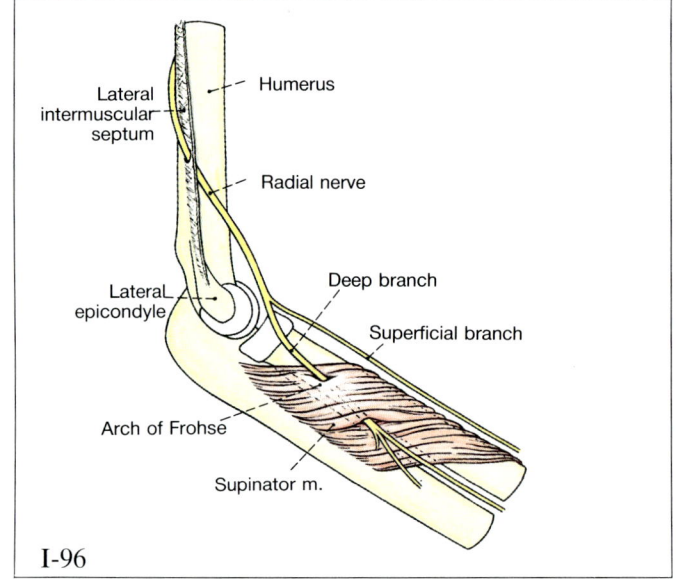

I-96

Head of Radius

Posterolateral Exposure

Indications

1. Irreducible fracture of the head of the radius
2. Resection of the head of the radius

Operative Steps

1. For exposure of the head of the radius only, a straight skin incision over the dorsolateral aspect of the elbow is sufficient. Begin the incision immediately behind the lateral epicondyle of the humerus and continue it downward for about 5 cm, at a distance of 1 cm from the lateral border of the olecranon (Fig. I-97).
2. Split the common origin of the extensor muscles of the hand longitudinally between the extensor carpi ulnaris and the extensor digitorum (Fig. I-98).
3. By reflecting the muscles, the capsule can be opened, leaving the annular ligament intact.
4. If a wider exposure is needed, detach the supinator muscle close to its ulnar origin.

Note

In step 4 avoid the deep branch of the radial nerve, which passes under the tendinous arch of the supinator muscle (arch of Frohse).

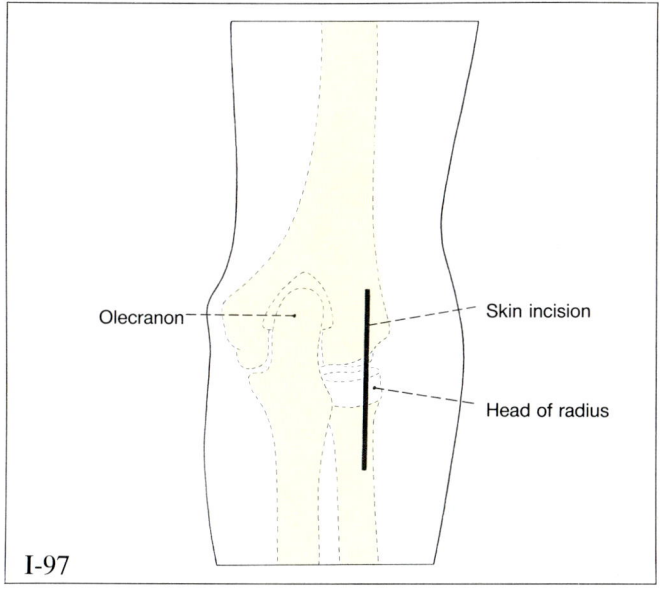

I-97

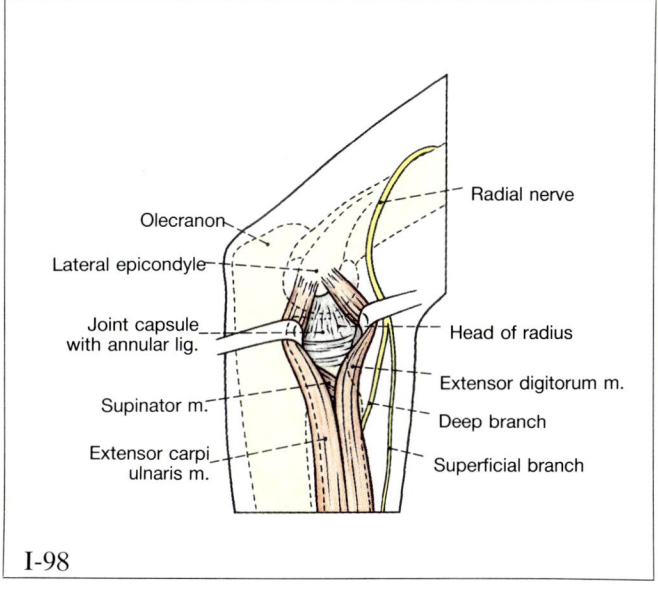

I-98

Elbow Joint (2)

Medial Exposure

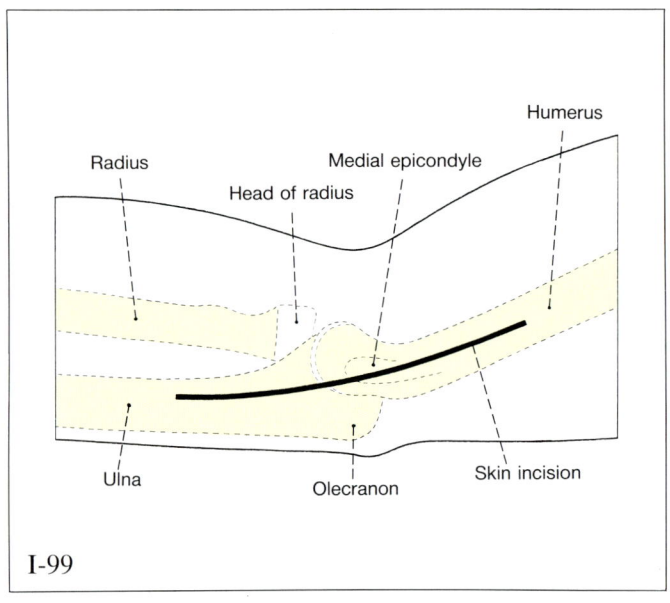

I-99

Indications

1. Inspection of all articular surfaces
2. Loose bodies in the joint cavity
3. Exploration of the ulnar nerve
4. Synovectomy (on the medial aspect)

Operative Steps

1. Make a skin incision over the medial epicondyle and extend it 5 cm both proximally and distally (Fig. I-99). This incision may be made at an obtuse angle if the elbow is flexed.
2. For a wider exposure, the course of the ulnar nerve should be fully appreciated. To be on the safe side, it may be helpful to expose different parts of it (Fig. I-100).
3. The need for further exposure of the ulnar nerve depends on the planned operative steps. If the ulnar nerve must be totally displaced from the field or may have to be brought forward, then it should be freed far enough proximal and distal to the ulnar sulcus to prevent kinking. This is especially important proximally, near the medial intermuscular septum. If necessary, the latter may be split.
4. Detach the tendinous origin of the flexor muscles from the medial epicondyle, or alternatively, remove the epicondyle using an osteotome. It is often sufficient to reflect part of the musculotendinous attachment by a short, longitudinal extension of the incision (Fig. I-101).

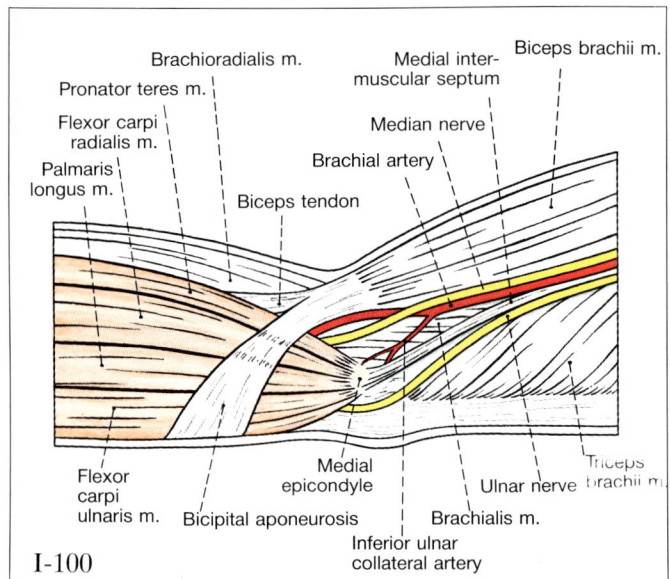

I-100

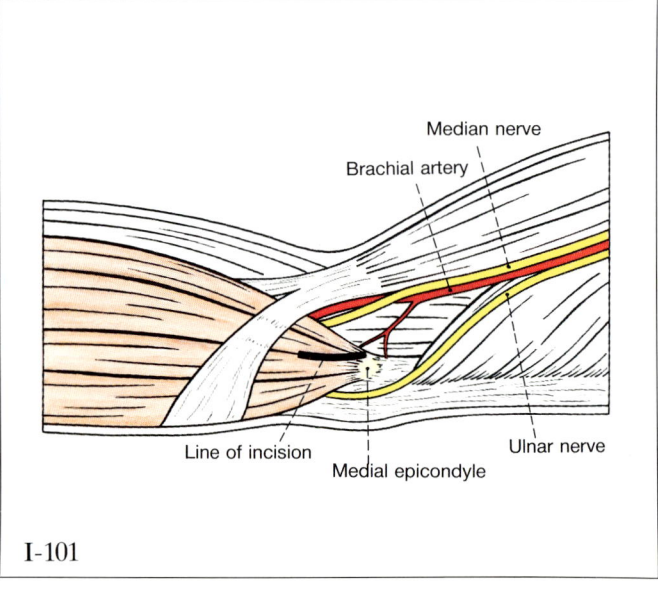

I-101

5. If the epicondyle is removed, reflect the fragment with the attached musculature distally (Fig. I-102). To facilitate reattachment later, leave some of the tendinous origins intact. Only gentle traction must be applied to these muscles to avoid injury to the branches of the median nerve that enter the muscle laterally.
6. Incise the capsule longitudinally and retract the cut edges forward and backward (Fig. I-102).
7. For a better exposure of the elbow joint, the capsule with the periosteum can be stripped off still farther. During this procedure the median nerve must be avoided as it lies over the anterior aspect of the joint.
8. The joint can be dislocated with the lateral part of the capsule serving as a hinge. For better visualization of the joint surfaces, the ulnar collateral ligament can be cut temporarily.

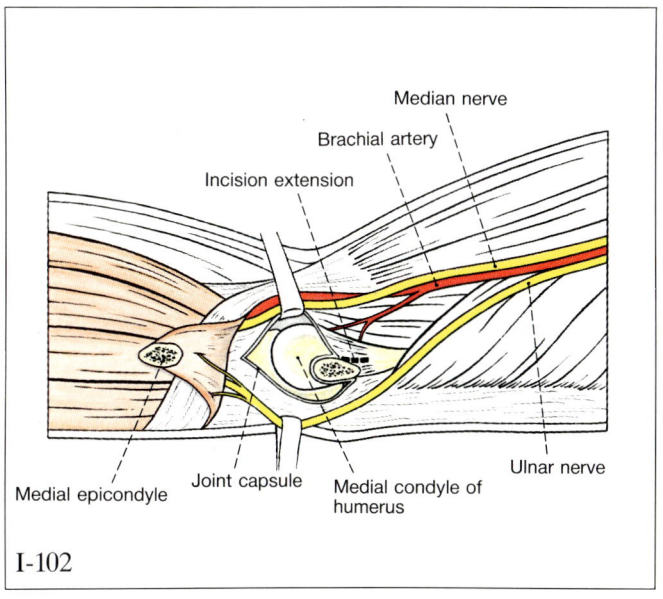

I-102

Notes

1. This approach is useful but cannot be performed with impunity because of the presence of the ulnar nerve in the operative field. The approach certainly affords a wide exposure of the elbow joint from the medial aspect as well as from the front and the back.
2. The dorsal aspect of the joint can be readily opened by retraction of the ulnar nerve and incision of the capsule behind the ulnar collateral ligament.
3. When the joint is opened in the back, it is important to note that the olecranon fossa is not accessible in an extended elbow because it is occupied by the olecranon. In the search for loose bodies, for example, the olecranon fossa is palpable only when the joint is flexed.

Posterolateral Exposure

Indications

1. Fractures of the ulna
2. Fractures of the head of the radius
3. Dislocation of the head of the radius
4. Fractures of the olecranon
5. Loose bodies in the posterior compartment of the joint
6. Arthroplasty of the elbow joint

Operative Steps

1. It is preferable to position the patient face down with the flexed elbow resting on a well-padded arm board. However, the operation may also be performed with the patient in a supine position and with a side table.
2. Make a slightly curved skin incision starting in the posterior midline 6–7 cm above the tip of the olecranon and continue it distally, lateral to the acromion, to a point 5 cm below the latter (Fig. I-103).
3. Alternative: Make a bayonet-shaped skin incision (Fig. I-104).

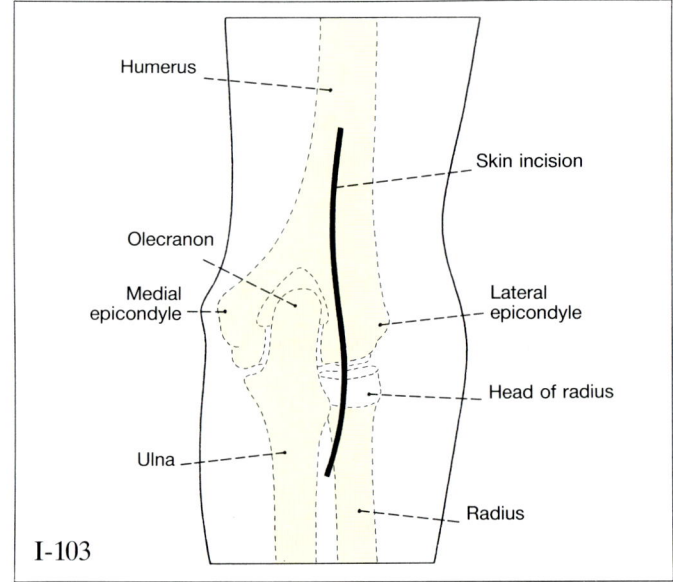

I-103

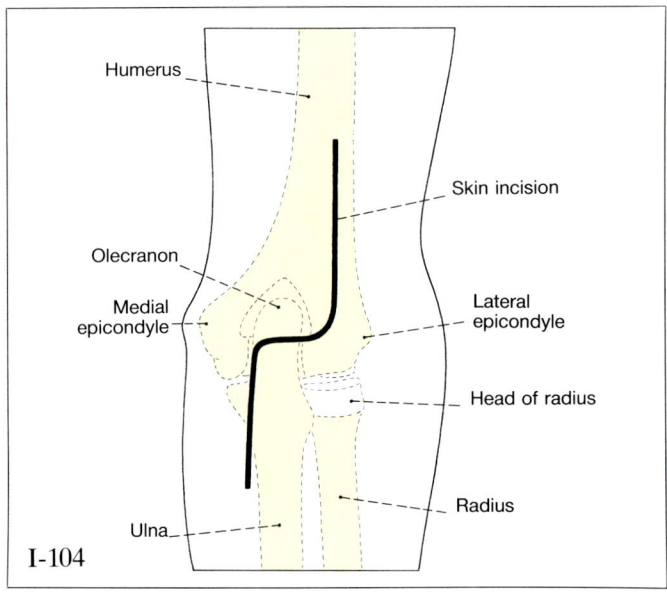

I-104

Elbow Joint — Posterolateral Exposure

4. Reflect the skin to reveal the triceps tendon and the tip of the olecranon (Fig. I-105).
5. Expose the distal end of the humerus and the posterior aspect of the joint capsule by splitting the triceps tendon down the middle and retracting the parts medially and laterally (Fig. I-106).
6. To gain an unobstructed view of the posterior aspect of the joint, retract the flexor carpi ulnaris muscle medially and the anconeus muscle laterally (Fig. I-106).

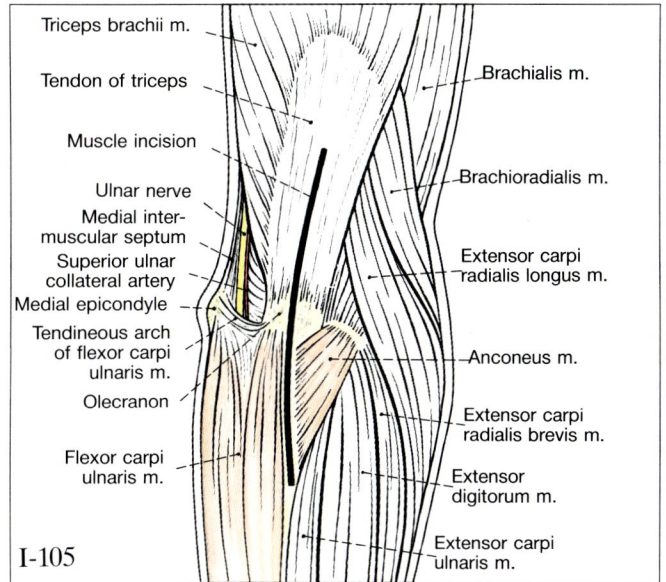

I-105

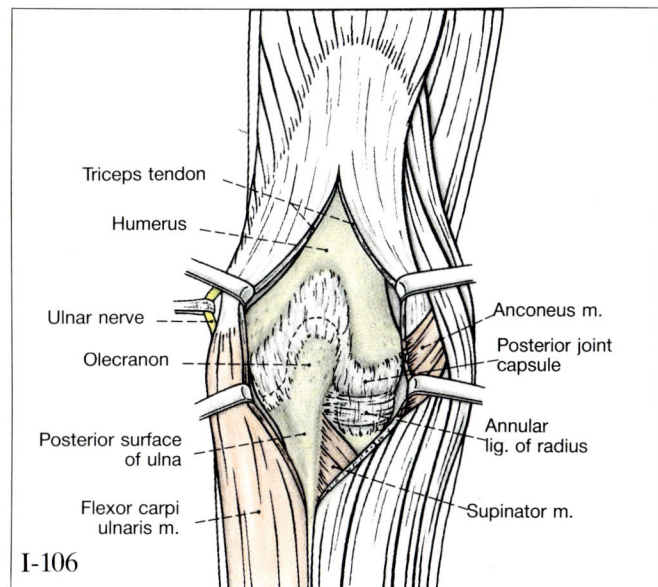

I-106

Posteromedial Exposure
Short Posterior Exposure

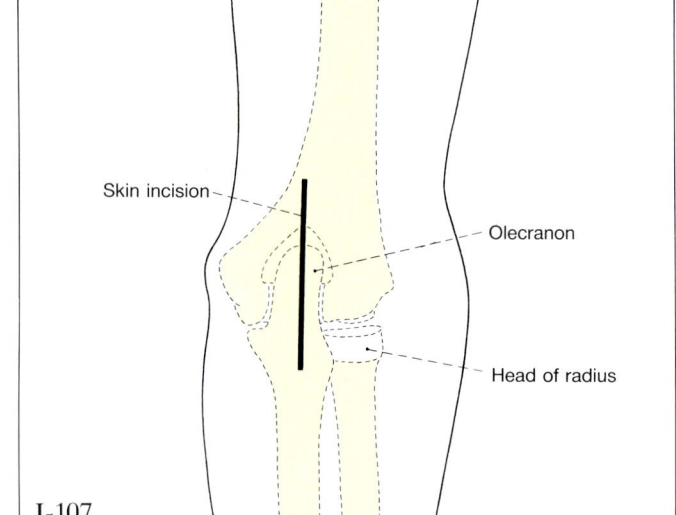

I-107

Indications

1. Fracture of the olecranon
2. Entry of the joint with temporary separation of the olecranon

Operative Steps

1. Place the patient in prone position with the forearm hanging over the edge of a side table.
2. Alternative: place the patient in supine position with the elbow flexed at a right angle and resting on the anterior chest wall.
3. Make a median longitudinal incision directly over the olecranon (Fig. I-107).
4. Prepare to open the joint by detaching the olecranon. Expose the ulnar nerve in the ulnar sulcus and protect the nerve by retracting it.
5. Drill two parallel canals in the olecranon with a 1.5-mm bit, for later reattachment by the AO technique (Fig. I-108).
6. Perform a transverse osteotomy of the olecranon with the oscillating saw in a vertical or slightly oblique plane (Fig. I-109).

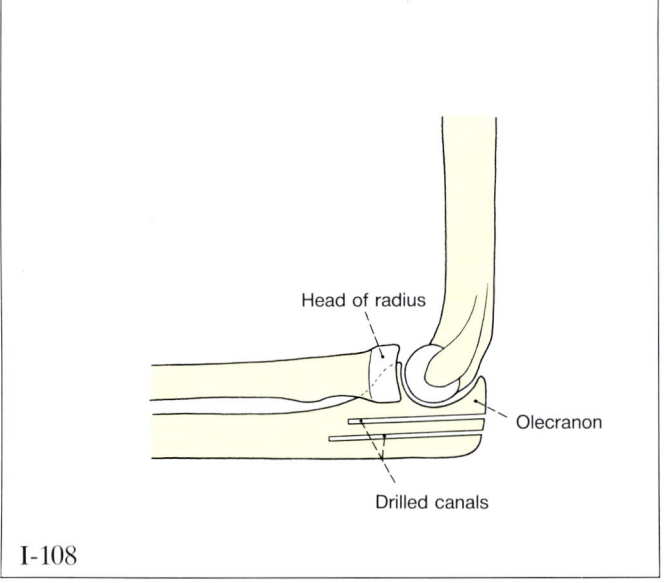

I-108

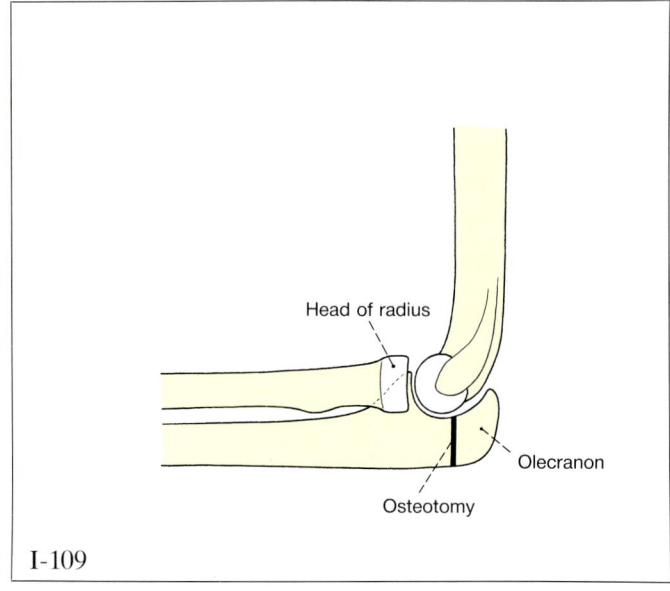

I-109

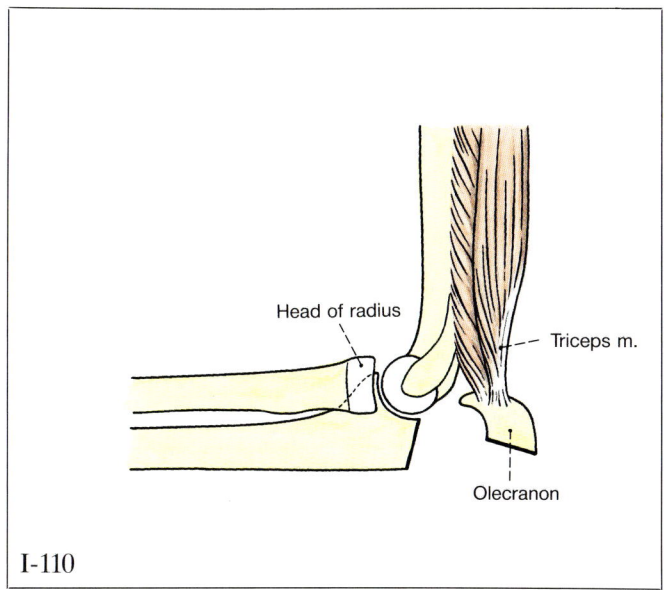

I-110

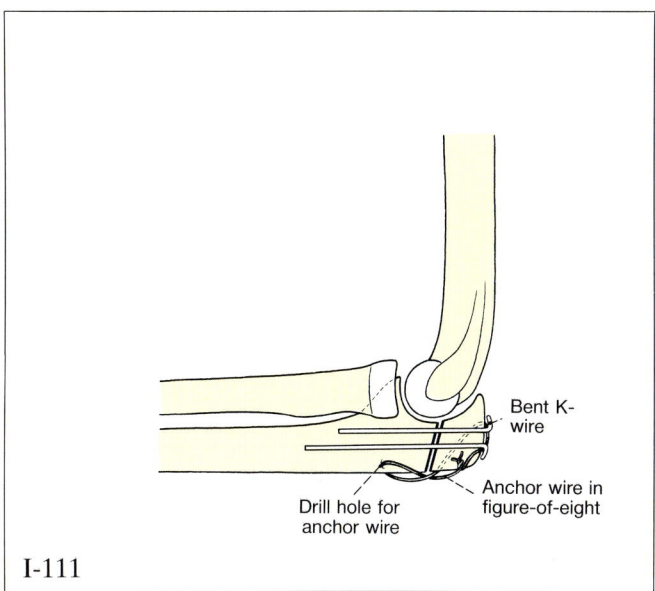

I-111

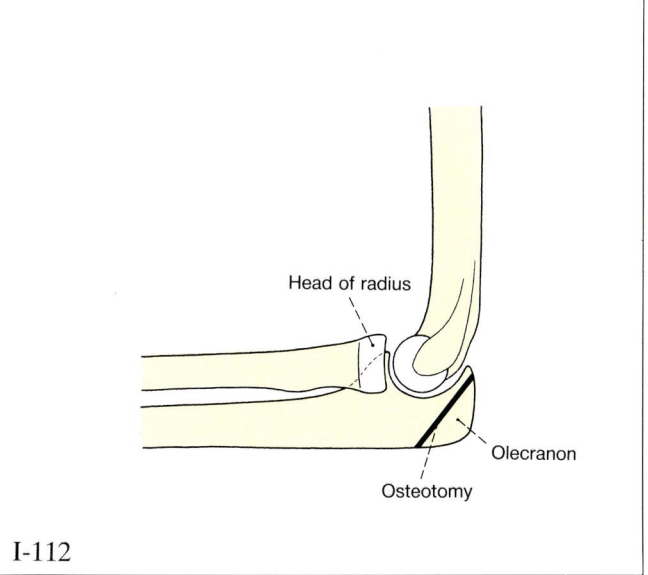

I-112

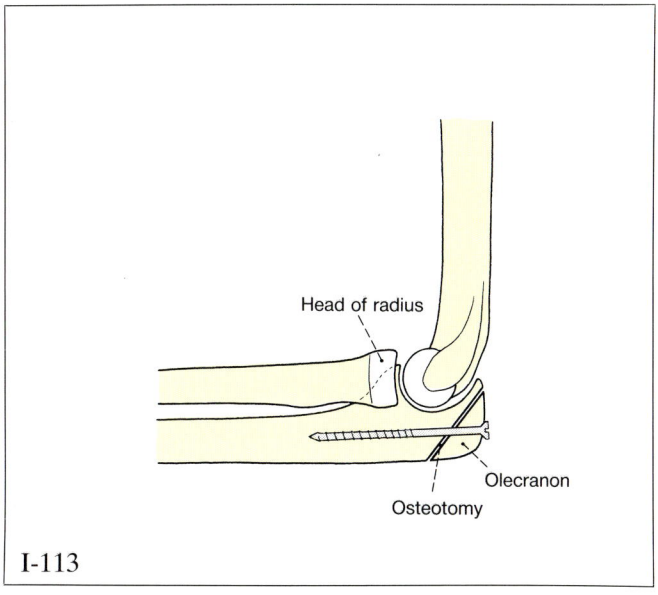

I-113

7. Reflect the separated olecranon with the attached triceps muscle (Fig. I-110). A good view of the articulation is obtained by flexing the elbow 140–150 degrees.
8. At the end of the operation, the olecranon is meticulously repositioned and attached with two Kirschner wires in the predrilled canals. Drill a hole for the fastening wire. Pull the wire through and apply it in a figure-of-eight. Tighten the wire. Bend the free ends of the Kirschner wires (Fig. I-111).
9. An oblique osteotomy of the olecranon outside the joint cavity offers a more conservative approach (Fig. I-112). Realignment of the bone is accomplished with a screw according to the AO-technique. The screw hole is made prior to the osteotomy (Fig. I-113). An additional application of an anchoring wire is highly recommended.

Posterior Exposure

Posterior Standard Exposure

Indications

1. Comminuted fractures of the elbow
2. Arthroplasty
3. Joint resection

Operative Steps

1. It is preferable to position the patient face down. The elbow lies flexed on a well-padded arm board. The operation may also be performed with the patient in a supine position with a side table.
2. Make the skin incision in the dorsal midline, beginning approximately 12 cm above the olecranon and continuing distally over the tip of the olecranon to a point 2–3 cm beyond it (Fig. I-114). The line of incision may be changed to pass lateral to the olecranon. A distal extension of the incision is possible (Fig. I-114).
3. When the skin is reflected, the triceps muscle, its attachments, and lateral tendon expansions are seen.
4. Free the ulnar nerve and move it carefully out of the way with a nerve retractor (Fig. I-115).
5. Cut the triceps tendon in the shape of a tongue, with the apex about 10 cm above the olecranon and the flared base at the level of the joint line (Fig. I-115).

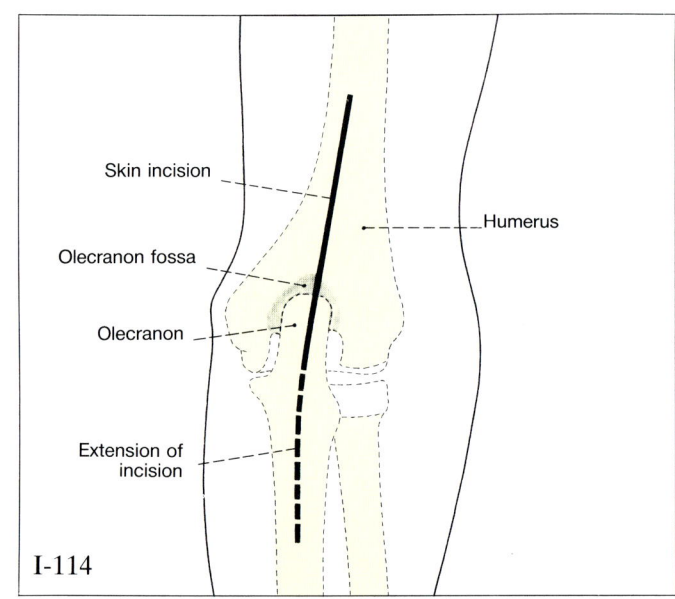

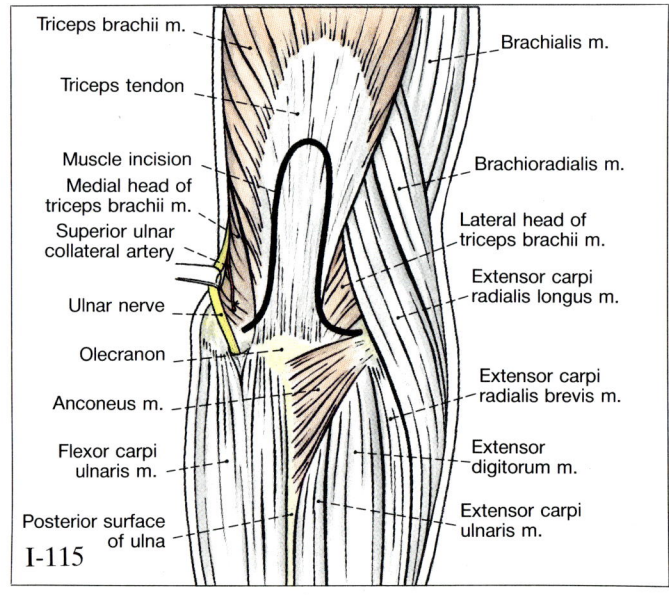

6. The upper consists of fascia and aponeurosis only, the middle portion of fascia, aponeurosis and muscle, and the base of the tongue contains the triceps tendon with all muscular attachments (Fig. I-116).
7. Make another median longitudinal incision through the remainder of the triceps muscle, the periosteum (down to the bone), and the posterior joint capsule.
8. Reflect the muscle, periosteum, and joint capsule to their respective sides so that the posterior surface of the distal humerus and the joint cavity are visible (Fig. I-117).
9. After the operation is completed, reunite the periosteum and the deepest layer of the triceps muscle with a few midline sutures.
10. Replace the tendinous tongue in its bed and suture it to the appropriate layers of tissue.

Note

This approach affords a wide operative field and is relatively safe.

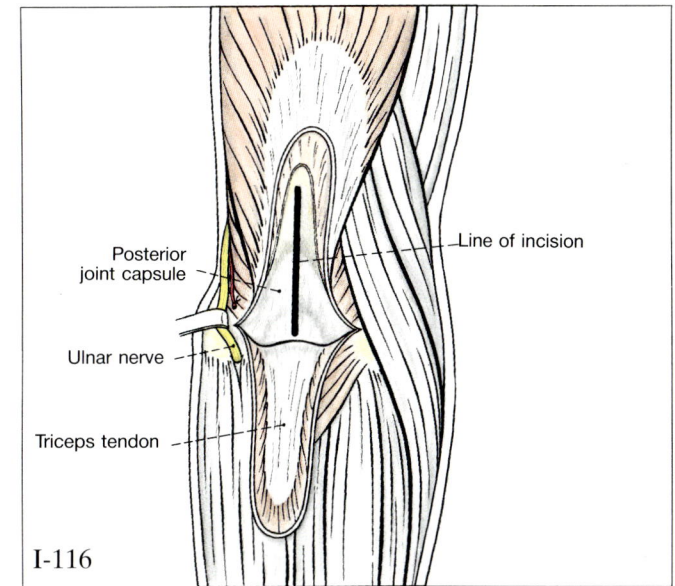

I-116

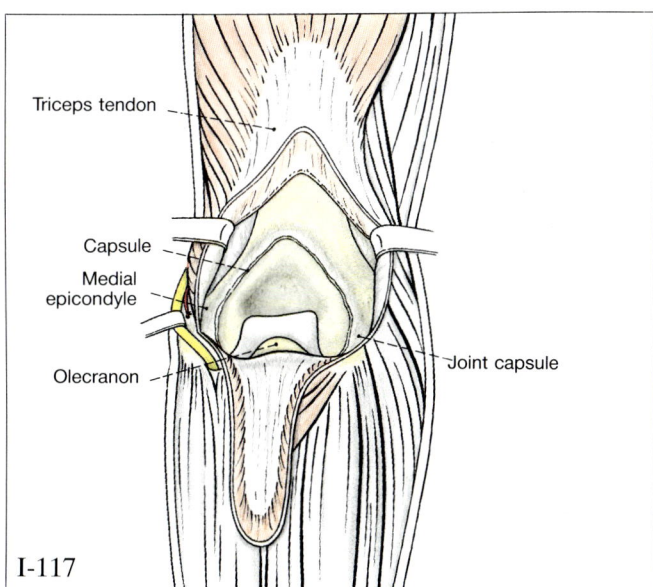

I-117

Elbow Joint — Posterior Curved Incision

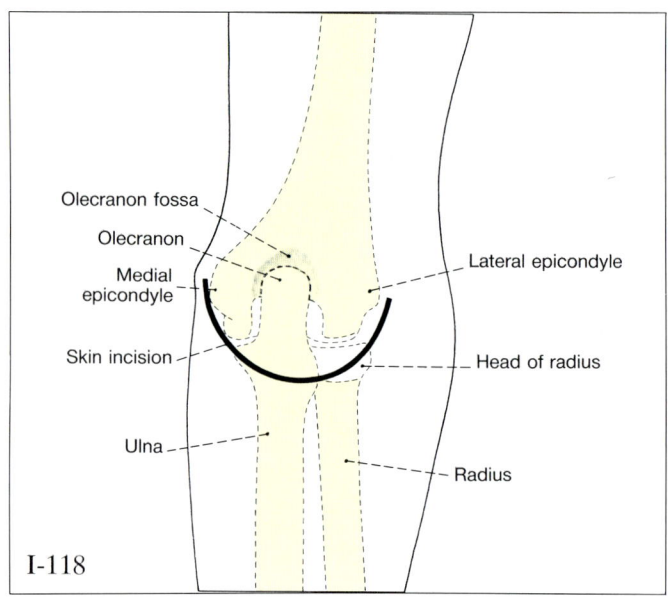

I-118

Posterior Curved Incision

Indications

1. Arthroplasty
2. Comminuted fracture of distal end of humerus

Operative Steps

1. Begin the dorsal "U"-shaped incision at the lateral epicondyle and extend it medially and distally, crossing the ulna at a point 5 cm below the tip of the olecranon. Then continue it medially and upward to the medial epicondyle (Fig. I-118).
2. Reflect the resulting skin flap proximally to bring into view the olecranon with the attached tendon of the triceps.
3. Free the ulnar nerve and carefully displace it medially with a nerve retractor.
4. Cut transversely through the subcutaneous tissue and the lateral retinacula of the triceps tendon down to the bone (Fig. I-119).
5. Resect the olecranon with an osteotome and pull the bony fragment upward with the attached muscle (Fig. I-120).
6. Strip off subperiosteally all muscles that attach medial and lateral to this area and reflect them. A wide exposure of the dorsal components of the elbow is now obtained.
7. A lateral extension of the incision is possible (Fig. I-120).

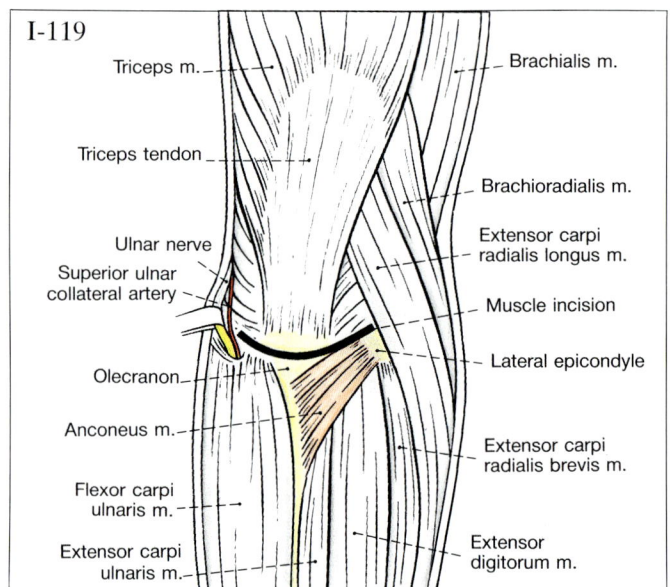

I-119

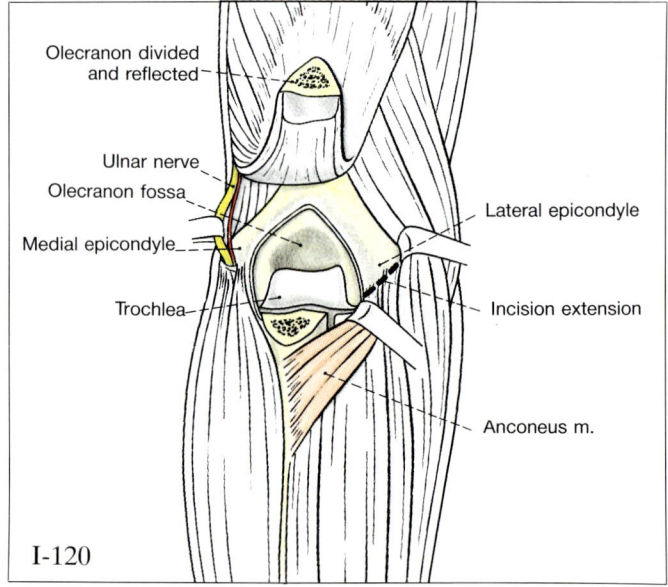

I-120

E. Forearm

Proximal Radius and Upper Fourth of Ulna

Elbow Joint –
Posterior Exposure

Indications

1. Fractures of the proximal third of ulna
2. Fracture of the head of the radius
3. Dislocation of the head of the radius

Operative Steps

1. Make a dorsal skin incision 2–3 cm above the elbow joint, closely following the lateral border of the triceps tendon. Continue the incision distally, lateral to the tip of the acromion, and along the lateral border of the ulna to about the junction of the upper and middle third of this bone (Fig. I-121).
2. Deeply incise the fascia between the ulna and the anconeus and extensor carpi ulnaris muscles (Fig. I-122).

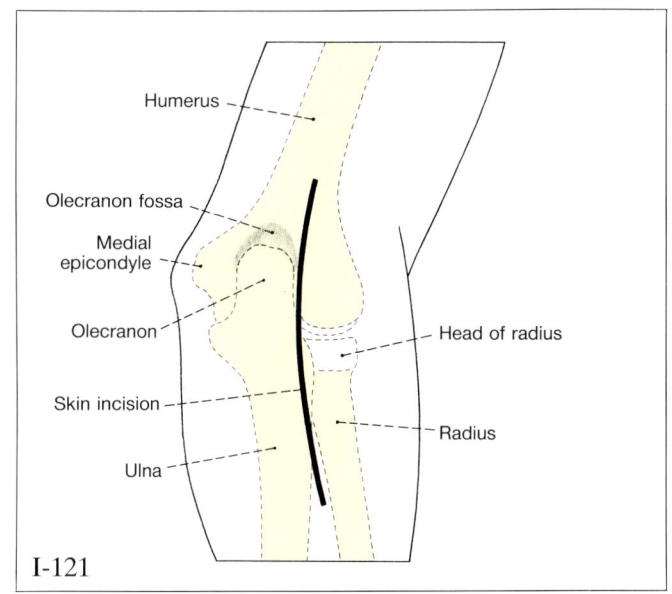

I-121

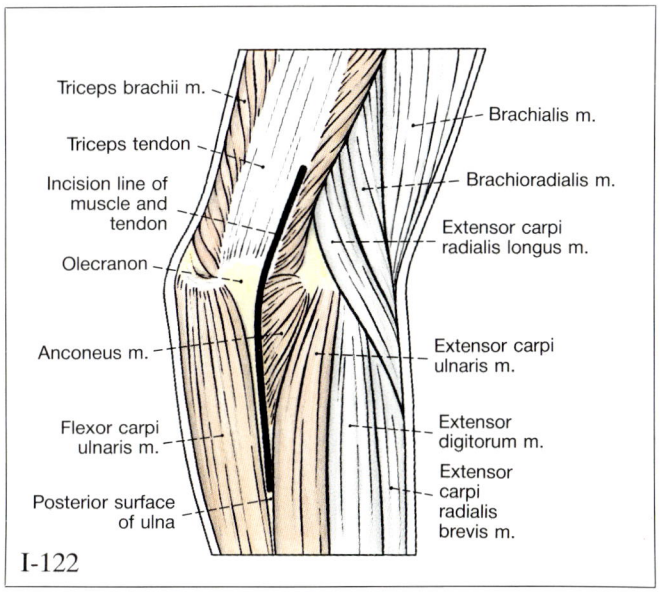

I-122

3. Detach the anconeus muscle subperiosteally from the bone in the upper part of the incision and reflect it laterally. The joint capsule that firmly embraces the head of the radius can now be seen, as well as the posterior joint capsule and the insertion of the supinator muscle (Fig. I-123).
4. Reflect the flexor carpi radialis muscle medially. The upper third of the ulna is now exposed.
5. Cut the proximal part of the supinator muscle close to its ulnar origin (Fig. I-123). By carefully reflecting the muscle laterally, the interosseous membrane and the upper fourth of the radius are seen (Fig. I-124).
6. The deep branch of the radial nerve, which runs embedded in the muscle, must be protected during this procedure.

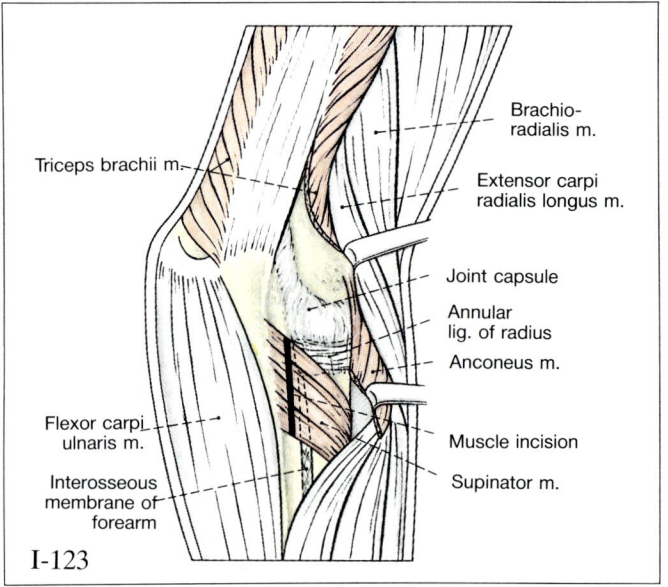

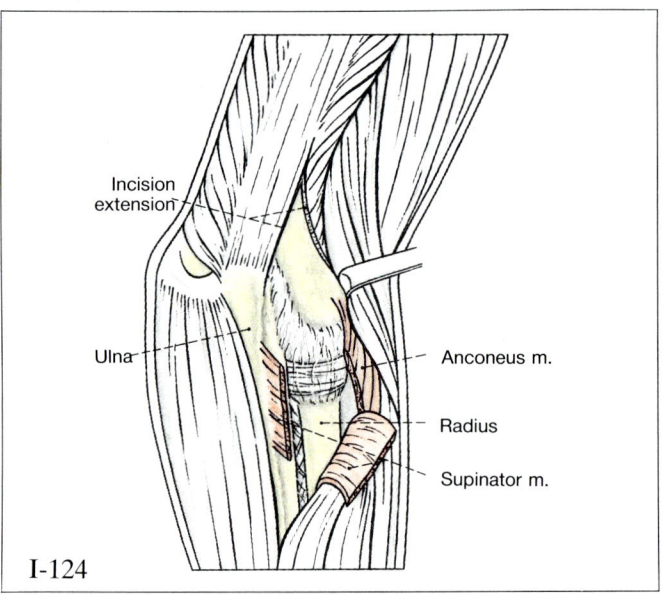

Radial Nerve – Supinator Arch

Lateral Exposure

Indications

Peripheral radial nerve compression – supinator syndrome

Operative Steps

1. The course of the radial nerve near the elbow joint and in the proximal forearm, and its division into superficial and deep branches are seen schematically in Fig. I-125.
2. Explore the radial nerve by making a 5-cm skin incision that begins about 3 cm distal to the lateral epicondyle in the forearm and follows the lateral border of the brachioradialis muscle (Fig. I-126). Ascertain the proper line of incision by palpating the depression between the brachioradialis and the extensor carpi radialis longus muscles (Fig. I-126).

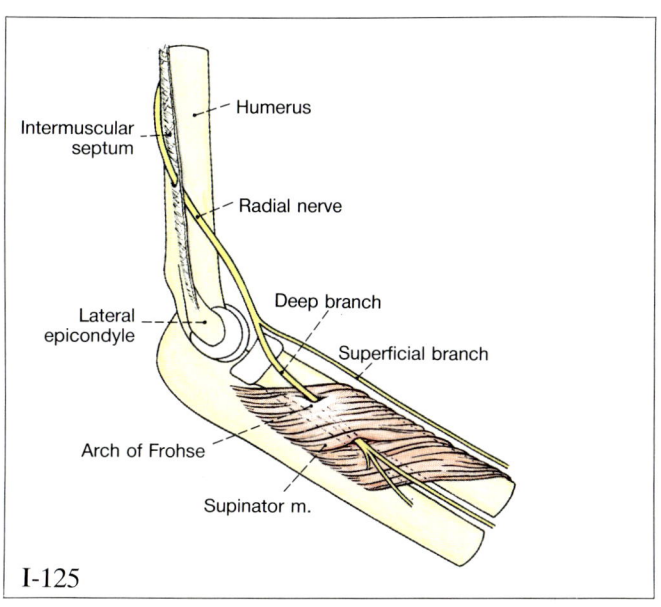

I-125

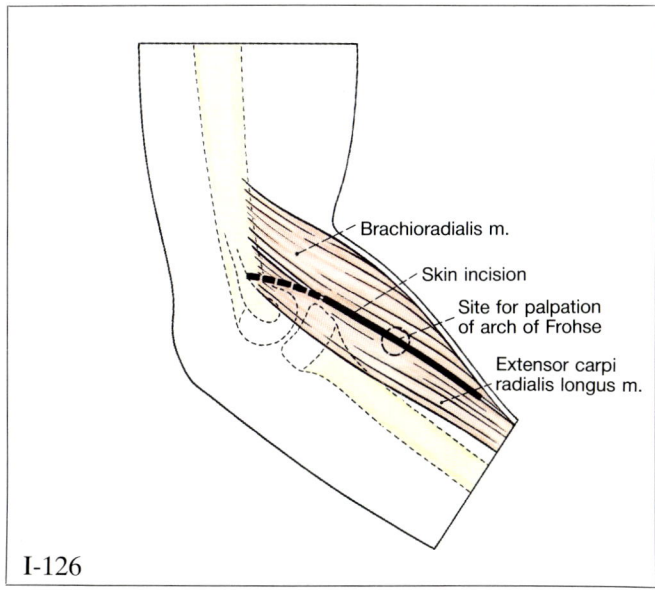

I-126

Radial Nerve – Supinator Arch — Lateral Exposure

3. To reach both branches of the radial nerve as well as the supinator arch, make a deep, blunt entry between the brachioradialis and extensor carpi radialis longus muscles (Fig. I-127).
4. The taut aponeurotic deep surface of the extensor carpi radialis brevis muscle can often interfere with the exposure of the radial nerve and may have to be cut across its fiber direction.
5. Extend the incision proximally (Fig. I-126) to expose the origin of the extensor muscles from the lateral epicondyle.
6. If necessary, make an additional upward extension of the incision to bring into view again the radial nerve where it pierces the lateral intermuscular septum (Fig. I-127, section B).
7. A distal continuation of the incision makes possible a view of the radial nerve as it emerges from the supinator muscle (Fig. I-127, section C).

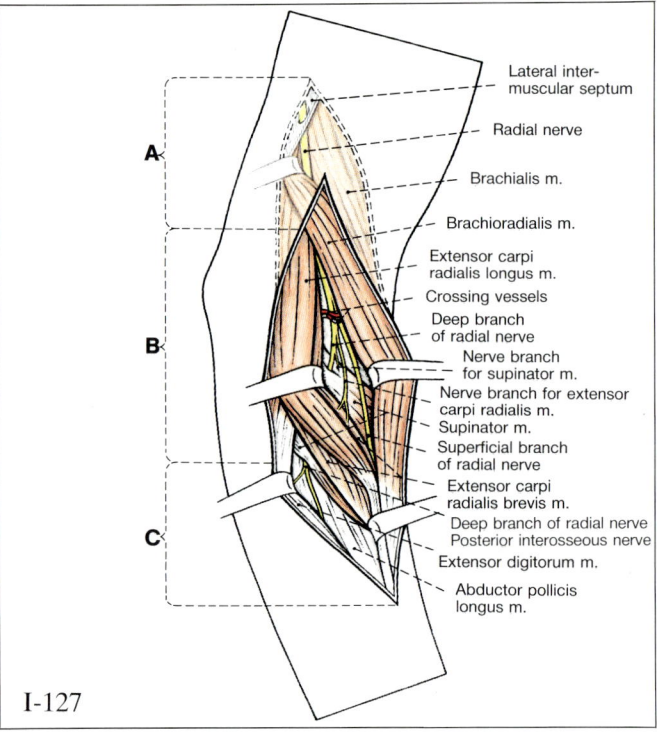

I-127

Notes

1. Dissection of the deep branch of the radial nerve must be performed with great care and preferably with some kind of ocular magnification because of the highly variable origins of the slender motor branches to the extensor carpi radialis brevis and the supinator muscles.
2. Blood vessels that cross the deep branch of the radial nerve should be isolated and cauterized with bipolar cautery.
3. Basically, a medial approach is also possible. In this case the line of incision follows the proximal medial border of the brachioradialis muscle. Both main divisions of the radial nerve are seen by retracting the brachioradialis muscle laterally.

Shaft of the Ulna

Posterior Exposure

Indications

1. Irreducible fractures
2. Inflammatory processes
3. Tumors
4. Ununited fractures

Operative Steps

1. Pronate the forearm and expose the shaft of the ulna by making a 15-cm skin incision from a point 5 cm distal to the olecranon and extend it along the dorsal surface of the ulna (Fig. I-128, skin incision A).

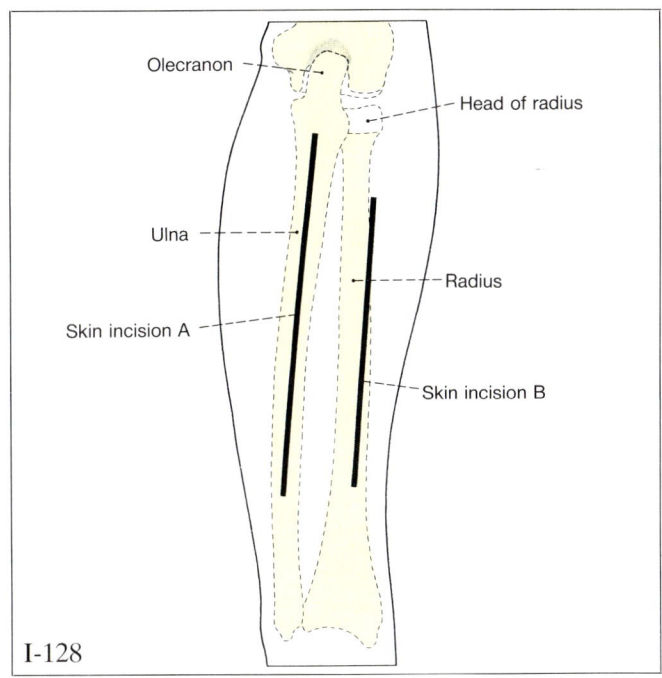

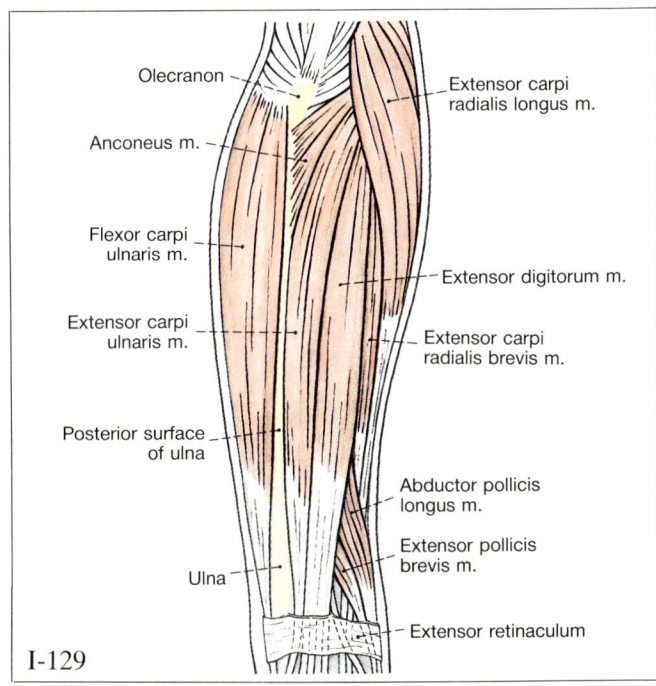

Shaft of the Ulna — Posterior Exposure

2. With a rasp, detach and reflect the flexor carpi ulnaris muscle and the extensor carpi ulnaris and anconeus muscles to their respective sides (Figs. I-129 and I-130).

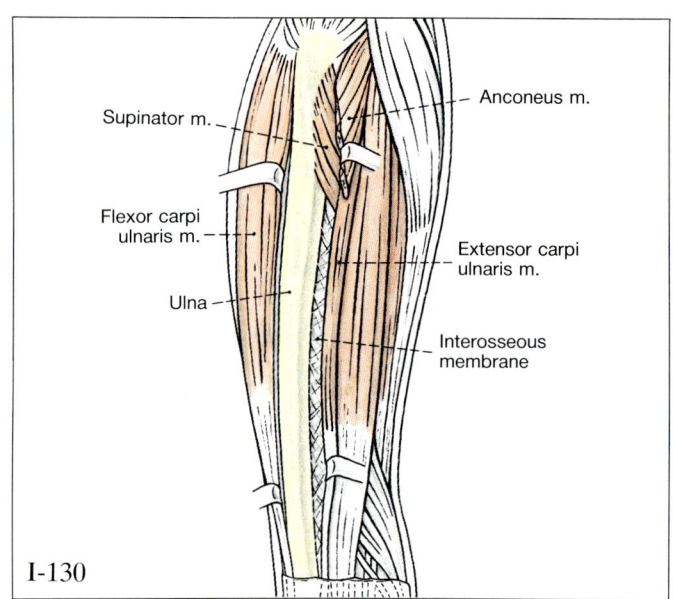

Shaft of the Radius

Posterior Exposure

Indications

See "Shaft of the Ulna"

Operative Steps

1. Expose the shaft of the radius by making a 15-cm incision on the dorsal aspect of the forearm, beginning about 4 cm below the head of the radius and continuing distally over the dorsal surface of the radius (Fig. I-128, skin incision B). Access to the shaft of the radius is gained between the extensor carpi radialis brevis and extensor digitorum muscles.
2. The extensor digitorum muscle is seen after cutting through the deep fascia. When the muscle is reflected laterally, the deep branch of the radial nerve can be identified where it pierces the upper portion of the supinator muscle (Fig. I-131).
3. Cut the supinator muscle along the lateral margin of the radius and reflect it toward the ulnar side with the thumb muscles (Fig. I-132). The shaft of the radius is now fully exposed.

Note

In this approach the patient may be in the supine position with a flexed elbow.

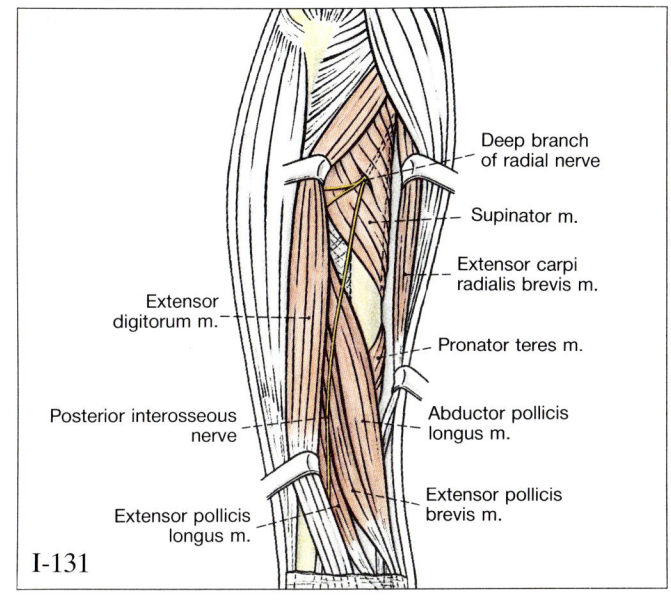

I-131

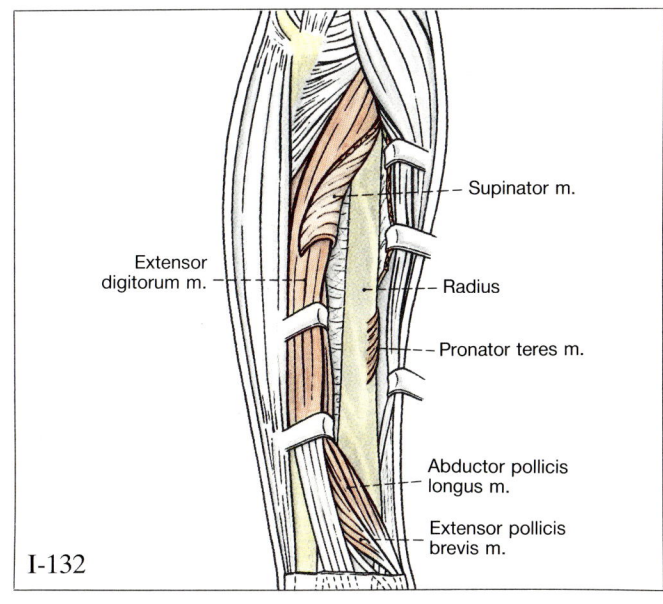

I-132

Shafts of the Radius and Ulna

Posterior Exposure

Indication

Multiple fractures

Operative Steps

1. A simultaneous approach to the shafts of both radius and ulna is achieved by means of an extensive curved incision on the dorsal aspect of the forearm.
2. Begin the skin incision behind the lateral epicondyle and pass over the lateral edge of the olecranon to the medial edge of the middle part of the ulna. Continue it laterally to the styloid process of the radius (Fig. I-133).
3. Begin the dissection proximally between the flexor carpi ulnaris muscle and the extensor group (Fig. I-134). Continue it by partially cutting the ulnar insertion of the anconeus muscle and the origin of the supinator muscle (Fig. I-134).
4. Expose the distal shaft of the radius between the extensor digitorum and extensor carpi radialis brevis muscles (Fig. I-134). Retract the abductor pollicis longus and extensor pollicis brevis muscles toward the ulnar side.

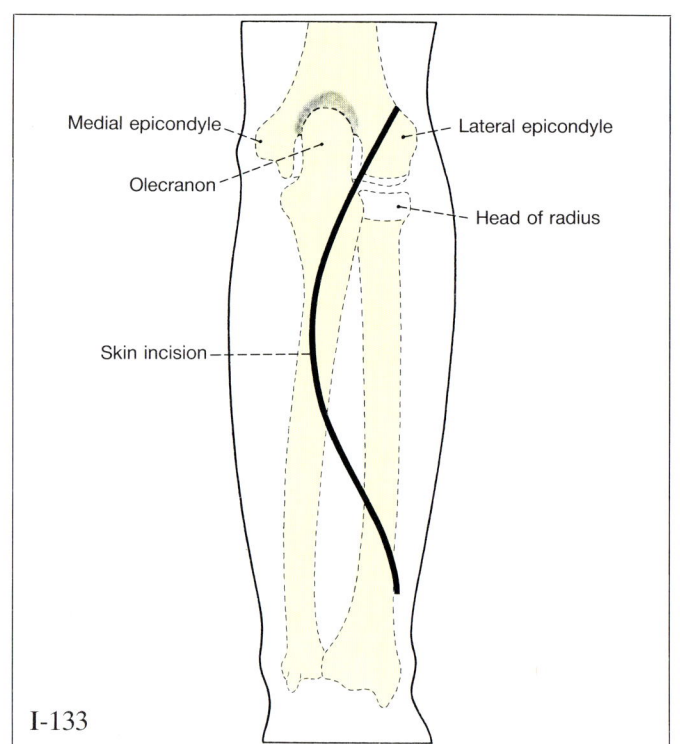

I-133

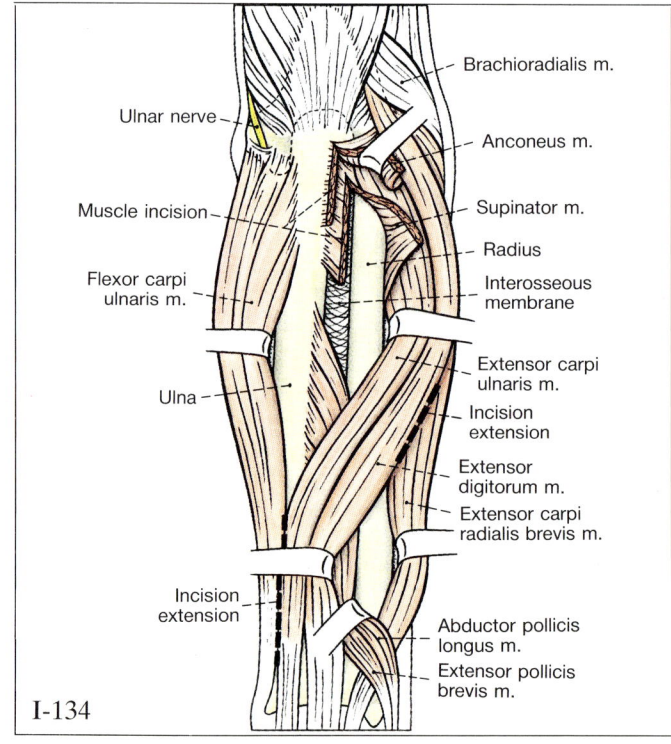

I-134

Median Nerve
(Exposure in the Forearm)

Volar Exposure

Indication

Exploration of the median nerve

Operative Steps

1. Make a skin incision on the volar side of the forearm, beginning close to the medial epicondyle and continuing straight distally to a point 2 finger breadths proximal to the wrist joint (Fig. I-135).
2. Expose the entire median nerve by extending the incision proximally to the elbow joint and distally to the wrist joint.
3. The plane between the superficial and deep muscle layers is now established so that the flexor digitorum superficialis and the flexor carpi ulnaris muscles can be retracted toward their respective sides (Fig. I-135).
4. The median nerve lies on the flexor digitorum profundus muscle.
5. The ulnar nerve accompanied by the ulnar artery is found near the ulnar edge of the field (Fig. I-135).

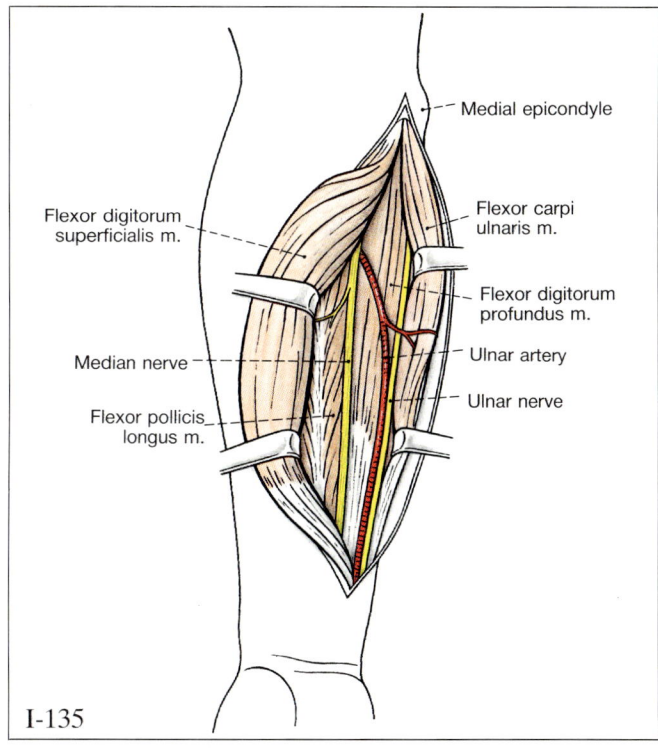

I-135

Distal Radius

Dorsal Exposure

Indications

1. Complicated fractures of the distal fourth of the radius
2. Inflammatory processes
3. Tumors

Operative Steps

1. Make a 7- to 8-cm dorsal skin incision, beginning at the styloid process of the radius and continuing proximally along the radius (Fig. I-136).
2. Incise the deep fascia and the extensor retinaculum (dorsal carpal ligament). This will expose the extensor digitorum muscle, the tendon of the extensor pollicis longus muscle, a small area of the radius, the abductor pollicis longus muscle, the extensor pollicis brevis muscle, and the tendon of the extensor carpi radialis brevis muscle (Fig. I-137).
3. Reflect the abductor pollicis longus and extensor pollicis brevis muscles to the radial side. Retract the tendons of the extensor carpi radialis longus and brevis and the extensor digitorum to the ulnar side. The distal fourth of the shaft of the radius is now exposed (Fig. I-138).

Note

The rami of the superficial branch of the radial nerve must be protected.

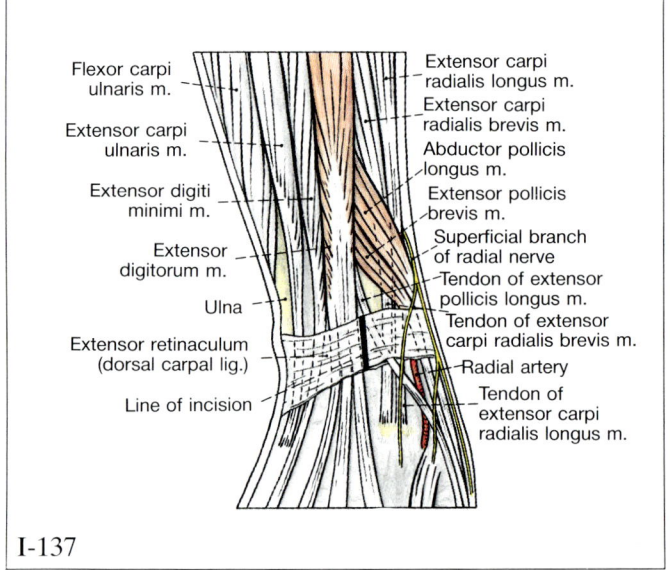

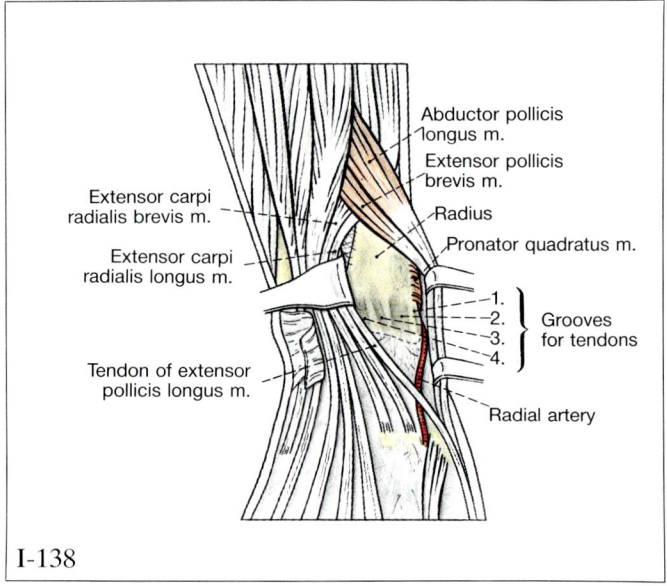

Volar Exposure

Operative Steps

1. Make a 6-cm volar longitudinal incision on the radial side of the flexor carpi radialis muscle, extending it proximally from the transverse skin crease of the wrist (Fig. I-139).
2. After splitting the antebrachial fascia, retract the tendons of the flexor carpi radialis and the flexor pollicis longus muscles toward the ulnar side, and displace the radial artery and accompanying veins radially.
3. Detach the radial origin of the pronator quadratus muscle and reflect it away from the radius (Fig. I-140).
4. The distal fourth of the radius is now seen.

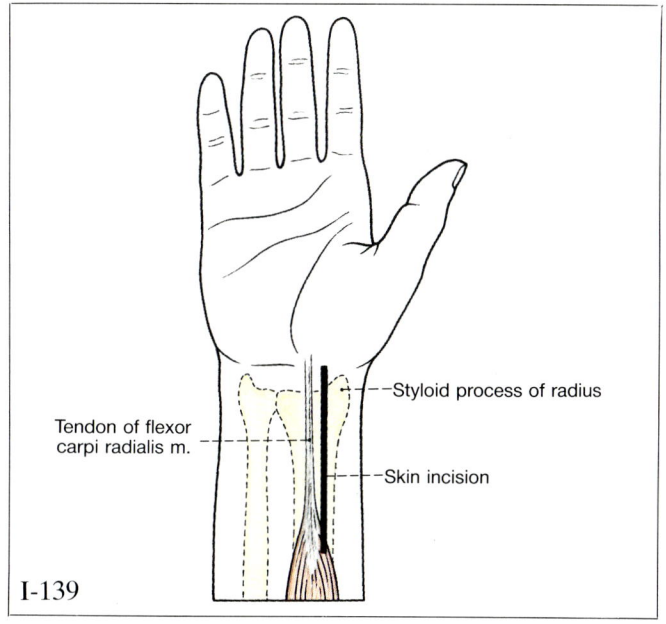

I-139

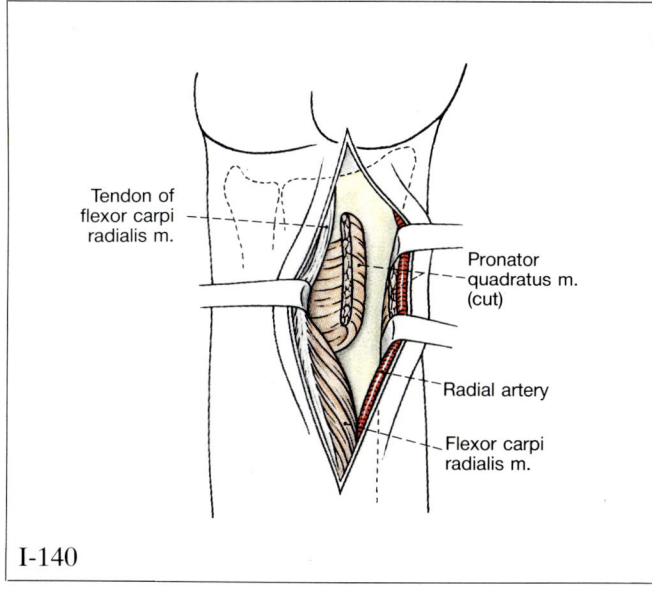

I-140

Palmar Tendon
(Tendon of Palmaris Longus Muscle)

Volar Exposure

Indication

Removal of palmar tendon for transplantation

Operative Steps

1. The palmar tendon lies close to the flexor carpi radialis muscle on its ulnar side (Fig. I-141).
2. Locate the palmar tendon by making superficial transverse skin incisions over its course at 5-cm intervals beginning at the flexor crease of the wrist (Fig. I-141).
3. Mobilize the tendon through the short skin incisions, cut it distally, and pull it out proximally (Fig. I-142).

Notes

1. The palmaris longus muscle originates from the medial epicondyle. The length of the tendon is variable.
2. Almost the entire length of the palmaris longus muscle may be tendinous.

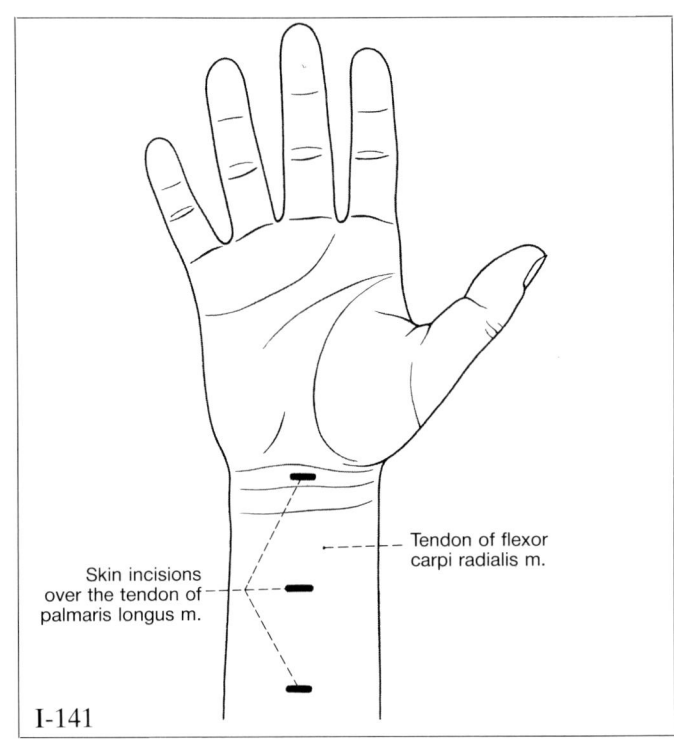

I-141

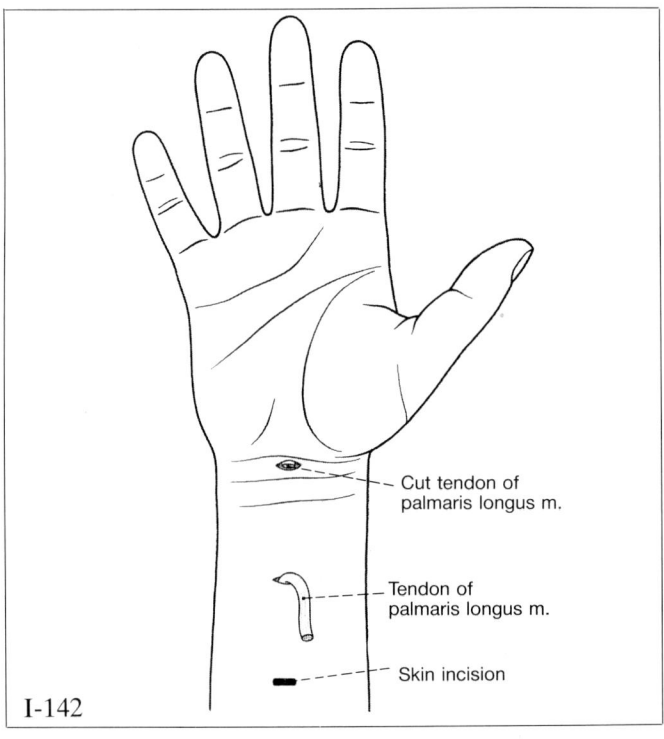

I-142

F. Wrist Region

Wrist Joint

Applied Anatomy

1. The topography of bony components of the wrist and hand is shown in a dorsal view in Fig. I-143.
2. The cutaneous nerves to the dorsum of the hand are seen in Fig. I-147.

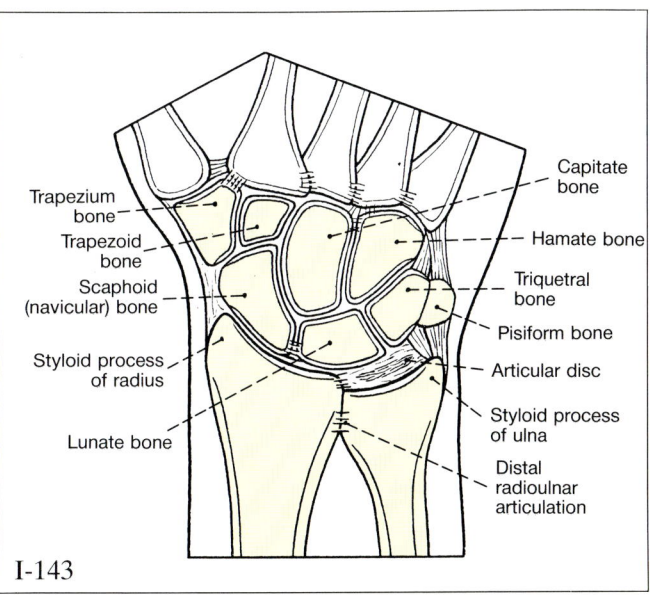

I-143

Wrist Joint

Dorsal Exposure

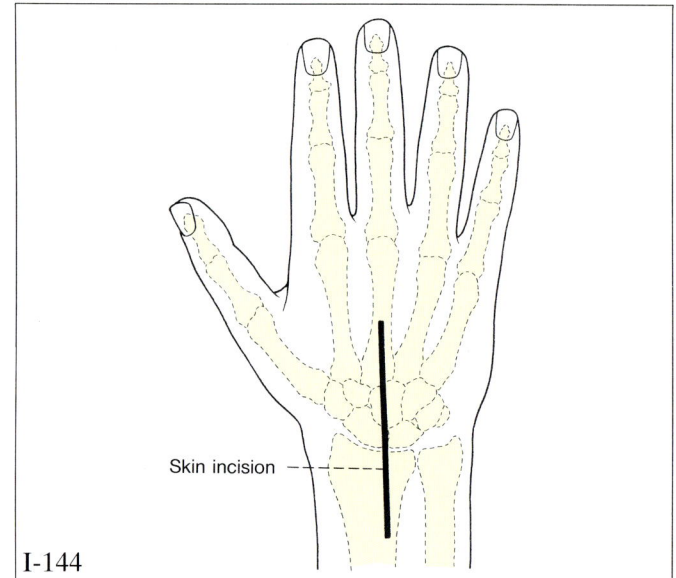

I-144

Indications

1. Irreducible fractures and dislocation of carpal bones
2. Ununited fractures of the wrist bones
3. Inflammatory processes
4. Tumors
5. Wrist joint arthrodesis
6. Wrist joint arthroplasty
7. Synovectomy and tenosynovectomy

Operative Steps

1. The dorsum of the wrist can be approached through a straight midline incision (Fig. I-144), through an S-shaped incision (Fig. I-145, skin incision A), or through a transverse cut (Fig. I-146).
2. A variation of the transverse incision that affords a wider exposure is illustrated in Fig. I-145, skin incision B.
3. When less extensive radial or ulnar exposure is indicated, longitudinally oriented lines of incisions also provide opportunities for expansion (Fig. I-147, skin incisions A and B).
4. The S-shaped skin incision begins on the dorsum of the hand, crosses the wrist joint, and terminates in the distal forearm (Fig. I-145, skin incision A).
5. The transverse incision follows the skin crease to prevent the formation of unsightly scar tissue later. The incision begins approximately 1.5 cm proximal to the styloid process of the radius and is slightly curved toward the styloid process of the ulna (Fig. I-146).

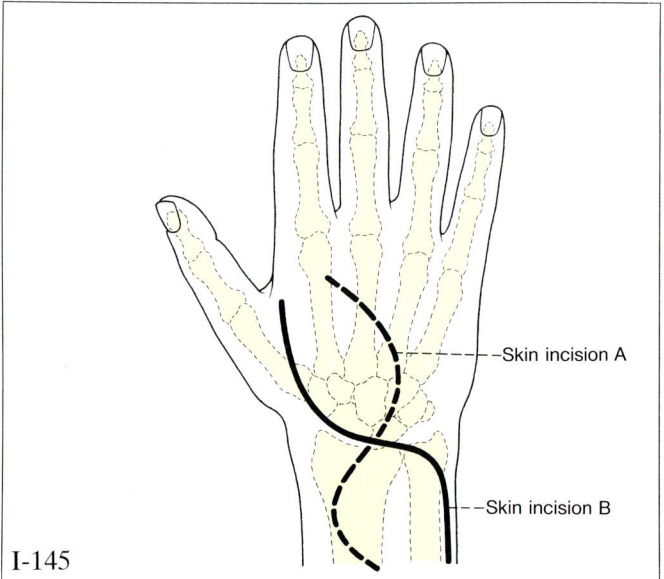

I-145

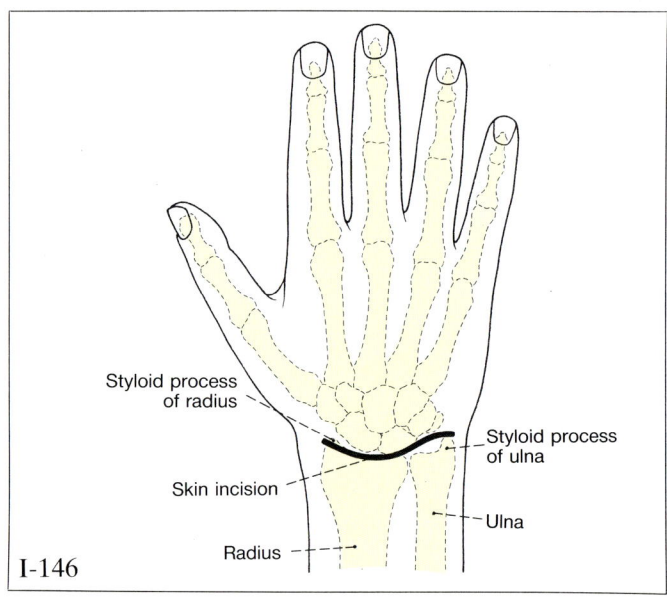

I-146

Wrist Joint — Dorsal Exposure

6. The midline straight skin incision is considered the standard approach (Fig. I-144). It is a 7- to 8-cm longitudinal incision that passes over the wrist joint and dorsum of the hand toward the middle finger.
7. Reflect the skin to expose the deep fascia and the extensor retinaculum (dorsal carpal ligament) (Fig. I-148). These are incised in a longitudinal direction (Fig. I-148).
8. Displace the underlying tendons of the extensor digitorum muscle toward the ulnar side, and retract the tendons of the extensor pollicis longus, extensor pollicis brevis, and abductor pollicis longus radially (Fig. I-149). The joint capsule is now exposed and may be incised wherever indicated.

Note

The midline longitudinal incision is usually preferred because the dorsal veins are protected.

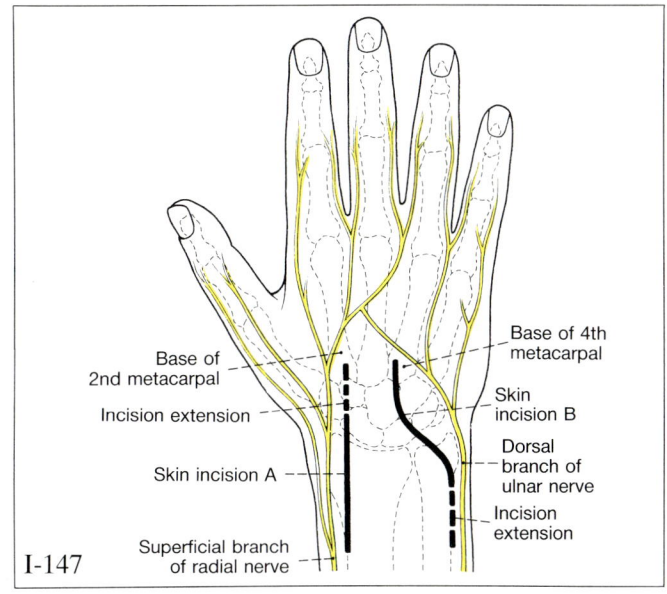
I-147

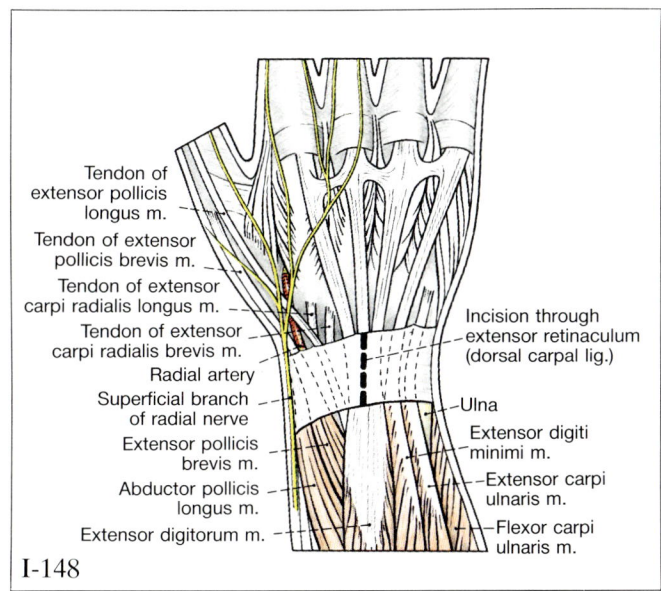
I-148

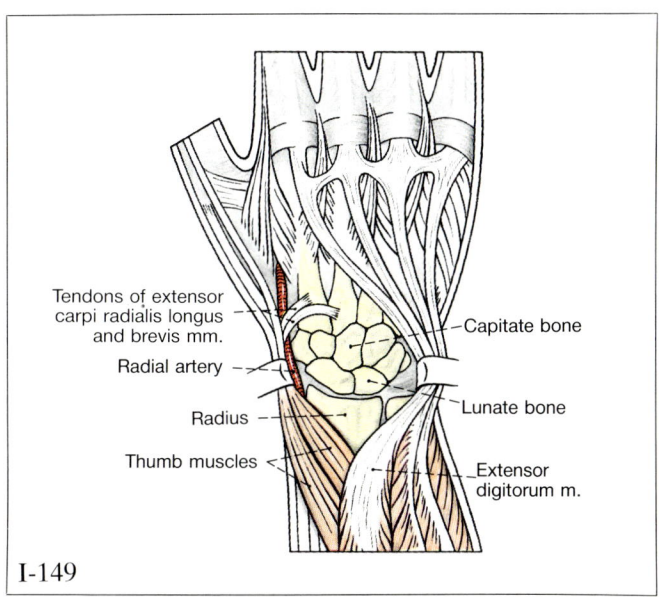
I-149

Wrist Joint – Palm

Applied Anatomy

Topography and Landmarks

1. The line of the wrist joint corresponds roughly to the middle flexor crease (Fig. I-150), while the distal crease overlies the proximal border of the pisiform bone and the tuberosity of the scaphoid bone (Fig. I-151).
2. The pisiform bone on the ulnar side and the tuberosity of the scaphoid bone are important palpable surface landmarks (Fig. I-151).
3. The intermediate crease is also known by other names such as the line of fortune and the axial line. It is directed toward the middle finger. The line has no anatomical significance.

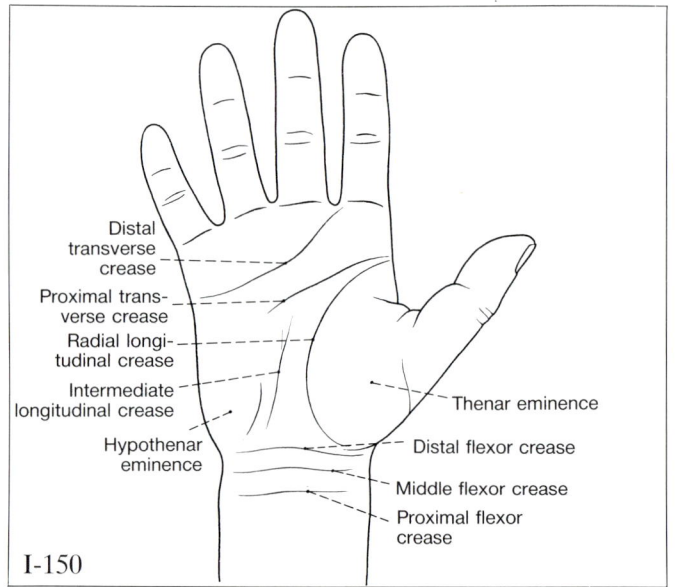

I-150

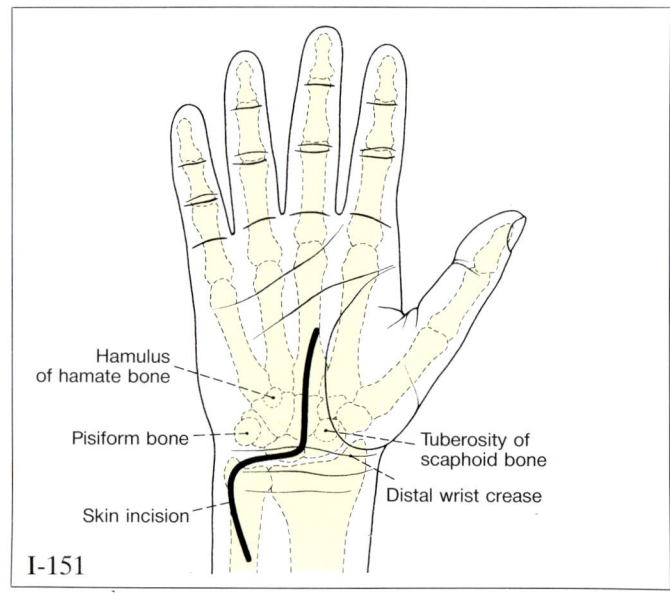

I-151

Carpal Tunnel – Wrist Joint

Volar Exposure

Indications

1. Carpal tunnel syndrome
2. Tenosynovitis of the flexor tendons
3. Dislocation of carpal bones
4. Ununited fractures of carpal bones
5. Tumors
6. Inflammatory processes

Operative Steps

There are five possible incisions:
1. A bayonet-shaped incision: Begin the incision on the radial side between the thenar and hypothenar eminences. Continue it parallel to the wrist skin crease and then curve it to end on the ulnar side (Fig. I-151).
2. A so-called gull-head incision: Run the incision parallel to the radial longitudinal crease and then curve it toward the ulnar side (Fig. I-152). This incision is particularly well suited for the exploration of the median nerve in the carpal tunnel syndrome, but it is also useful for tenosynovectomy and exploration of the ulnar nerve.
3. A 4-cm longitudinal skin incision: Begin between the thenar and hypothenar eminences and continue proximally, slightly toward the ulnar side (Fig. I-153).
4. A transverse incision in the distal wrist crease: It passes from the styloid process of the radius to the styloid process of the ulna (Fig. I-154).
5. An S-shaped incision (Fig. I-155).
6. Reflect the skin to reveal the deep fascia and the flexor retinaculum (transverse carpal ligament).

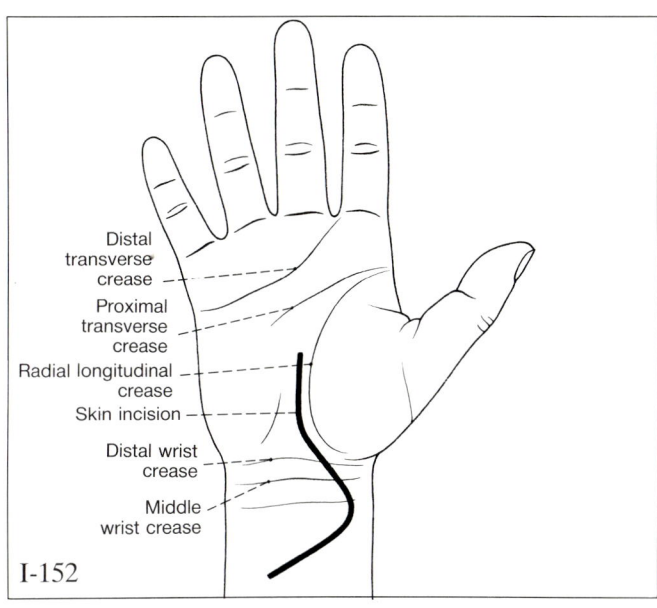

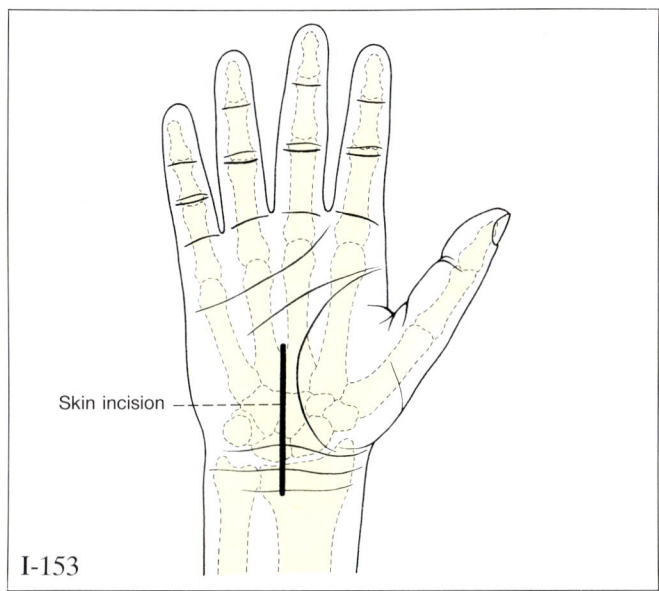

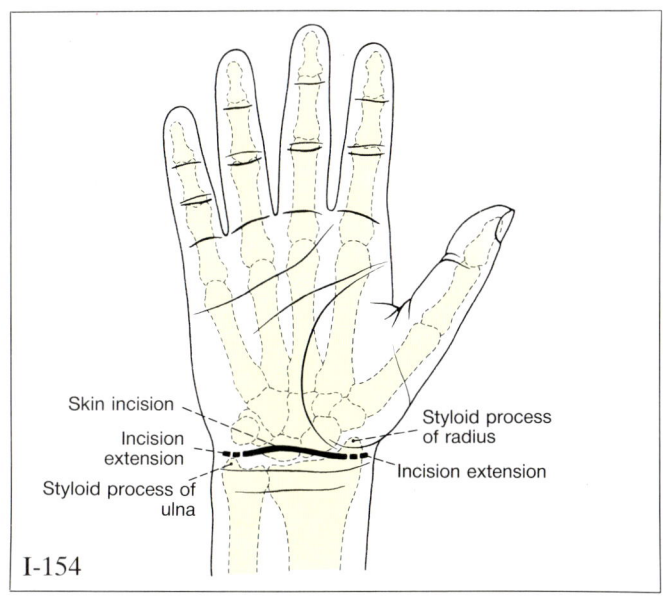

Carpal Tunnel – Wrist Joint — Volar Exposure

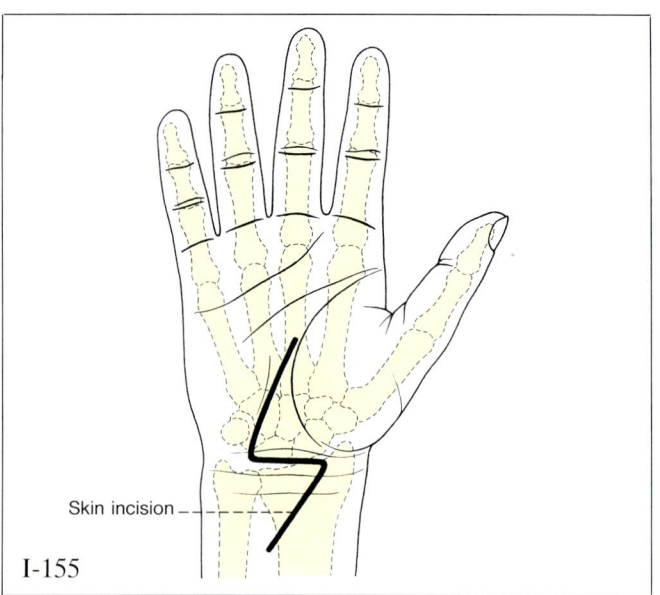

I-155

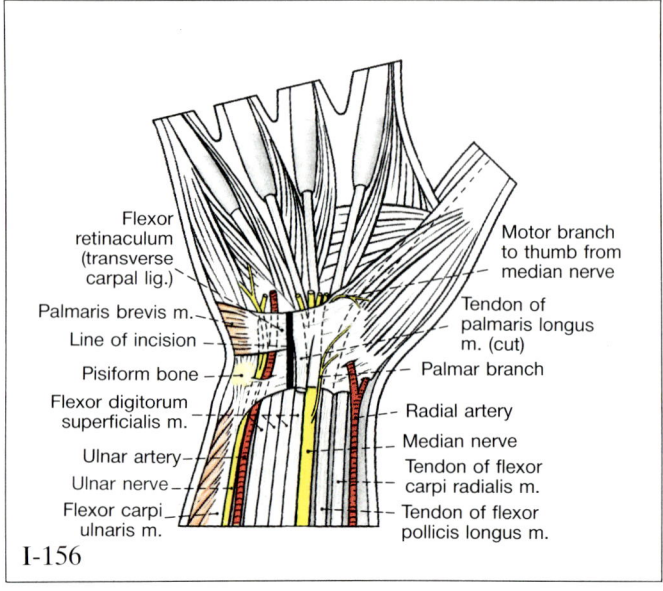

I-156

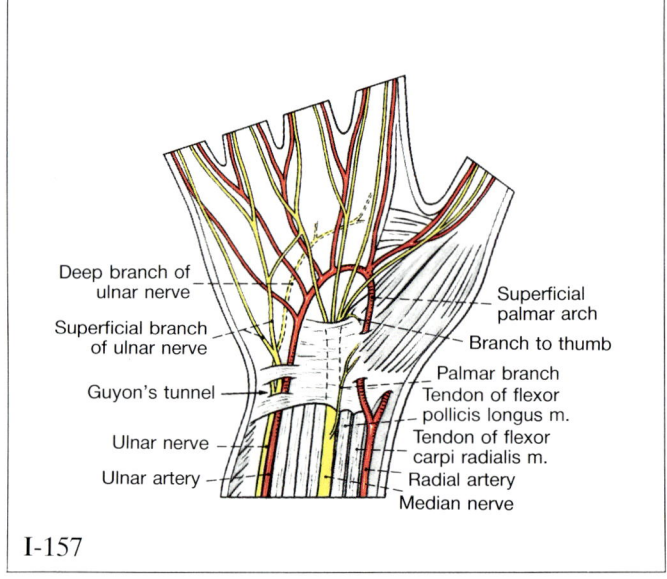

I-157

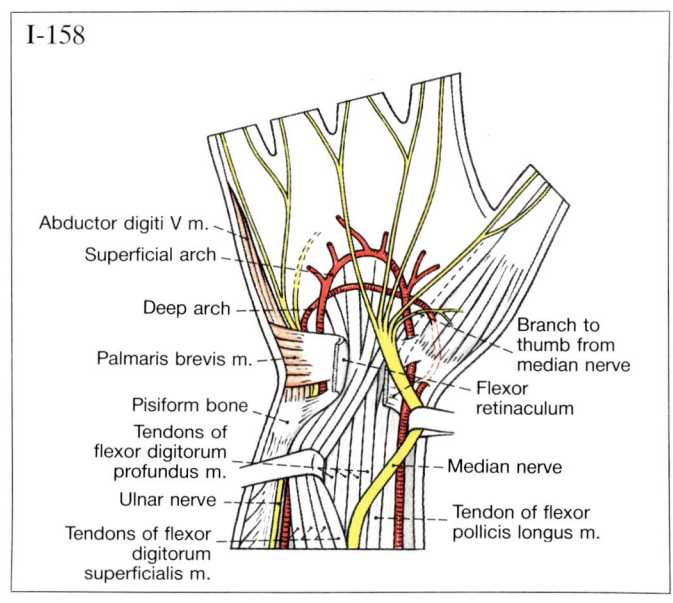

I-158

7. Incise these longitudinally (Fig. I-156) and reflect them toward the ulnar side to prevent injury to the palmar branch of the median nerve. The palmar branch (see Fig. I-156) and its rami pierce the radial portion of the flexor retinaculum. Expose the carpal tunnel with the median nerve and the flexor tendons by cutting through the flexor retinaculum.
8. The nerves and arteries of the palm are shown in Fig. I-157.
9. Reflect the tendons of the flexor digitorum superficialis muscle to the ulnar side, and displace the median nerve radially (Fig. I-158). This brings into view the deep flexor tendons (flexor digitorum profundus muscle), which are retracted to the radial side to expose the volar aspect of the joint capsule.
10. Careful subcutaneous dissection and the cutting of some fiber extensions of the antebrachial fascia (volar carpal ligament) on the ulnar side, outside the carpal tunnel, will reveal the ulnar nerve and its branches in Guyon's tunnel.

Notes

1. The bayonet incision and the gull-head incision are standard approaches. They afford wide exposures and are usually preferred over the longitudinal incision. The latter, if used, should be kept very short (to prevent scar contracture) and slightly S-shaped.
2. The palmar branch of the median nerve should be protected when making the skin incision and during the dissection.

3. Particular attention must be paid to the motor branch to the thumb, which has a quite variable course. It leaves the carpal tunnel independently through its own radially located point of exit near the distal edge of the flexor retinaculum.
4. In the hand and finger regions, subcutaneous sutures should not be used when closing the wound.

Flexor Retinaculum

1. The customary description of the flexor retinaculum (transverse carpal ligament) is too schematic and therefore misleading, a fact to which every surgeon will testify.
2. The flexor retinaculum of the carpal tunnel consists in reality of two transverse bands that blend into one another (Fig. I-180).
3. Older anatomical accounts described and illustrated two components of the flexor retinaculum, which was advantageous from a surgeon's point of view.
4. The ring-shaped thickening of the antebrachial fascia, the volar carpal ligament, lies proximal to the pisiform bone and attaches to the outer surface of the radius and the styloid process of the ulna. It bridges the flexor tendons. The volar carpal ligament consists of two layers (deep and superficial).
5. The transverse fibers of the deep layer are continuous distally with the true transverse carpal ligament.
6. The transverse carpal ligament is suspended between the tuberosity of the scaphoid bone and the pisiform bone proximally, and the tuberosity of the trapezium and the hamulus of the hamate bone distally.
7. The entire thickness of the flexor retinaculum must be cut, of course, to enter the carpal tunnel.

Palmar Branch of the Median Nerve

1. The delicate palmar branch (Figs. I-156 and I-157) supplies a skin area in the proximal part of the palm. The nerve is easily injured when making a skin incision. This may lead to the formation of a small painful neuroma and dysesthesia of the palm.
2. With a carefully made incision, the risk of injuring the palmar branch may be decreased. The skin incision over the flexor retinaculum can be made somewhat toward the ulnar side (approximately along the axis of the ring finger). A corresponding incision is made in the fascia and through the ulnar part of the flexor retinaculum. In this case, the palmar branch will lie in the subcutaneous tissue of the intact skin flap over the radial aspect of the retinaculum.
3. The palmar branch is also readily injured by an unnecessary resection of the radial part of the transverse ligament or by mobilizing the tendon of the palmaris longus muscle where it is continuous with the palmar aponeurosis.
4. Alternatively, the palmar branch can be exposed and protected proximal to the wrist crease. It arises from the main trunk of the median nerve 1–1.5 cm proximal to the upper edge of the flexor retinaculum (although this is variable). It may unwittingly be mistaken for the motor branch to the thumb, which forks off farther distally and also should be protected (Figs. I-156 and I-157).
5. In a special case, when injury to the palmar branch can not be avoided, it should be sharply separated from the median nerve at its origin. This will prevent the formation of a superficial neuroma in the palm.

Distal Ulnar Nerve

Guyon's Tunnel

Volar Exposure

Indication

Compression of the ulnar nerve and its branches in Guyon's tunnel

Operative Steps

1. The readily palpable pisiform bone is a good landmark.
2. Make a bayonet-shaped skin incision radial to the pisiform bone (Fig. I-159, skin incision A).
3. An alternative, make a short longitudinal incision immediately radial to the pisiform bone (Fig. I-159, skin incision B).
4. Carefully dissect the neurovascular bundle by cutting the fiber extensions of the antebrachial fascia (volar carpal ligament). The flexor retinaculum forms the floor of the tunnel (Fig. I-160).

Notes

1. Dissection of the slender branches of the ulnar nerve may at times require ocular magnification.
2. The dissection of the distal ulnar nerve in Guyon's tunnel in connection with a carpal tunnel syndrome does not require any additional skin incisions.

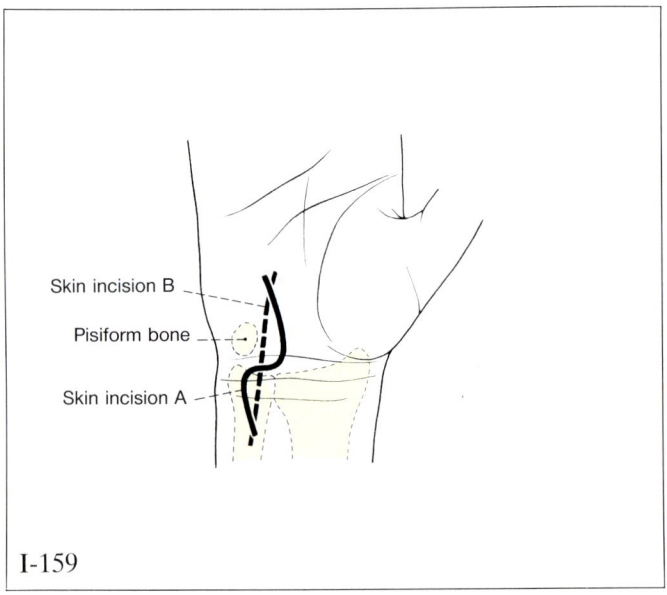

I-159

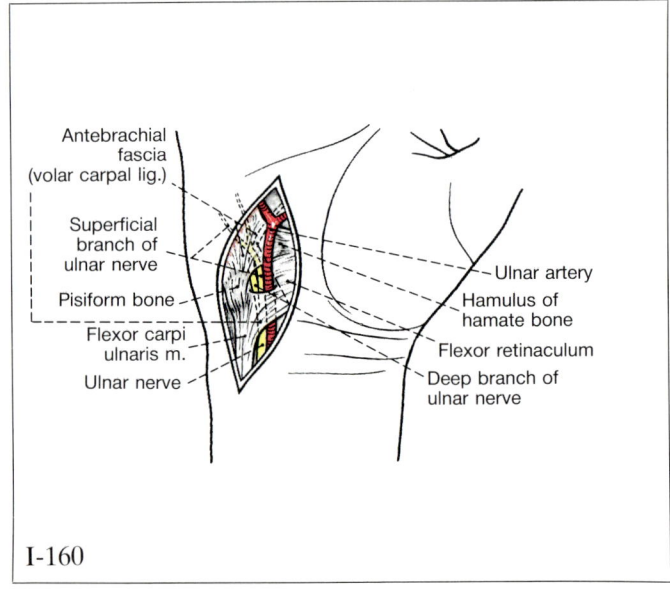

I-160

Radial Wrist Region – Anatomical Snuff Box (Radial Fovea)

Applied Anatomy

Topographical relationships of important structures in the radial wrist region are shown in Fig. I-161.

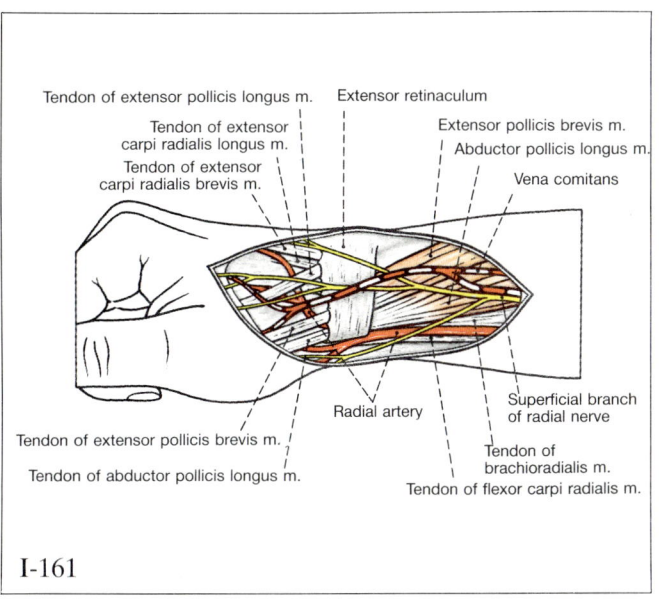

I-161

Anatomical Snuff Box – Extensor Tendons of Thumb

Indications

1. Quervain's disease
2. Tenosynovitis of extensor pollicis longus muscle
3. Ruptured tendons

Operative Steps

1. Incise the skin longitudinally on the outside of the distal radius along the tendons of the thumb (Fig. I-162, skin incision A).
2. An alternative transverse incision can be made at the level of the radial expansion of the extensor retinaculum (Fig. I-162, skin incision B).
3. Split the extensor retinaculum longitudinally (Fig. I-163). Expose the tendons to the thumb, which may be identified by passive traction.

Notes

1. The transverse incision is often preferred.
2. The tendons of the abductor pollicis longus and extensor pollicis brevis muscles lie in the first compartment. There can be some variations at this point. The important thing is to open all subdivisions that may at times exist in the first compartment.
3. The tendon of the extensor pollicis longus muscle lies in the third compartment. It frequently leaves the compartment through a separate opening in the extensor retinaculum shortly after it curves around Lister's tubercle (anatomically: dorsal tubercle of radius), a site where it is often injured.
4. Subcutaneous sutures are not used during closure because branches of the radial nerve may be injured.

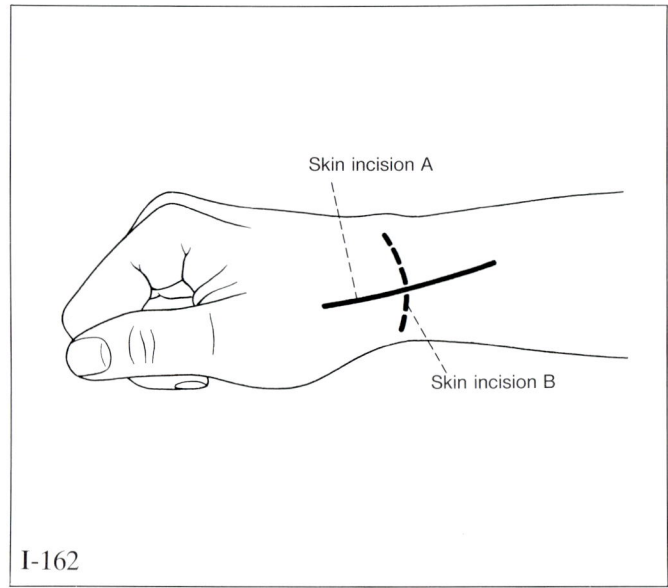

I-162

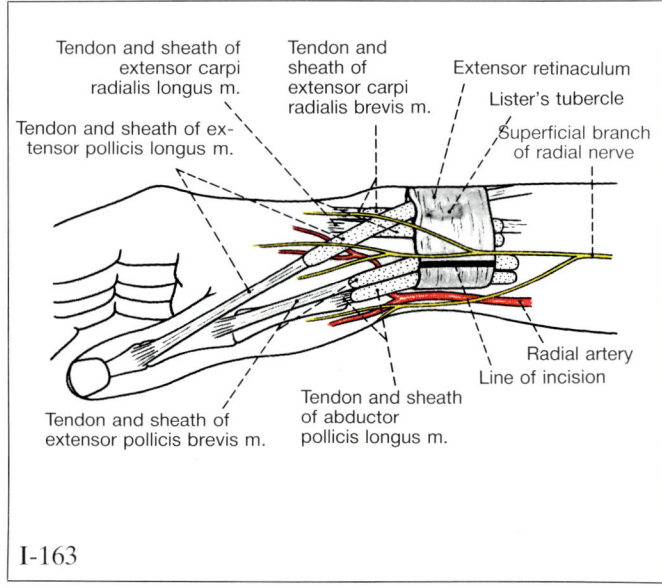

I-163

G. Hand

Carpus

Applied Anatomy

The topography of bony components of the wrist joint and carpus is shown in a dorsal view in Fig. I-164.

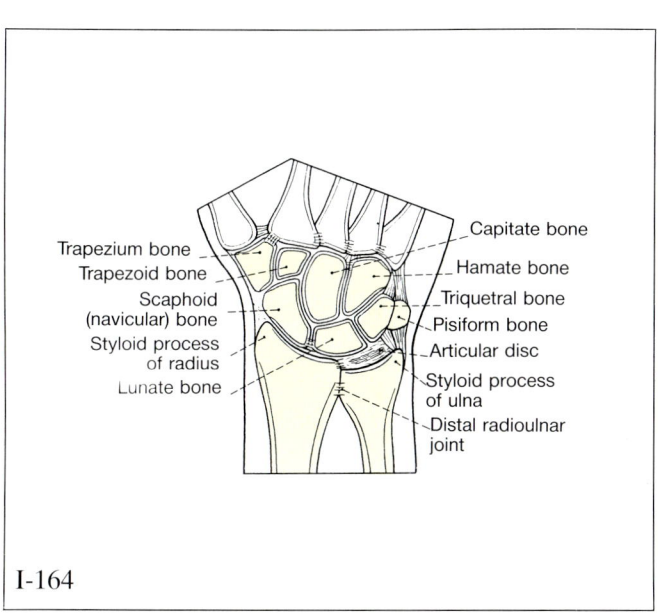

I-164

Scaphoid Bone (Navicular Bone)

Medial Exposure

Indications

1. Fractures of the scaphoid bone
2. Dislocation of the scaphoid bone
3. Pseudoarthrosis of the scaphoid bone

Operative Steps

1. Make an approximately 5-cm skin incision on the radial side of the wrist joint between the tendons of the extensor pollicis longus and extensor pollicis brevis muscles in the anatomical snuff box. The midpoint of the incision should be over the tuberosity of the scaphoid bone (Fig. I-165).
2. Alternatively, a curved incision in the snuff box may be chosen with a transverse radial extension (Fig. I-166).
3. Reflect the skin to reveal the deep fascia and the extensor retinaculum (dorsal carpal ligament). Incise these to bring into view the underlying extensor pollicis brevis and abductor pollicis longus muscles.
4. Retract the tendons and the radial artery toward the palm (Fig. I-168). Displace the tendon of the extensor pollicis longus toward the dorsum of the hand (Fig. I-168).
5. Cut the capsule longitudinally to expose the lateral aspect of the wrist joint.
6. Identify the scaphoid bone (perhaps radiologically).

Notes

1. The sensory fibers of the superficial branch of the radial nerve must be protected in the snuff box area.
2. The line of incision can also follow the dorsoradial margin.

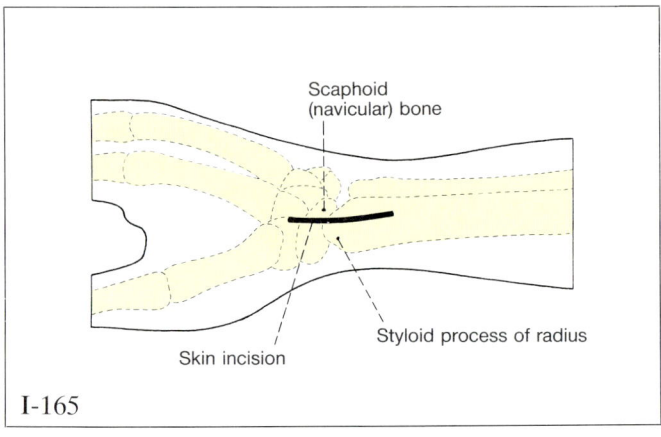

I-165

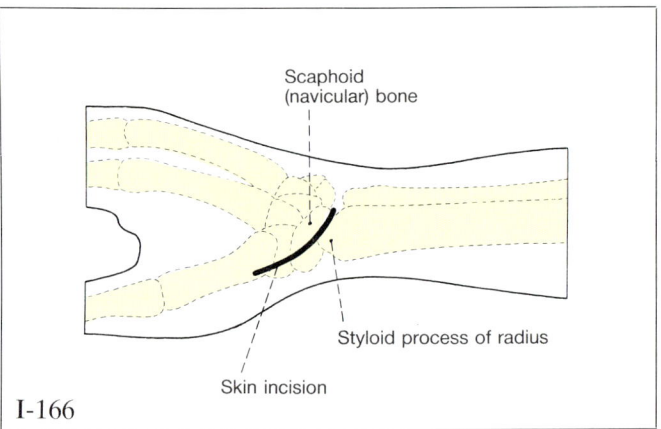

I-166

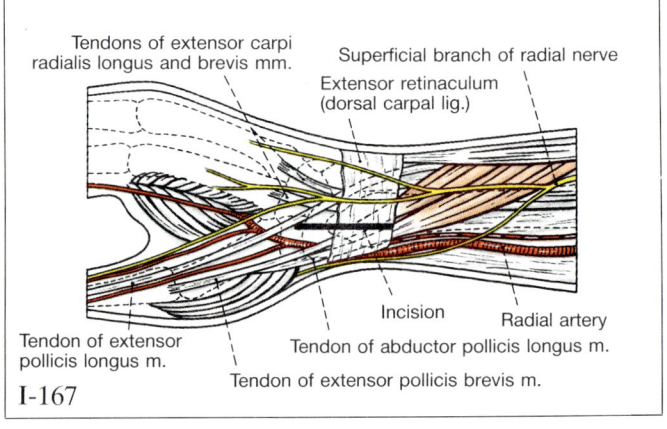

I-167

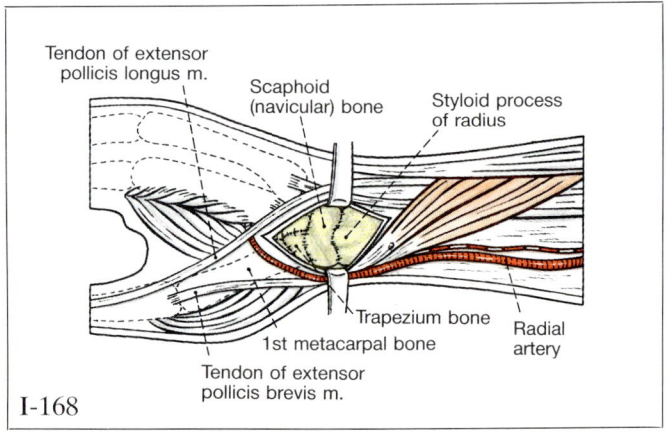

I-168

Scaphoid Bone — Volar/Transverse Exposures

Volar Exposure

Indications

Same as for the medial exposure

Operative Steps

1. Make a short straight incision over the volar aspect of the wrist joint on the radial side of the flexor carpi radialis muscle. Curve it toward the ulnar side and terminate it between the thenar and hypothenar eminences (Fig. I-169).
2. Reflect the tendon of the flexor carpi radialis muscle and the radial artery laterally, and retract the flexor tendons and the median nerve toward the ulnar side (Fig. I-170).
3. Open the wrist joint by a longitudinal cut through the capsule.
4. Identify and expose the scaphoid bone.

Alternative Transverse Exposure

1. The scaphoid bone can also be exposed by a transverse incision at the level of the tip of the styloid process of the radius (Fig. I-171).
2. Cut the tendon of the flexor carpi radialis muscle by using a Z-shaped incision (Fig. I-171).
3. Detach the capsule of the wrist joint between the styloid process of the radius and the scaphoid bone.
4. Occasionally, the styloid process of the radius may be osteotomized after detachment of the radial collateral ligament. The tendons of the abductor pollicis longus and extensor pollicis brevis muscles are retracted after opening the first osteofibrous compartment.

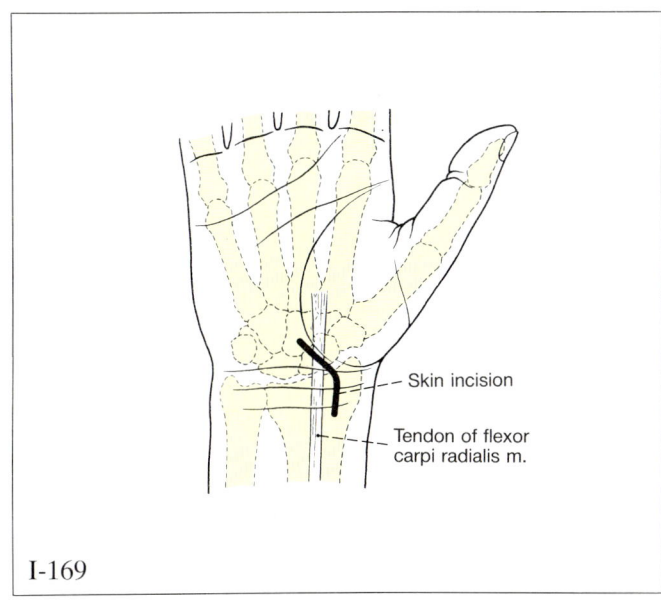

I-169

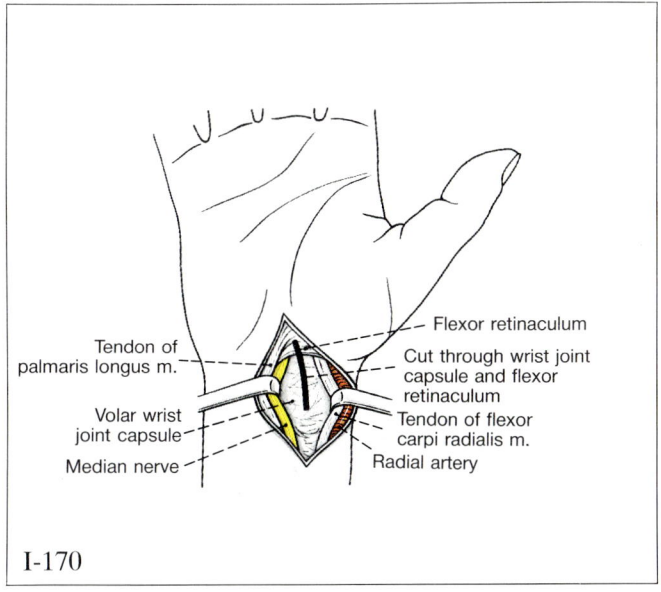

I-170

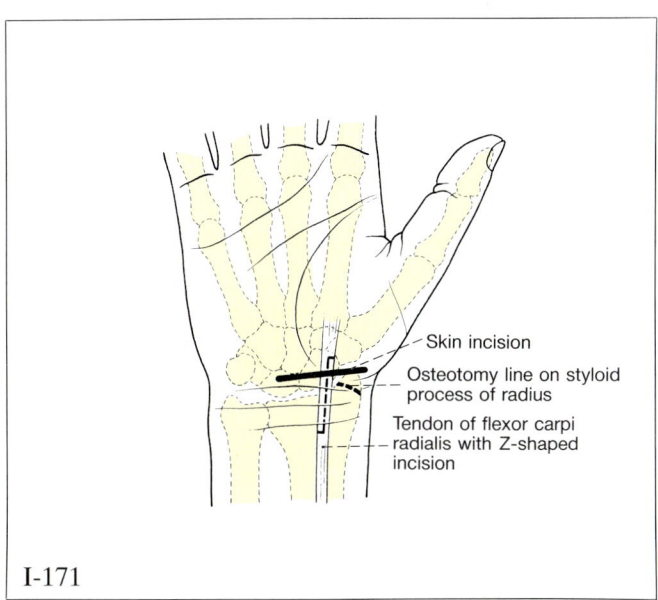

I-171

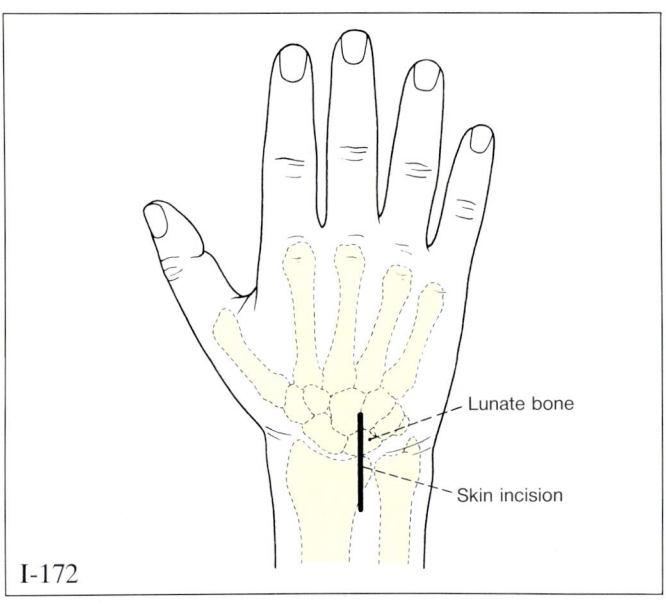

I-172

Lunate Bone

Dorsal Exposure

Indications

1. Infection of lunate bone
2. Lunate bone prosthetics
3. Capitate bone osteoplasty

Operative Steps

1. Make an approximately 5-cm-long longitudinal incision aimed at the web between the third and fourth fingers (Fig. I-172). This is similar to the dorsal approach to the wrist joint.
2. Retract the extensor tendons and enter the space between the extensor pollicis longus and extensor digitorum muscles.
3. Make a transverse incision of the capsule with a hinged flap extension distally. Capsular parts should be overlapped during closure.

the styloid processes of the radius and ulna (Fig. I-173).
2. Split the antebrachial fascia. Retract the tendon of the flexor carpi radialis muscle radially. Displace the long flexor tendons toward the ulnar side after splitting the proximal portion of the flexor retinaculum.
3. The lunate bone is exposed when the volar aspect of the joint capsule is opened.

Note

Compare with the approach to the carpal tunnel.

Alternative Volar Exposure

Indications

1. See dorsal exposure
2. Perilunar dislocation

Operative Steps

1. Make a straight transverse or slightly curved transverse skin incision in the distal wrist crease between

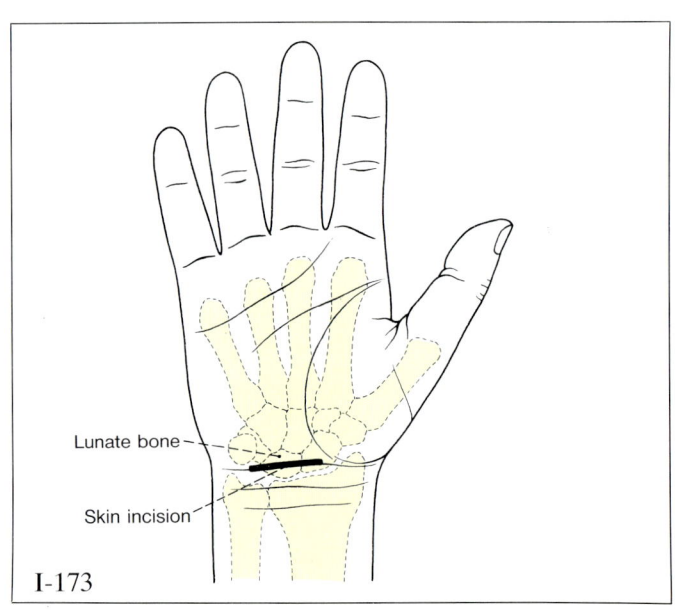

I-173

Trapezium Bone – Saddle Joint of Thumb (Greater Multangular Bone)

Dorsal Exposure

Indications

1. Arthrodesis
2. Resection arthroplasty
3. Prosthetics

Operative Steps

1. Make an approximately 5-cm-long incision in the snuffbox, parallel to the course of the abductor pollicis longus and extensor pollicis brevis tendons (Fig. I-174).
2. Carefully identify and handle rami from the superficial branch of the radial nerve and small blood vessels.

Notes

1. Compare this with the exposure for the anatomical snuff box.
2. See the volar exposure to the first metacarpal bone ("Metacarpal I").

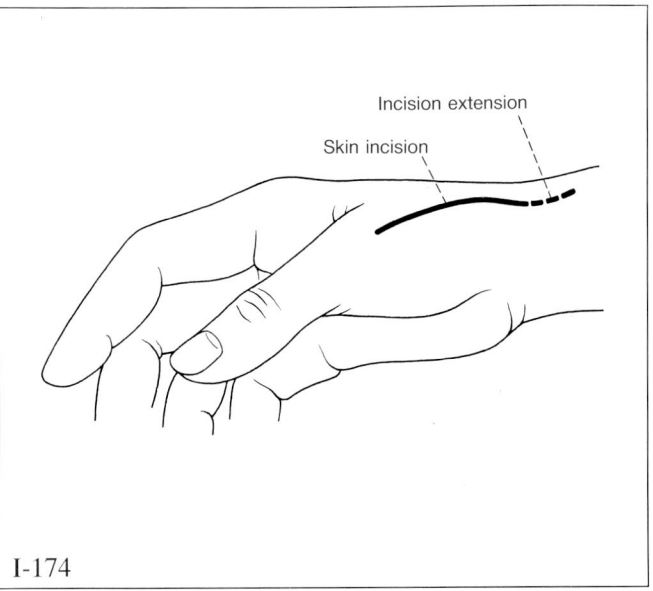

I-174

Metacarpal I – Saddle Joint of Thumb

Volar Exposure

Indications

1. Fractures of first metacarpal bone
2. Bennett's fracture
3. Tumors
4. Arthrodesis, prosthetics

Operative Steps

1. Make a curved volar-radial incision, as shown in Fig. I-175.
2. Extension of incision is possible both proximally and distally.
3. To free the thumb musculature, make a longitudinal periosteal incision along the radial surface of the first metacarpal. Reflect the thumb muscles toward the palm (Fig. I-176).
4. The tendons of the abductor pollicis longus and extensor pollicis brevis muscles are seen along the dorsolateral (radial) edge.

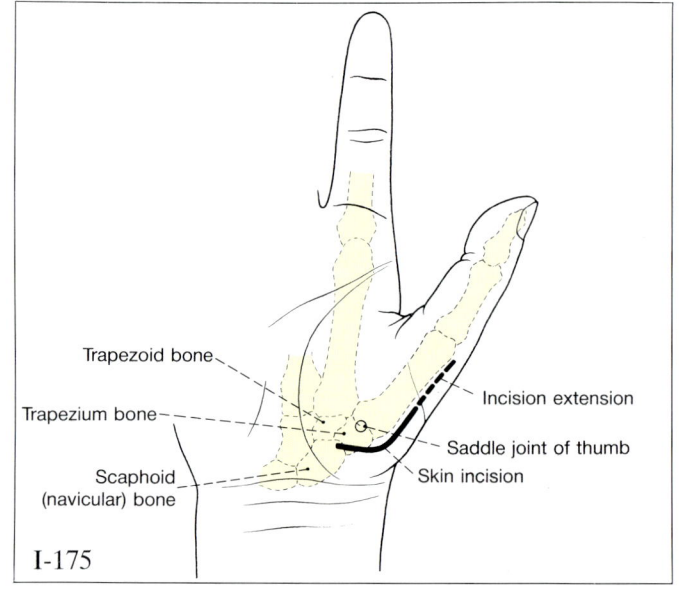

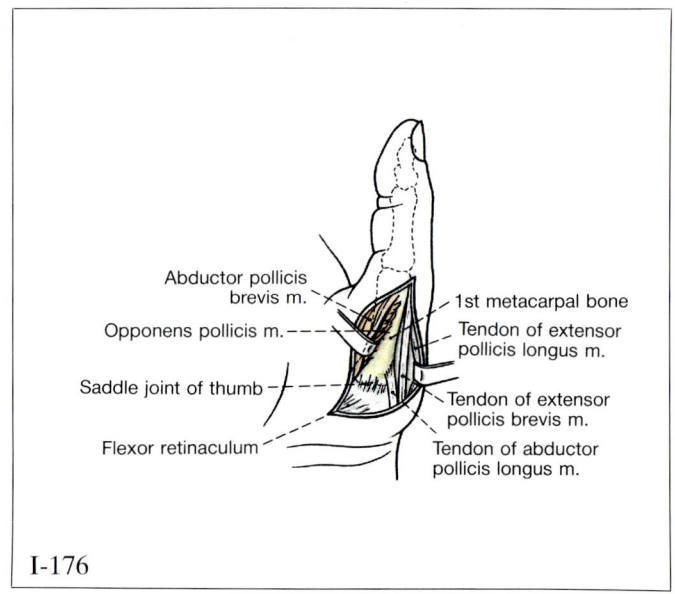

Long Flexor Tendons of Thumb

Volar Exposure

Indications

1. Trigger thumb
2. Frozen thumb

Operative Steps

1. Make short transverse skin incisions over the volar aspect of the first metacarpophalangeal joint (Fig. I-177), if possible, over the usually palpable tendon of the flexor pollicis longus muscle.
2. The wound must be very shallow because even the skin incision may injure the adjacent medial or lateral neurovascular bundles (Fig. I-178).
3. Split the circular reinforcement of the fibrous tendon sheath (annular ligament; pars anularis vaginae fibrosae) and open the latter wide along its extent.

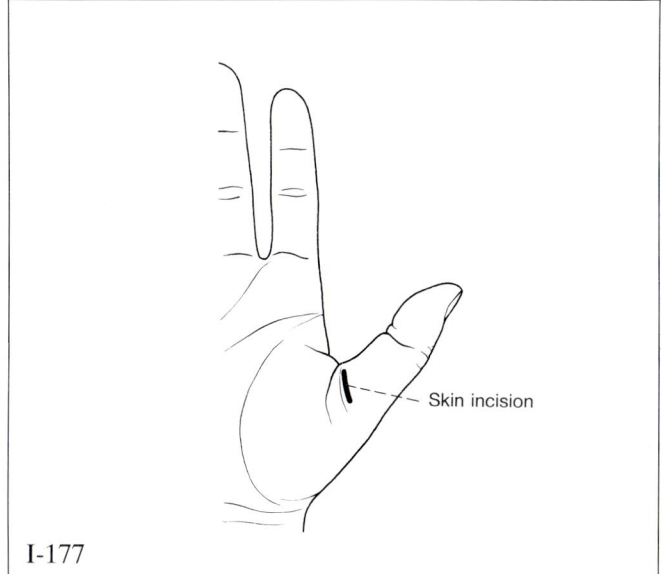

I-177

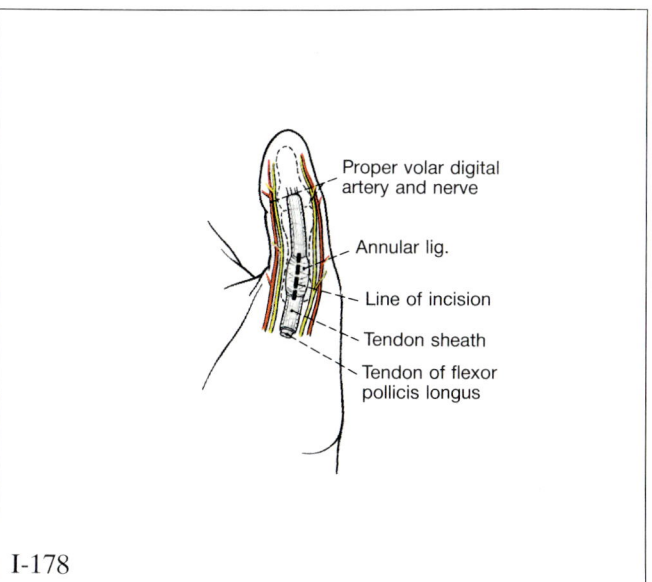

I-178

Tension Lines of the Palm

1. Skin incisions in the palm should, if at all possible, follow the tension lines (Fig. I-179). The flexor creases of the palm and fingers are even more important in this respect.
2. Regard for the tension lines is rewarded by a cosmetically less conspicuous scar and will not cause undesirable tissue contracture later. An incision parallel to the tension lines is the most desirable.

3. If crossing the tension lines (and the flexor creases of the palm and fingers) can not be avoided, the incision should not be at a right angle to the line or crease but rather oblique, in a zig-zag fashion.
4. Deep dissection away from the skin incision should not involve undermining of the skin. Aside from the fact that little is gained by separating the subcutaneous fat from skin, the latter may undergo necrosis.
5. Subcutaneous sutures are undesirable when closing wounds in the hand or on the fingers.

Palmar Aponeurosis

Applied Anatomy

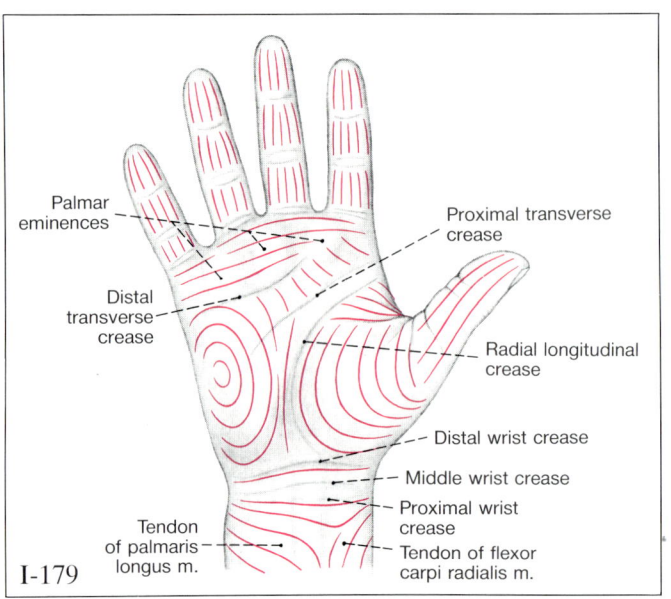

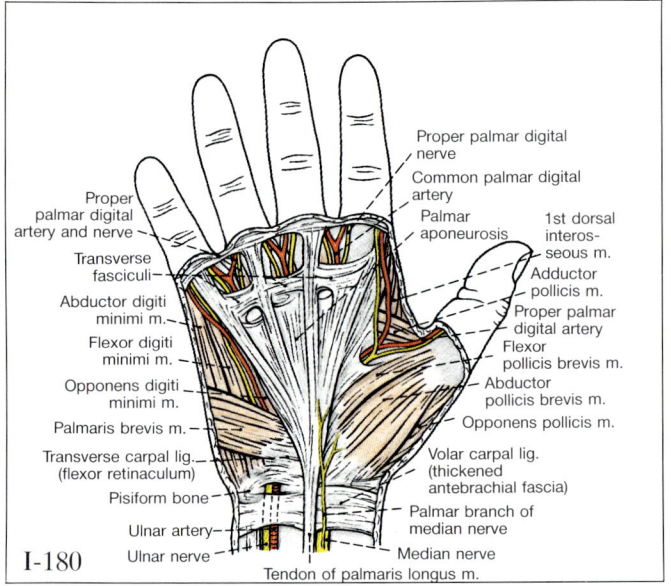

1. The topographic anatomy of the second layer is illustrated in Fig. I-180.
2. The palpable tendon of the palmaris longus muscle on the ulnar side of the flexor carpi radialis muscle is a superficial landmark.
3. The flexor retinaculum lies in a plane deep to the palmaris longus muscle and the palmar aponeurosis.
4. The "flexor retinaculum" consists of two layers whose names, unfortunately for the surgeon, are no longer recognized in the new Nomina Anatomica. (See flexor retinaculum in connection with the carpal tunnel.)
5. Proximally there is a circular reinforcement of the fascia of the forearm, the volar carpal ligament, whose superficial fibers attach to the tendon of the palmaris longus muscle. Distally the transverse carpal ligament extends from the radial side to the pisiform bone and the hamulus of the hamate bone (Fig. I-180).

Palm – Palmar Aponeurosis

Digitopalmar Zig-Zag Incision of *Bruner*

Indications

1. Dupuytren's contracture – partial or radical fasciectomy
2. Exploration of flexor tendons

Operative Steps

1. The longitudinal zig-zag incision is the standard approach (Fig. I-181). This "VW-incision" takes into consideration Langer's lines (Fig. I-179) and makes possible a wide exposure of the palmar aponeurosis and its digital expansions (Fig. I-180).
2. Carefully avoid the neurovascular bundles in the finger region when the direction of the skin incision is changed.
3. Confine the angles of the incision to the ends of the flexor creases.
4. Only part of the incision can be used for a limited exposure.
5. A bayonet incision may serve as a proximal extension over the carpal tunnel (Fig. I-182).

Notes

1. The zig-zag incision allows a wide exposure without loss of sensation or scar formation if the neurovascular bundles along the sides of the fingers are protected.
2. The zig-zag incision may be performed using angles *(Bruner)* or rounded corners *(Littler)*.

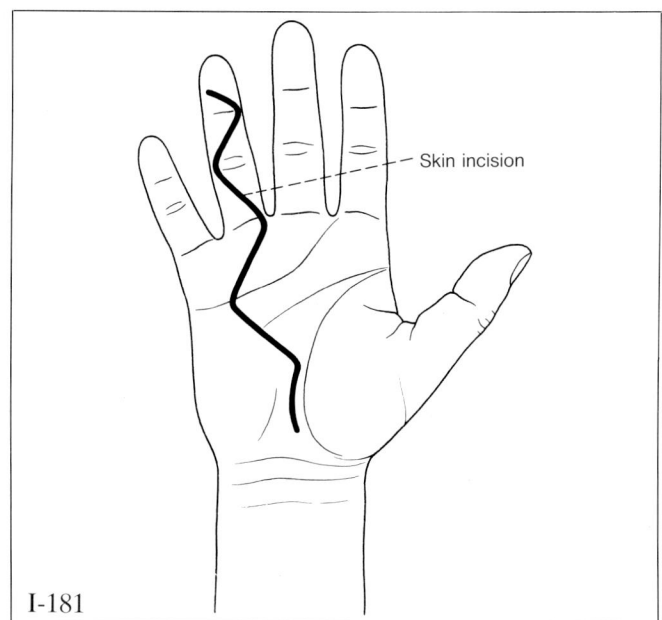

I-181

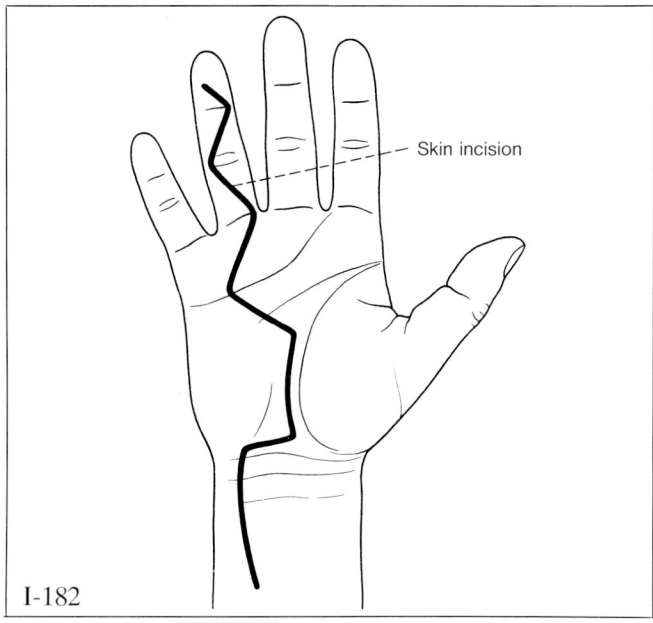

I-182

Alternative
Y-Incision of *Millesi*

Operative Steps

1. In the palm of the hand, the Y-incision (Fig. I-183) is an alternative. This incision takes into account the fact that the blood supply reaches the skin of the palm from the periphery, thus decreasing the danger of necrosis in cases of marginally maintained skin.
2. Digital extension is possible with zig-zag incisions (Fig. I-184).

Notes

1. In the palm, the Y-incision, the VW-incision, and the multiple Z-incisions can be used interchangeably.
2. The Z-incision of Iselin is rarely indicated. It may, however, be used to advantage in the fingers, particularly over the joints in cases of contracture. Good quality skin is a prerequisite.

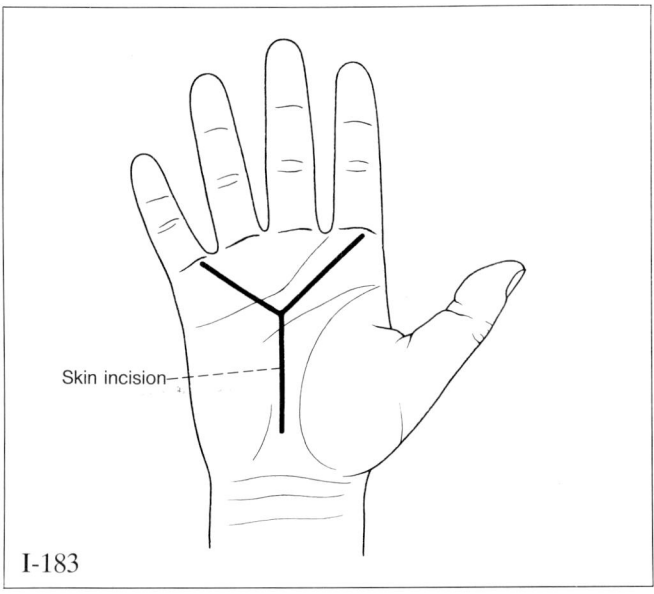

I-183

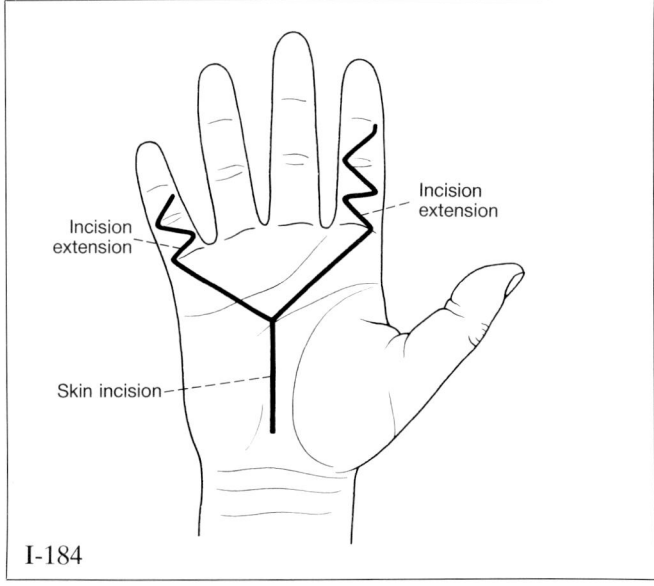

I-184

Additional Volar Exposures
Overview

Fig. I-185, Nos. *1–7*

1. Incision at the base of the thumb.
2. Radial midaxial incision of thumb (see also finger incision).
3. Skin incision for exposure of the flexor tendon sheath of the thumb, as for example in the case of trigger thumb. Care must be taken to avoid the neurovascular bundle on the side. (See also the long flexor tendon of the thumb.)
4. Skin incision for approach to structures of the thenar eminence.
5. Skin incision for exposure of structures in the middle of the palm.
6. Bayonet incision with distal extension for wide exposure of the palm and carpal tunnel.
7. Transverse skin incision for exposure of the distal palmar aponeurosis. This is justifiable only when the "open palm" technique is employed in Dupuytren's contracture, i.e., when the wound edges are not approximated and the standard digitopalmar approach is used.

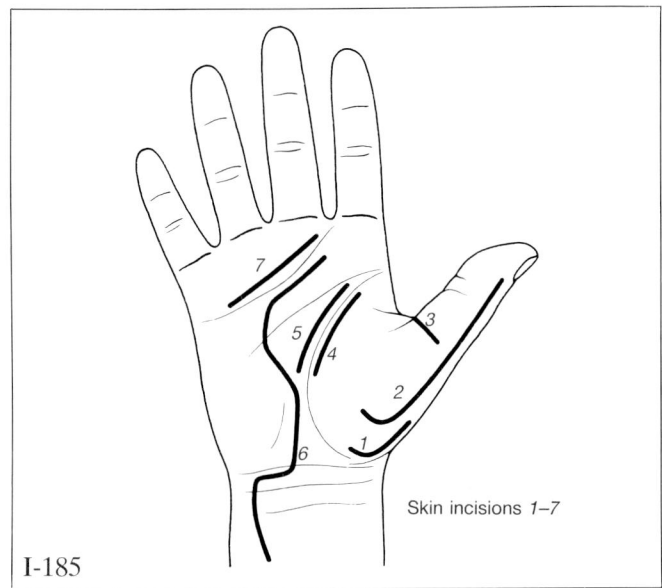

I-185   Skin incisions *1–7*

Palm

Wide Volar Exposure of *Kanavel*

Indications

1. Bacterial tendovaginitis
2. Tuberculous hygroma

Operative Steps

1. An extensive exposure with a wide overview is possible with this particular bayonet incision in which the distal part of the cut is continued into a slightly curved transverse incision (Fig. I-186).
2. In this manner two flaps are created, a proximal and a distal, each being mobilized and reflected to the radial and ulnar sides, respectively, as indicated by arrows (Fig. I-186).
3. The thickness of the skin flaps should not be reduced. The subcutaneous tissue must remain with the flap. This is particularly important in areas at some distance from the incision due to danger of skin necrosis.

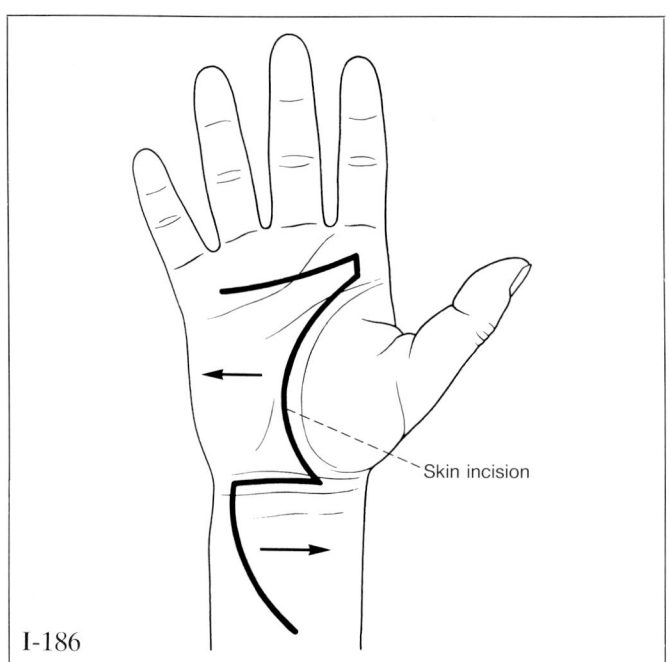

Distal Palm

Transverse Exposure

Indications

1. Trigger finger
2. So-called ganglion of annular ligament

Operative Steps

1. Make a transverse skin incision half-way between the proximal flexor crease of the finger and the distal flexor crease of the palm (see Fig. I-187, skin incision A).
2. Carefully prepare the fibrous sheath of the digital flexor tendon to avoid damage to the adjacent neurovascular bundles on the sides (Fig. I-188).
3. Split the fibrous sheath as in Fig. I-188. Frequently there are proximal and distal circular fibers of the tendon sheath (annular part of the fibrous sheath), which also should be split.

Alternative

An angular incision that crosses the flexor crease medially or laterally is useful for an augmented exposure (Fig. I-187, skin incision B).

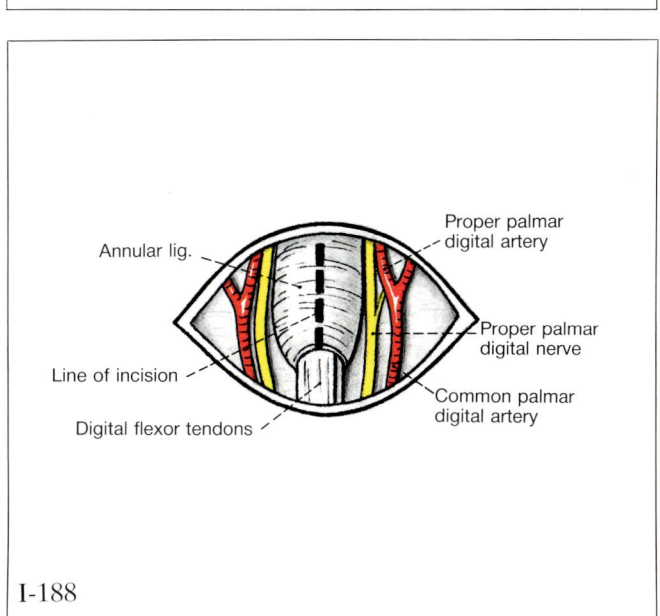

I-187

I-188

Dorsum of Hand

Tension Lines of the Skin

1. The pattern of the tension lines is seen in Fig. I-189.
2. The incisions on the dorsum of the hand should, if at all possible, follow the tension lines.
3. Incisions parallel to the tension lines induce negligible scar formation.
4. If it becomes necessary to cross the tension lines, it should be done obliquely, not at a right angle.

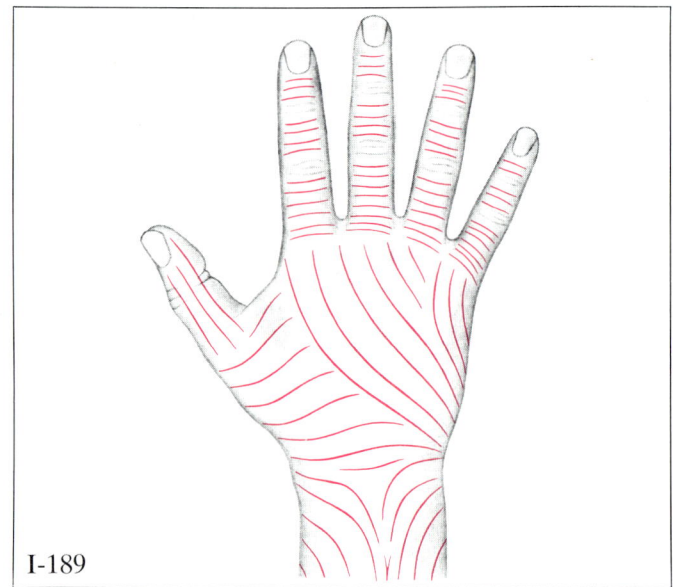

I-189

Metacarpals II–V

Dorsal Exposure

Indication

Fractured metacarpals

Operative Steps

1. Make longitudinal lines of incision on the dorsum of the hand, as shown in Fig. I-190.
2. The incision makes possible simultaneous exposure of two adjacent metacarpals.
3. Approach to the metacarpophalangeal joint is possible with an angular hinged-flap extension of the incision.

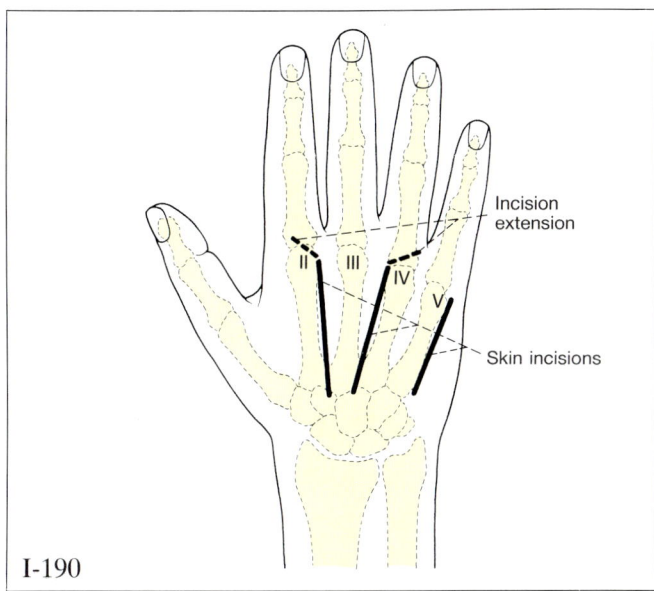

I-190

Dorsum of Hand

Dorsal Exposures

Overview

Fig. I-191, Nos. *1–6*

1. Midaxial ulnar skin incision of the thumb.
2. Skin incision on the base of the index finger.
3. Short radial transverse incision for exposure of the extensor tendons of the thumb and the tendon of the abductor pollicis longus muscle.
4. Curved transverse skin incision for approach to the metacarpophalangeal joint. A C-shaped incision is sufficient for exposure of a single joint.
5. Longitudinal incision for exposure of one metacarpal bone.
6. Zig-zag incision.

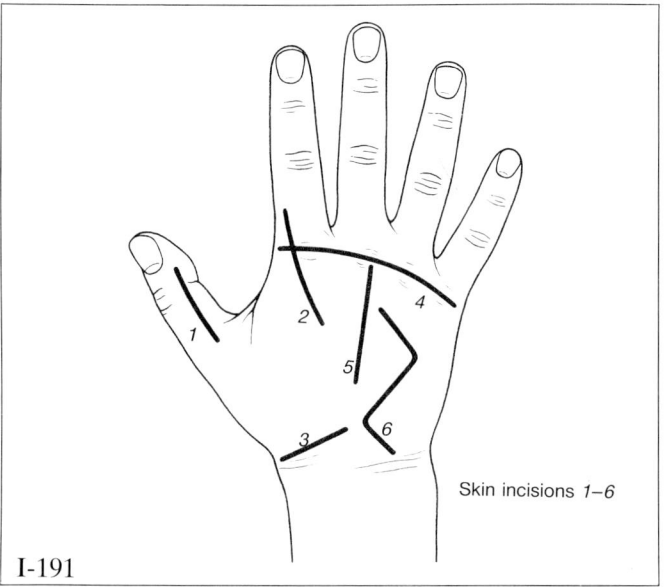

Skin incisions *1–6*

I-191

H. Finger

Volar Exposure

Zig-Zag Incision

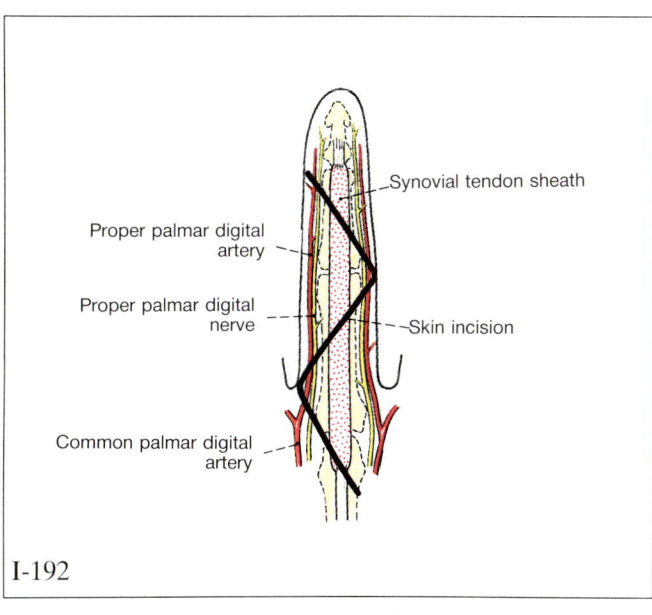

I-192

Indications

1. Tendovaginitis – tenosynovectomy
2. Exploration of flexor tendons
3. Dupuytren's contracture involving the fingers

Operative Steps

1. The zig-zag incision (Fig. I-192) is the standard approach with optional extension into the distal palm.
2. The laterally situated neurovascular bundles should be carefully observed.
3. If possible, the end of the oblique incision should be at the level of the joint flexor crease so that with later reflection of the skin flaps, the transverse limb of the incision lies over the flexor crease.
4. Mobilize the skin flaps with the vascular subcutaneous tissue.
5. The bilateral neurovascular bundles must be handled with care.

Alternative

Digitopalmar Z-Incision of *Iselin*

Indication

Dupuytren's contracture involving the fingers

Operative Steps

1. Make a midline incision over the palpable contracture (Fig. I-193).
2. For the Z-incision, make multiple oblique extensions, each at about a 60-degree angle to the main incision, as indicated in Fig. I-193.

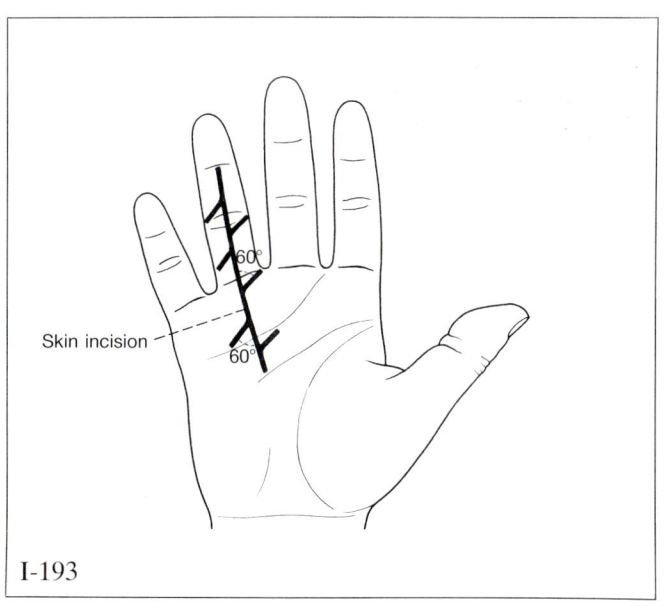

I-193

Volar Digital Exposures

Overview

a) Fig. I-194, Nos. *1–6*

1. S-shaped incision at the base of the finger.
2. L-shaped angular incision at the base of the finger.
3. *and* 4. Zig-zag incision over the phalanges.
5. *and* 6. Hinged-flap incision for exposure of the flexor tendons. The incision begins distal to the flexor crease of the terminal phalanx and ends, in the case of the index and little fingers, at the distal palmar crease. On the middle and ring finger it ends at the proximal finger crease (Fig. I-195, No. 4) in order to protect the web of the fingers. The volar neurovascular bundle remains on the finger when the flap is elevated.

b) Fig. I-195, Nos. *1–6*

1. Z-incision.
2., *4.*, 6. Angular cuts from lateral longitudinal incisions.
3. Short longitudinal incision along the edge.
5. Large hinged-flap incision as seen in Fig. I-194, No. 5 and 6.

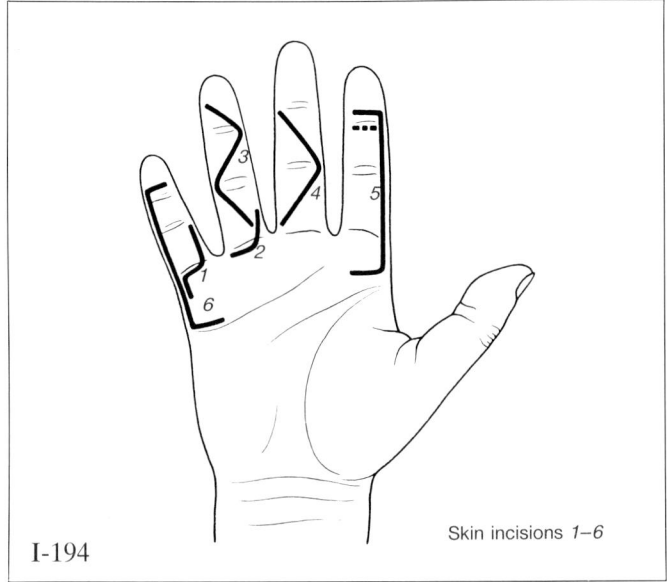

I-194 — Skin incisions *1–6*

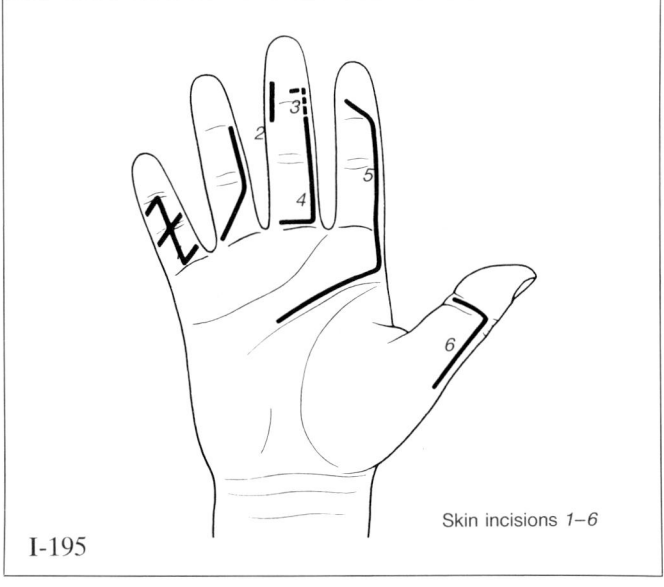

I-195 — Skin incisions *1–6*

Finger — Volar Digital Exposures

c) Fig. I-196, Nos. *1–5*

1. Long digitopalmar incision of Tubiana.
2. Short S-shaped incision.
3. Short Z-incision. The acute angles are approximately 60 degrees.
4. Short oblique incision between two flexor creases corresponding to a portion of the zig-zag incision.
5. Radial incision of the thumb.

d) Fig. I-197, Nos. *1–7*

1. Short angular incision.
2. S-shaped incision with extension into the palm (no. 8).
3. Short transverse incision in the proximal finger crease.
4. Short Z-incision.
5. Short angular incision.
6. Short limb of a zig-zag incision.
7. Wide volar exposure of the thumb.

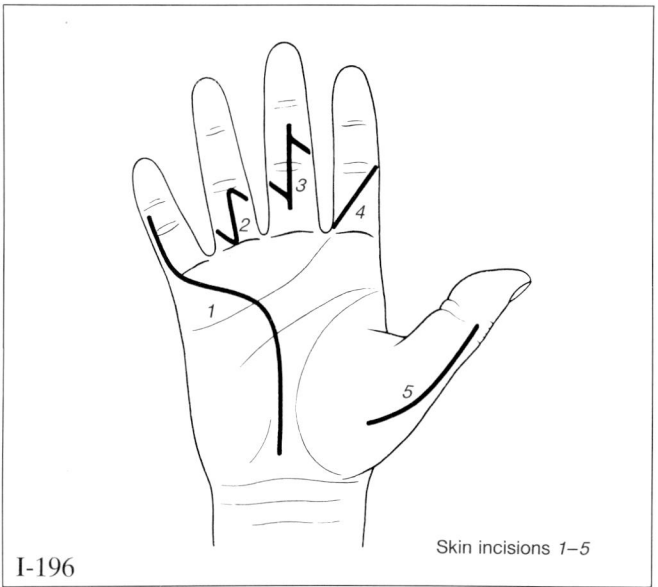

I-196 Skin incisions *1–5*

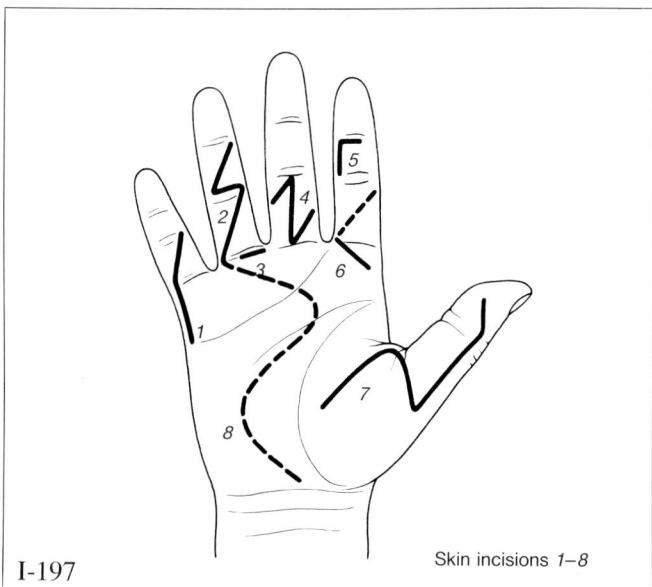

I-197 Skin incisions *1–8*

Dorsal Exposures

Overview

a) Fig. I-198, Nos. *1–6*

1. C-shaped incision for synovectomy of finger joints.
2. Inverted V-incision for arthrodesis of distal interphalangeal joint.
3. S-shaped incision for exposure of the distal end of the extensor tendon.
4. S-shaped incision for exposure of the extensor aponeurosis.
5. Zig-zag incision for wide exposure of the extensor apparatus.
6. Short oblique incision over a phalanx.

b) Fig. I-199, Nos. *1–6*

1. Hinged flap on the thumb.
2. Zig-zag incision with rounded corners for complete exposure of the extensor apparatus of the finger.
3. Hinged flap over a phalanx.
4. C-shaped incision for exposure of a metacarpophalangeal joint.
5. C-shaped incision for exposure of a proximal interphalangeal joint.
6. Hinged-flap incision on the little finger.

Note

With the hinged-flap incision the neurovascular bundle remains on the finger when the flap is mobilized.

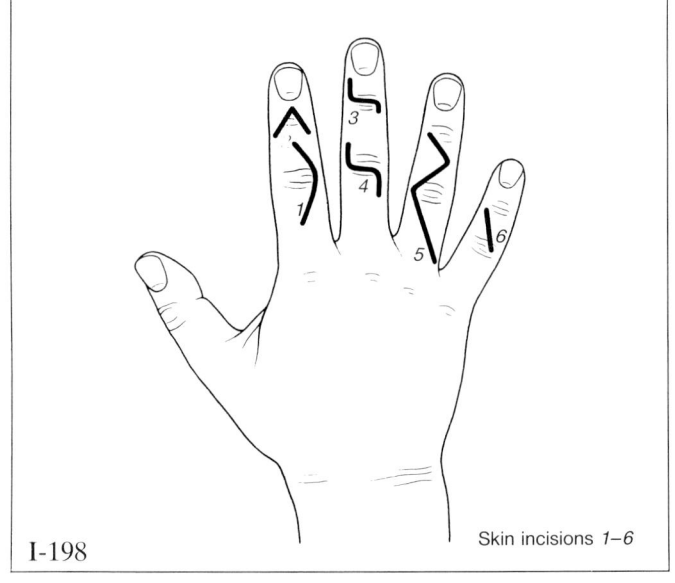

I-198 — Skin incisions *1–6*

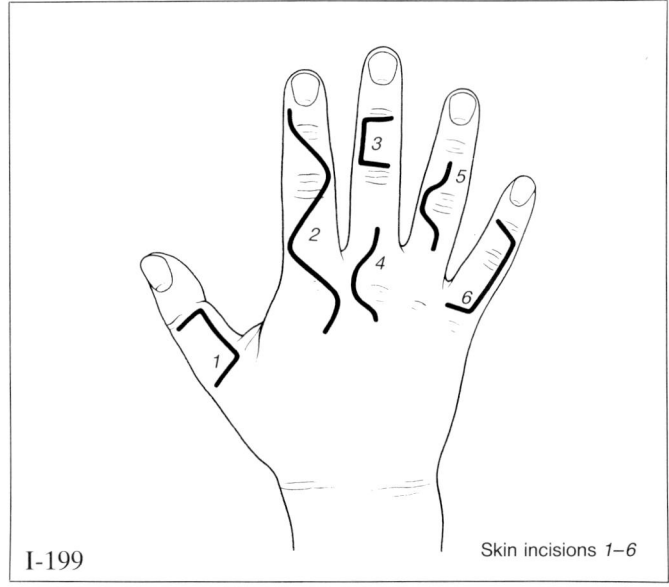

I-199 — Skin incisions *1–6*

Dorsolateral Exposure

1. Make an incision on the radial or ulnar side of the finger, with modified hinged-flap extensions (Fig. I-200, skin incision A).
2. Alternative: Make a lazy S-shaped line of incision on the dorsel espect (Fig. I-200, skin incision B).
3. Mobilize the skin flap. The dorsolateral neurovascular bundle remains on the finger.
4. Split the extensor apparatus longitudinally and expose the phalanx by means of Hohmann elevators (Fig. I-201).

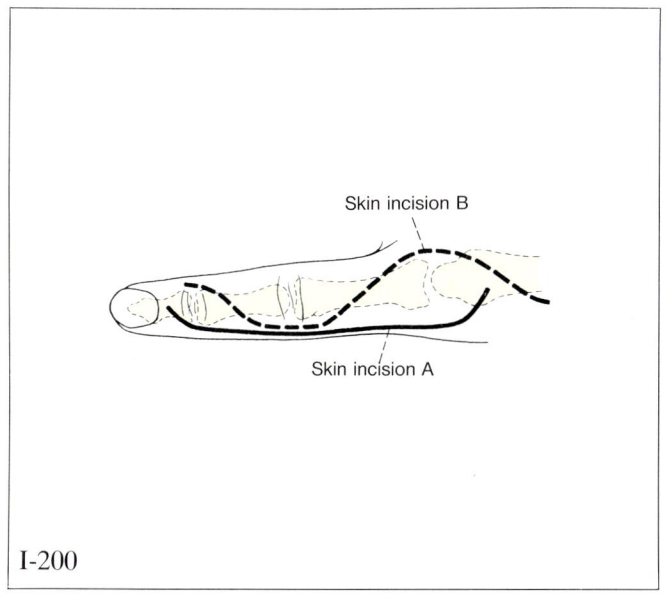

I-200

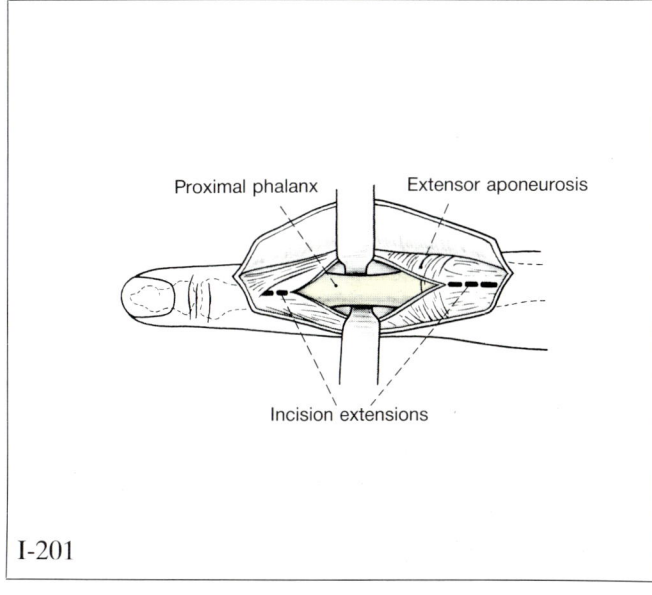

I-201

Terminal Phalanx/Fingertip — Exposures

Terminal Phalanx – Nail Bed

Exposures

Skin incisions A–C for paronychia (Fig. I-202).

Fingertip

Exposures

Skin incisions A and B for paronychia (Fig. I-203).
A. Lateral hockey stick incision.
B. Hockey stick incision into tip of finger.
C. Hockey stick incision with gaping wound.

Notes

1. The similarity to a hockey stick is only seen when the wound edges are separated.
2. It is important that the incision on the tip of the finger is near the nail to prevent the formation of touch-sensitive scar tissue.
3. The "Froschmaul" incision is obsolete on the fingertip.

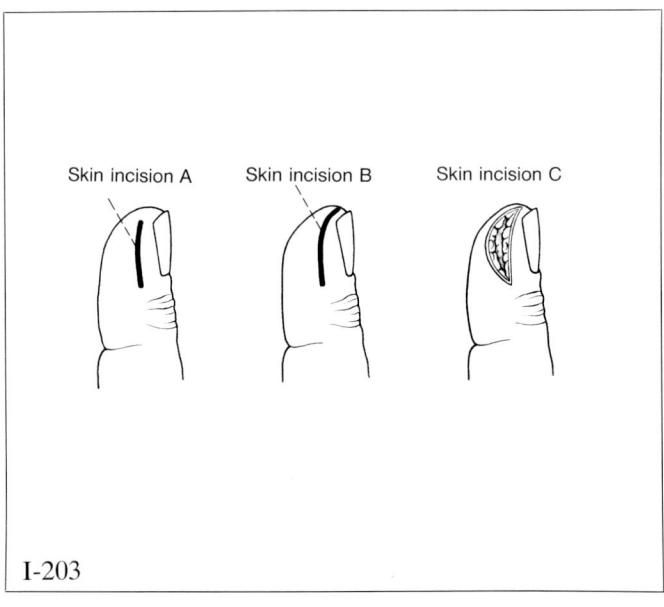

I-202

I-203

Finger

Midaxial Exposure
Midlateral Exposure

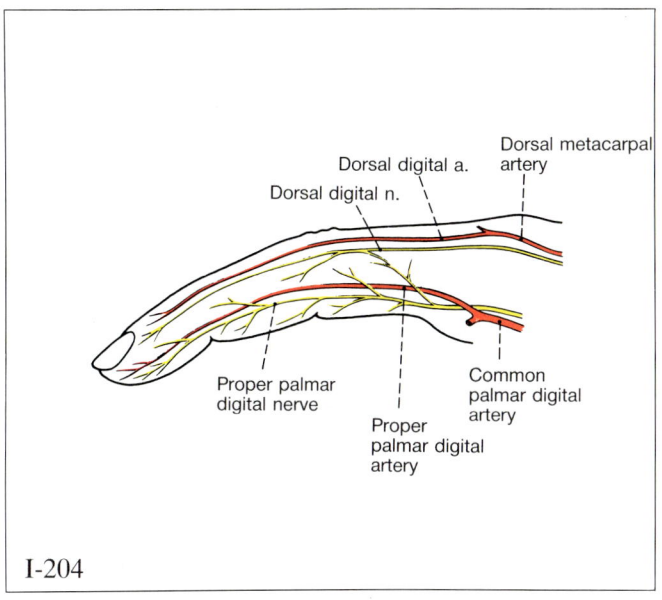

I-204

1. Applied anatomy: The bilateral volar and dorsal locations of the neurovascular bundles leave an area on the side of the finger devoid of nerves except for some very fine branches. An incision can be made in the middle of this area (Fig. I-204).
2. The relationships of the neurovascular bundles can be observed in cross section in Fig. I-205.
3. The midaxial incision is placed in the "neutral" zone on the side of the finger and passes through the ends of the flexor creases. Thus, the line of incision is slightly toward the dorsal aspect (Figs. I-206 and I-207).

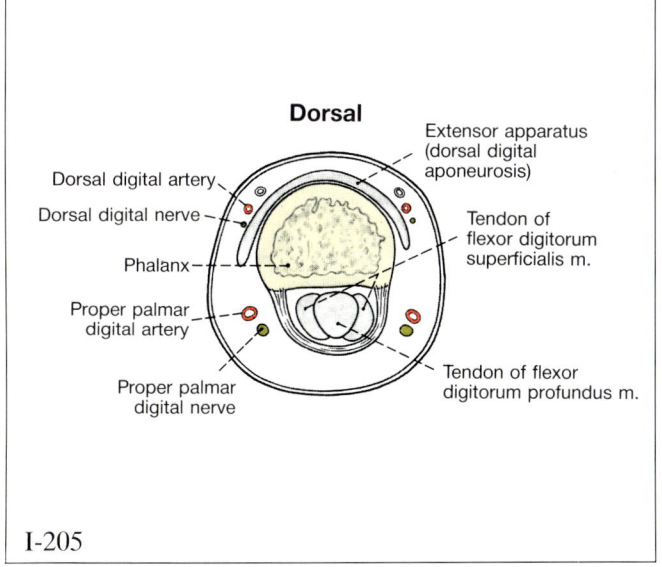

I-205

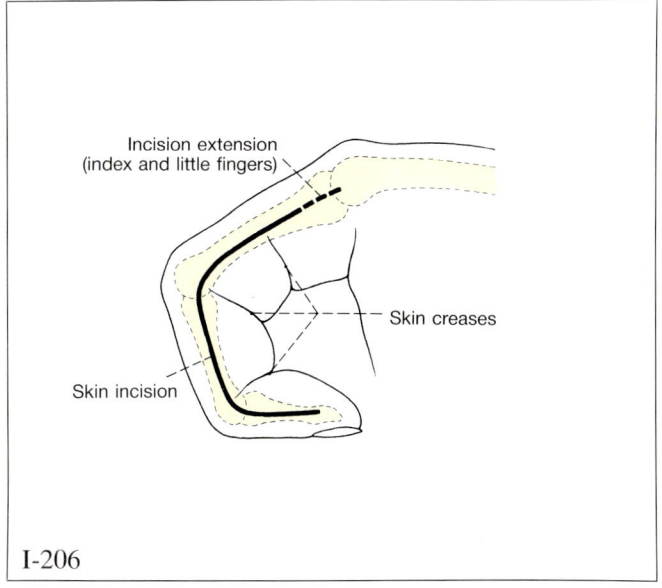

I-206

Finger — Midaxial Exposure

4. The topographical relationships are illustrated in Fig. I-208.
5. The approach to the middle phalanx is shown in Fig. I-209.

Notes

1. This incision often fails to give a good overview.
2. Furthermore, the small blood vessels to the flexor tendons are easily injured.
3. In general, the zig-zag incision of *Bruner* is preferred.

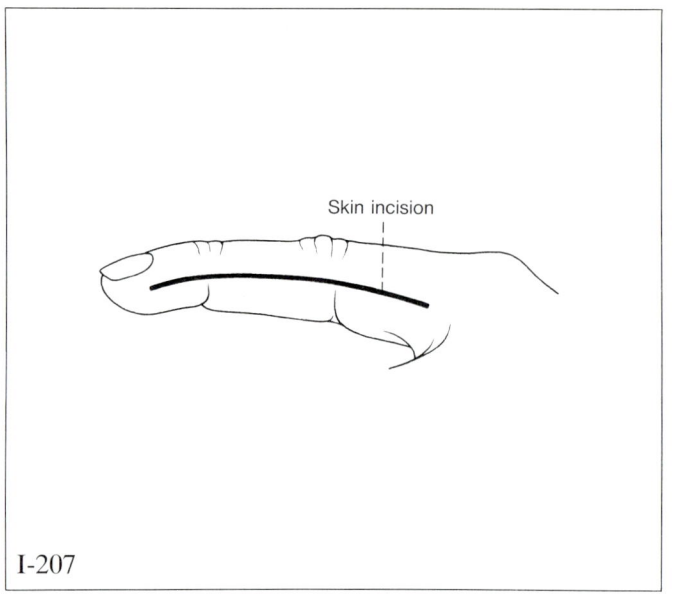

I-207

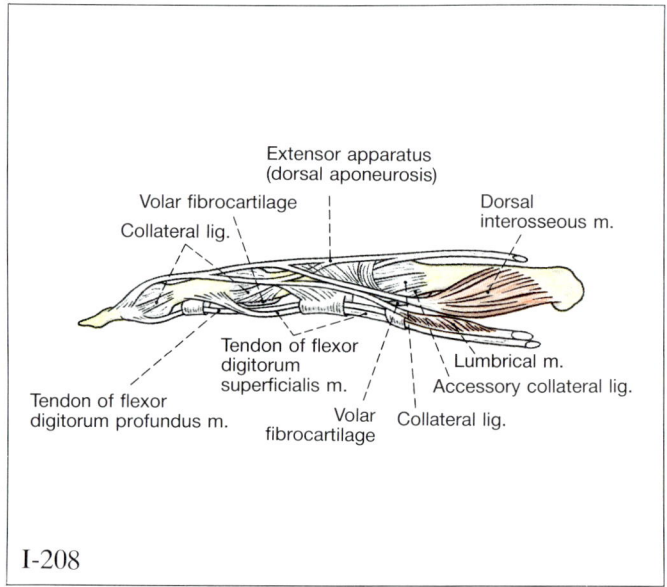

I-208

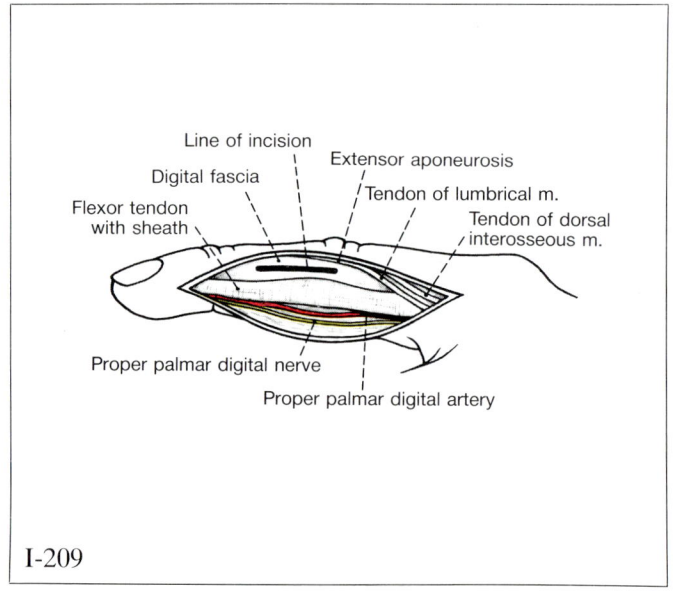

I-209

Alternative
Midaxial Hinged Flap
Midlateral Hinged Flap

1. This incision makes possible an approach to the flexor tendons (Fig. I-210).
2. However, the approach has considerable drawbacks. It can easily lead to sensory deficits on the palmar aspect of the finger.
3. Therefore, the digitopalmar zig-zag incision of *Bruner* is preferred.

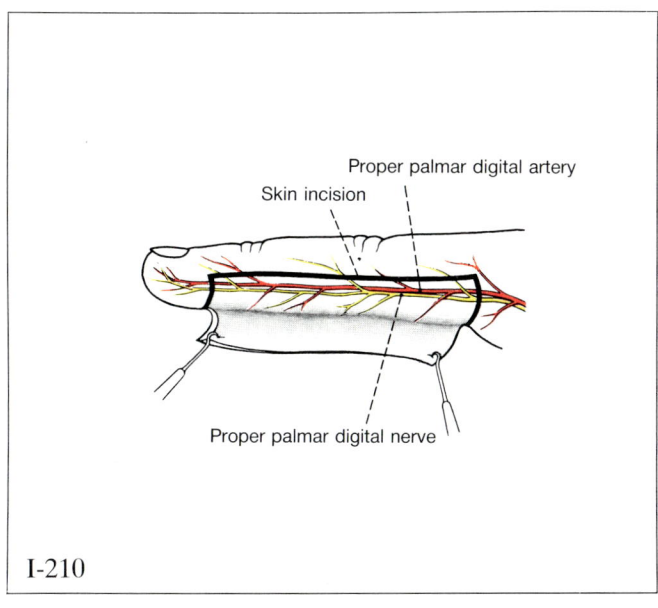

I-210

Syndactyly of the Fingers

Zig-Zag Incision
of *Blauth*

1. Dorsal and volar zig-zag incisions are compatible with subsequent requirements for skin coverage and function (Fig. I-211a).
2. At the base of the finger, the incision on the palmar side is saddle-shaped for later coverage of the commissure (Fig. I-211b).

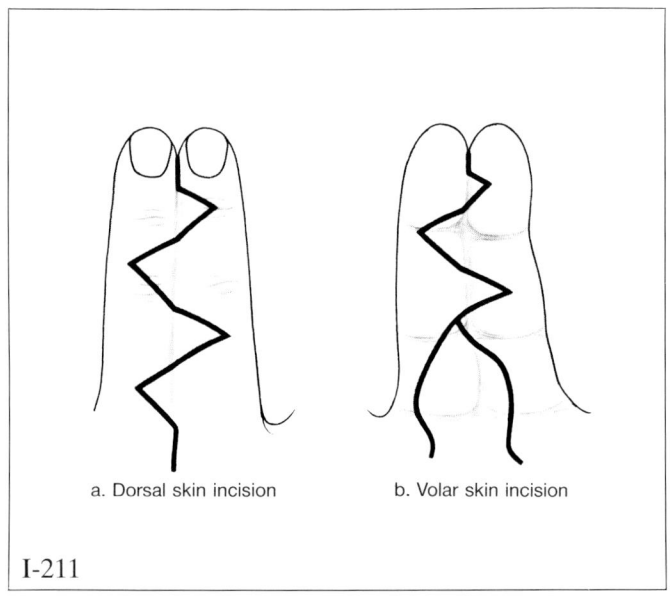

a. Dorsal skin incision   b. Volar skin incision

I-211

Amniotic Syndactyly

Z-incision
of *Iselin*

1. The multiple Z-incisions aligned in a row make possible the excision of the adhesion without risk of residual problems (Fig. I-212).
2. The incision is also well suited for adhesions in other locations.

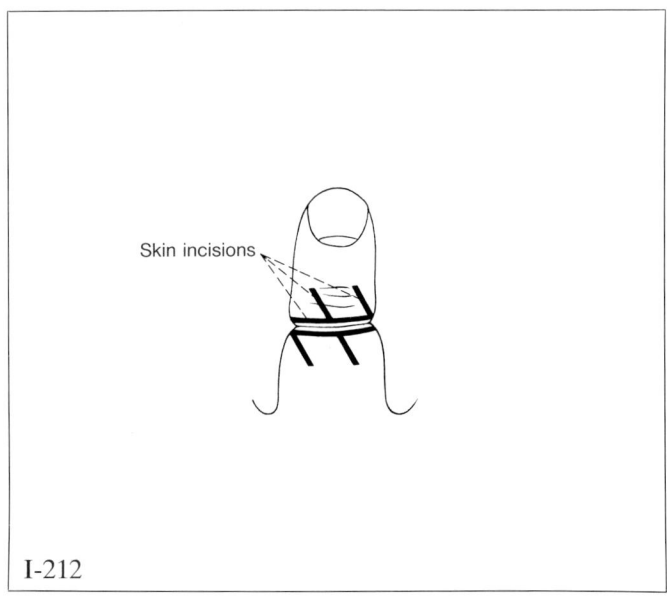

I-212

Part II
Neck and Trunk

Contents Part II

Neck and Trunk

A. Introduction 112
    Applied Anatomy 112
    Practical Considerations in
    the Prone Position 113

B. Neck – Cervical Spine 114
    Cervical Spine 114
        Extension of the Head 114
    Upper Cervical Spine 115
        Transoral Exposure 115
    Occiput to T1 117
        Posterior Exposure 117
    C3 to T1 119
        Anteromedial Exposure 119
        Variation for the Vertebral Artery
        – Spinal Nerve Root 122
    Superficial Cervical Lymph
    Nodes – Lateral Triangle of the Neck 123
        Transverse Exposure 123
    Cervical Rib 124
        Anterior Exposure 124

C. Thoracic Spine 126
    Posteromedial Exposure 126
    Posterolateral Exposure 128

D. Lumbar Region 130
    Lumbar Spine 130
        Posteromedial Exposure 130
        Laminoplasty 134
        Lumbar Transversectomy 135
    Lumbosacral Junction 136
        Anterior Exposure 136
        Transverse Incision 137
    Sacroiliac Joint 138
        Posterolateral Exposure 138
    Lumbosacral Zygapophyseal Joint
    and Ipsilateral Sacroiliac Joint 139
        Posterior Exposure 139
    Bilateral Lumbosacral Zygapophyseal
    Joints and Both Sacroiliac Joints 140

E. Pelvis 141
    Ilium – External Surface 141
        Lateral Exposure 141
    Iliac Fossa 142
    Iliac Crest 144
        Anterolateral Exposure 144
        Posterior Exposure 145
        Exposure of *Louis* 146
    Ischium 147

A. Introduction

Applied Anatomy

Topography of superficial muscles of the back (Fig. II-1).

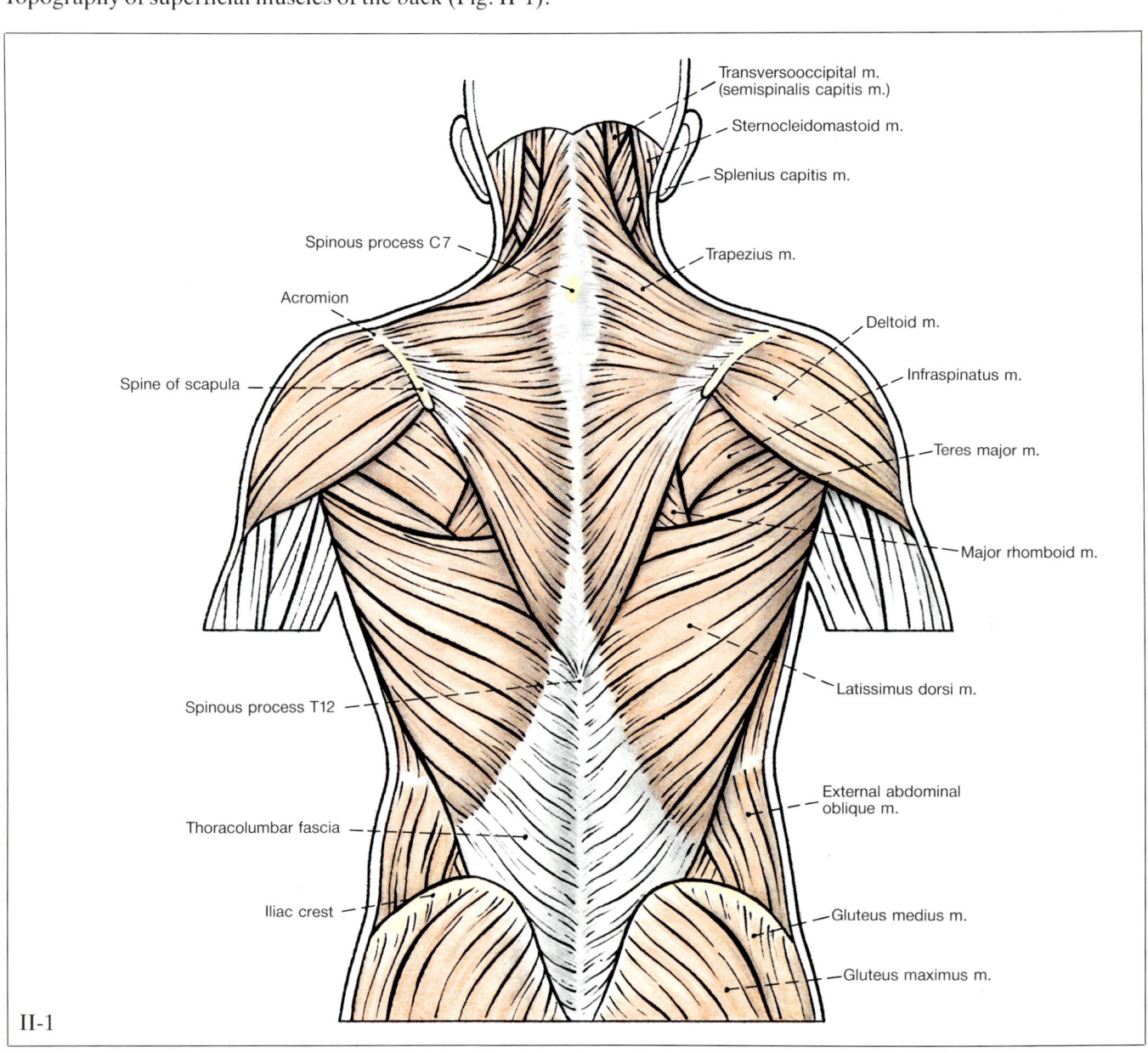

II-1

Practical Considerations in the Prone Position

1. In the prone position, venous stasis should be prevented by making certain that the abdomen is not compressed.
2. The moderately reclined position of the operating table facilitates venous drainage from the operative field. In operations on the neck and the thoracic spine, the head end of the table is elevated. This is opposite of what is desirable in operations on the lumbar spine.
3. Placement of a pillow directly beneath the shoulders ensures freedom of movement of the thoracic cage.
4. The endotracheal tube should be firmly secured to prevent it from slipping out. During operations on the neck and the thoracic spine, the tube can only be reached with great difficulty.
5. The support for the forehead must be adequately padded. This is also true for the chin in the anteflexed position.
6. The eyes should be prepared preoperatively to prevent dryness.
7. Lack of pressure on the eyes should also be ascertained prior to the operation.
8. The position must make possible the frequently required use of intraoperative radiographic imaging.

B. Neck – Cervical Spine

Cervical Spine

Extension of the Head
(with the Crutchfield Tong)

Indications

1. Cervical dislocation
2. Cervical fracture dislocations

Operative Steps

A hole is drilled (with a special bit) through the outer table of the calvaria at a point above the external acoustic meatus on a line that passes 1–1.5 finger breadths above the eyebrow (Fig. II-2). The hole is about 6–8 cm over the external acoustic meatus.

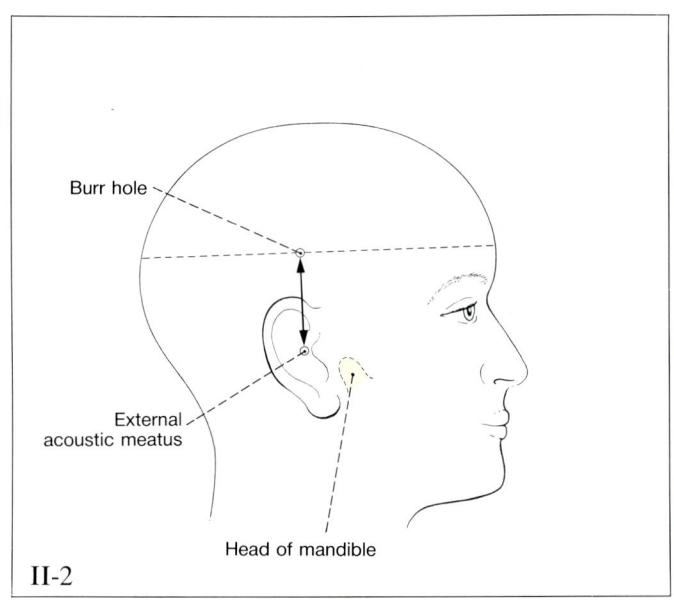
II-2

Upper Cervical Spine

Atlas-Axis-C3

Transoral Exposure

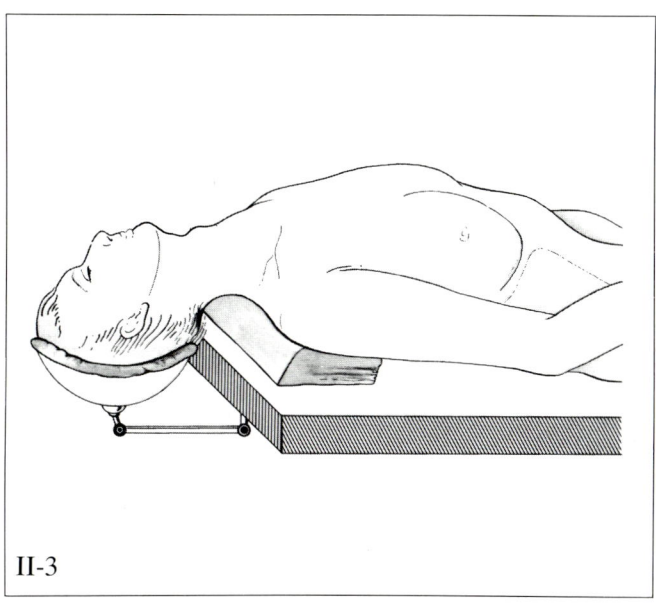

II-3

Indications

1. Tumors
2. Inflammatory processes
3. Fusion operations

Operative Steps

1. Place the patient's head in a slightly hyperextended position (Fig. II-3).
2. Use a self-retaining ENT-retractor to keep the mouth open. This retractor is supported on the upper and lower dental arches and simultaneously depresses the tongue with a curved spatula.
3. Elevate the soft palate with a thin rubber tube that is introduced through the nose and retrieved from the mouth. A retractor can also be used to accomplish the same.
4. Fig. II-4 illustrates the topographical relationships.
5. Pack the hypopharynx with gauze to prevent blood and lavage from entering the trachea.
6. After identifying the anterior tubercle of the arch of the atlas by palpation, start a median longitudinal incision at that point and continue it down the posterior pharyngeal wall for about 5 cm to C2 or C3 (Fig. II-5). With this incision four layers are penetrated:
   1) mucosa (with the muscularis and connective tissue of the posterior pharyngeal wall),
   2) the superior pharyngeal constrictor muscle,
   3) the prevertebral fascia, and
   4) the anterior longitudinal ligament.

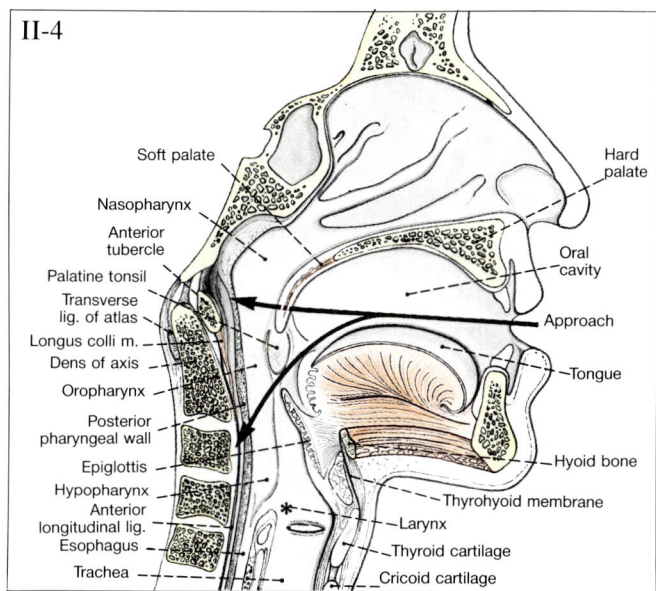

II-4

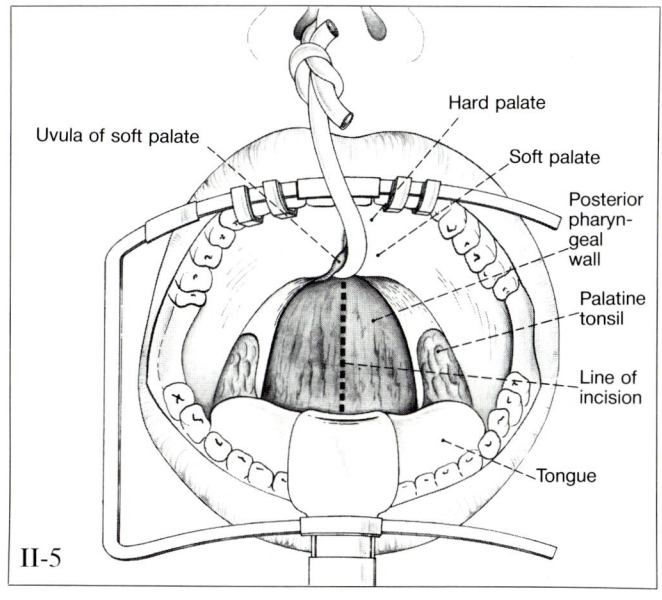

II-5

7. Retract the soft tissues bilaterally and bluntly. Control hemorrhage at the base of the dens of the axis by bipolar cautery.
8. Exposure can be achieved laterally for approximately 2 cm, or to the zygapophyseal joints (Fig. II-6).
9. The longus colli muscle inserts on the anterior tubercle of the arch of the atlas and can be detached.
10. Reflect the pharyngeal wall to both sides and hold it there by superficial stay sutures or by means of small retractors.

Notes

1. A preoperative inspection of the teeth for caries and the need for restoration is mandatory.
2. In the interest of safety, the pharyngeal wall should be swabbed and a culture obtained 2 days before the operation and intraoperatively before the start of the procedure.
3. With a transoral approach it is frequently deemed necessary to do a tracheotomy. In fact, it is quite feasible to operate next to an indwelling tube; this is particularly true for an endonasal-tracheal tube.
4. The gauze pack in the hypopharynx should not be forgotten. As a safety factor, a thread may be attached to it, exteriorized, and tagged.
5. The oral cavity and oropharynx may be sprayed with Hexoral preoperatively. Whether this is advantageous or not has not been determined.
6. Perioperative systemic antibiotic prophylaxis is recommended.
7. Intraoperative x-ray equipment with an image intensifier for identification of proper levels should be readied prior to the operation.
8. Before the incision is made in the posterior pharyngeal wall, a submucosal injection of a commercially available local anesthetic (0.5%–1%) with epinephrine to control bleeding is useful.
9. At the level of C3 and the lower border of C2, it is advisable not to dissect laterally more than 10 mm to prevent injury to the vertebral artery.
10. The wound in the posterior pharyngeal wall is closed in two layers with absorbable sutures.
11. After major transoral operative procedures, there should be parenteral feeding for 2–3 days, followed by liquid and soft foods.

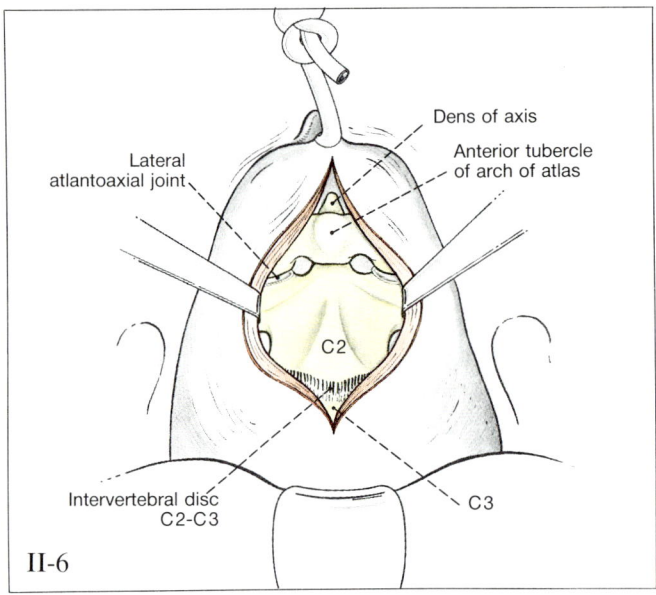

II-6

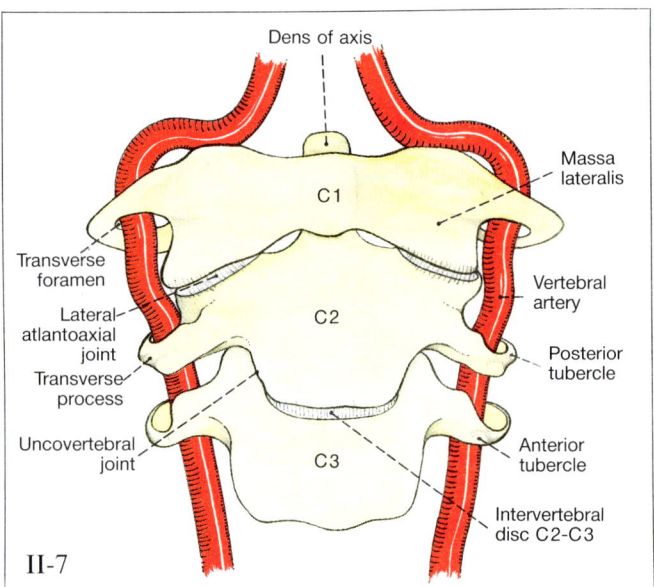

II-7

Occiput to T1

Posterior Exposure

Indications

1. Posterior fusion operation
2. Operation for prolapsed disc
3. Hemilaminectomy – laminectomy
4. Exploration of fractures and dislocations

Operative Steps

1. Make a midline longitudinal incision over the spinous processes from the base of the occipital bone and approximately 12 cm long to the prominent spinous process of C7 (Fig. II-8).
2. If only a portion of the incision is needed, refer to Fig. II-8 in which subdivisions are indicated by broken lines.
3. Reflect the skin and incise the exposed ligamentum nuchae (Fig. II-9).
4. Split the ligamentum nuchae down to the spinous processes. Then with a wide rasp or a straight chisel, displace the neck musculature to both sides of the spinous processes and the arches of the vertebrae.
5. Reflect the musculature to achieve a wide exposure of the vertebral arches including the laterally situated zygapophyseal joints, whose articular facets overlap like tiles on a roof.
6. Subsequent steps depend on the purpose of the operation.
7. To expose the nerve roots, create a window between two adjacent vertebral arches close to the zygapophyseal joints (hemilaminotomy). This is achieved by carefully placing holes in a circular pattern with an air drill and punching out the connecting bony bridges until an adequate opening is established. If the vertebral arches are spread apart properly, the punch rongeur alone can be used for this procedure. Start with the upper lamina.

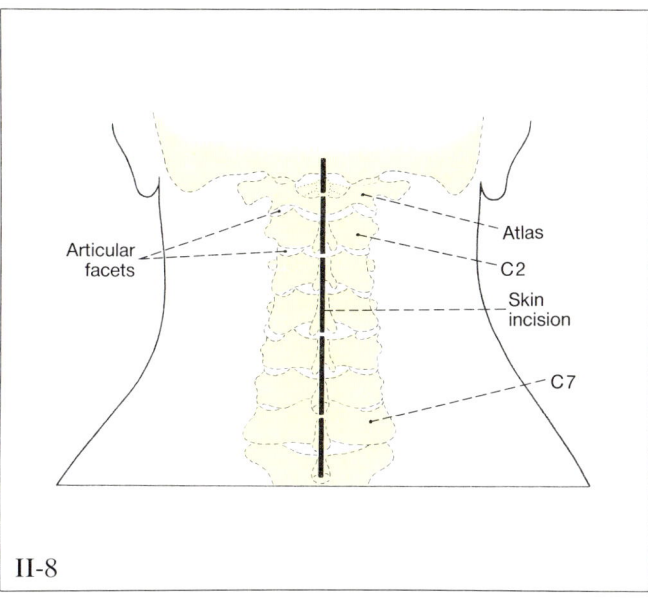

II-8

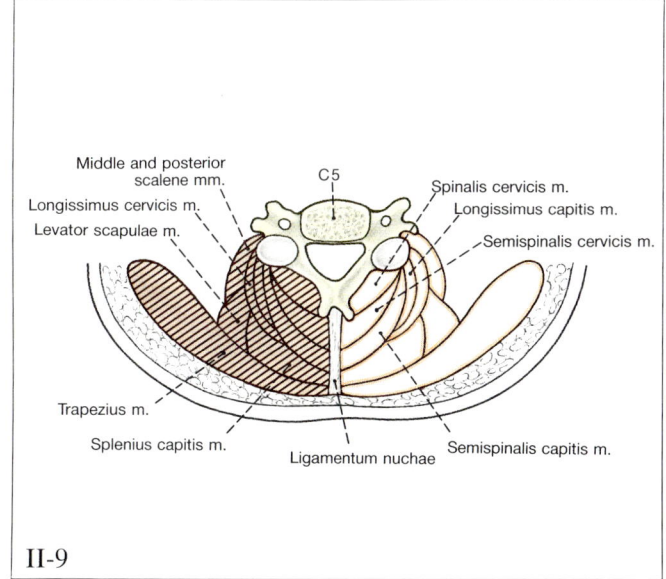

II-9

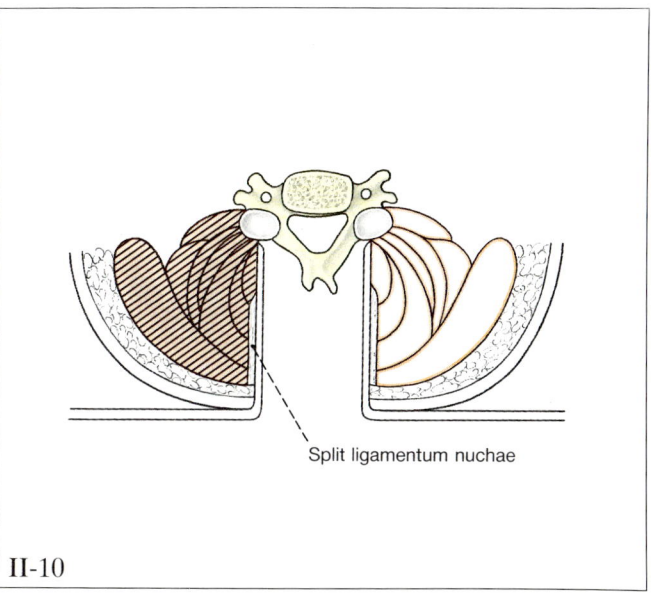

II-10

8. Elevate the underlying yellow band (ligamentum), incise it very carefully with a pointed knife, and remove it with the punch rongeur. Preparation of the window is now complete (Fig. II-11).
9. Expose the dura mater and the spinal nerve root by displacing the epidural fat (with epidural veins, Fig. II-11).
10. Commensurate with need, the field can be augmented by performing a hemilaminectomy, a foraminectomy, and a facetectomy (Figs. II-12 and II-13).

Notes

1. Usually the spinous processes and the vertebral arches separate if the head is moderately or maximally anteflexed in both the prone and the sitting positions.
2. When the patient is lying down, the head and upper part of the trunk should be elevated to promote venous drainage. In the sitting position there is a danger of cerebral hypoxia; the risk of venous air emboli is also increased.
3. The midline incision is also well suited for an approach to the occipitocervical region (occiput-atlas-axis). Lateral extension of the incision can be made with angular or T-shaped incisions for reflection of neck musculature.
4. A paraspinal longitudinal incision is adequate for a unilateral approach to the cervical spine. The soft tissues are then reflected to one side.
5. If the rasp used for detachments of soft parts is too narrow, the tip of the instrument may break off in the interlaminar space and cause injury to the sensitive nervous structures.
6. In a fusion operation, which is planned at multiple levels, special attention should be focused on the functional position of the cervical spine (adequate for daily life activities). To obviate intraoperative repositioning in these cases, the head should only be placed in a slight anteflexion.

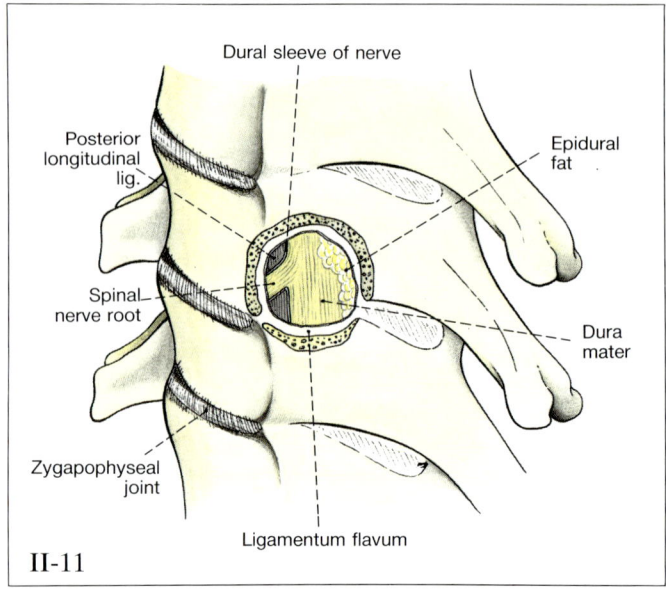

II-11

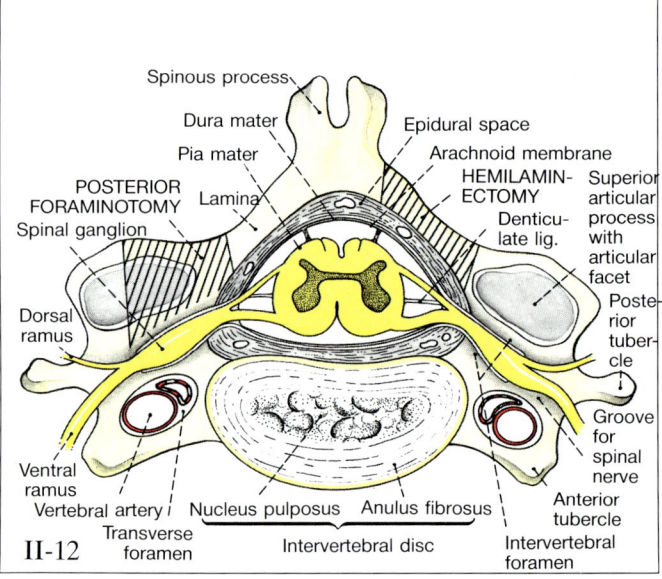

II-12

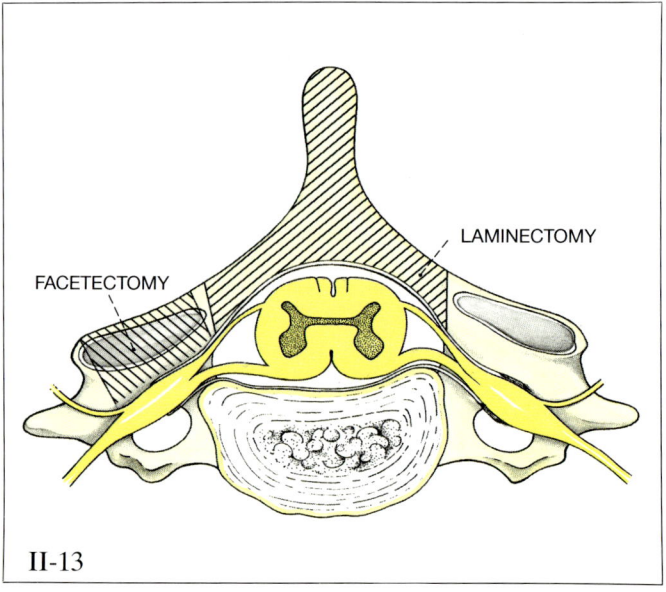

II-13

C3 to T1

Anteromedial Exposure

Indications

1. Inflammatory processes or tumors of the body of the cervical vertebra
2. Degenerative changes – prolapsed disc, bony spurs, compression of vertebral artery
3. Anterior fusion operations
4. Exploration of fractures and dislocations

Operative Steps

1. Support the head in slight to moderate hyperextension with the chin rotated away from the side of the operation.
2. Prepare the operative field from the surface of the mandible above to well below the clavicle.
3. In general, it is preferable to approach the area from the left side to prevent injury to the recurrent nerve.
4. Make an 8- to 10-cm transverse incision in a skin crease at the level of the cricoid cartilage (Fig. II-14, skin incision A). See also point 1 under Notes. The anterior jugular vein and its cross-anastomoses should be protected. Begin the incision in the midline and continue it over the belly of the sternocleidomastoid muscle.
5. Alternatively, a longitudinal skin incision can be placed along the medial (anterior) border of the muscle. This incision is definitely more conspicuous later from a cosmetic viewpoint (Fig. II-14, skin incision B).

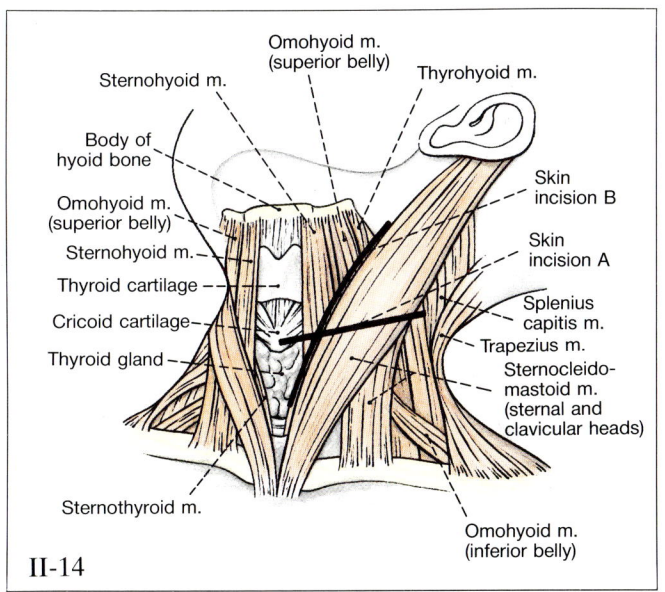

II-14

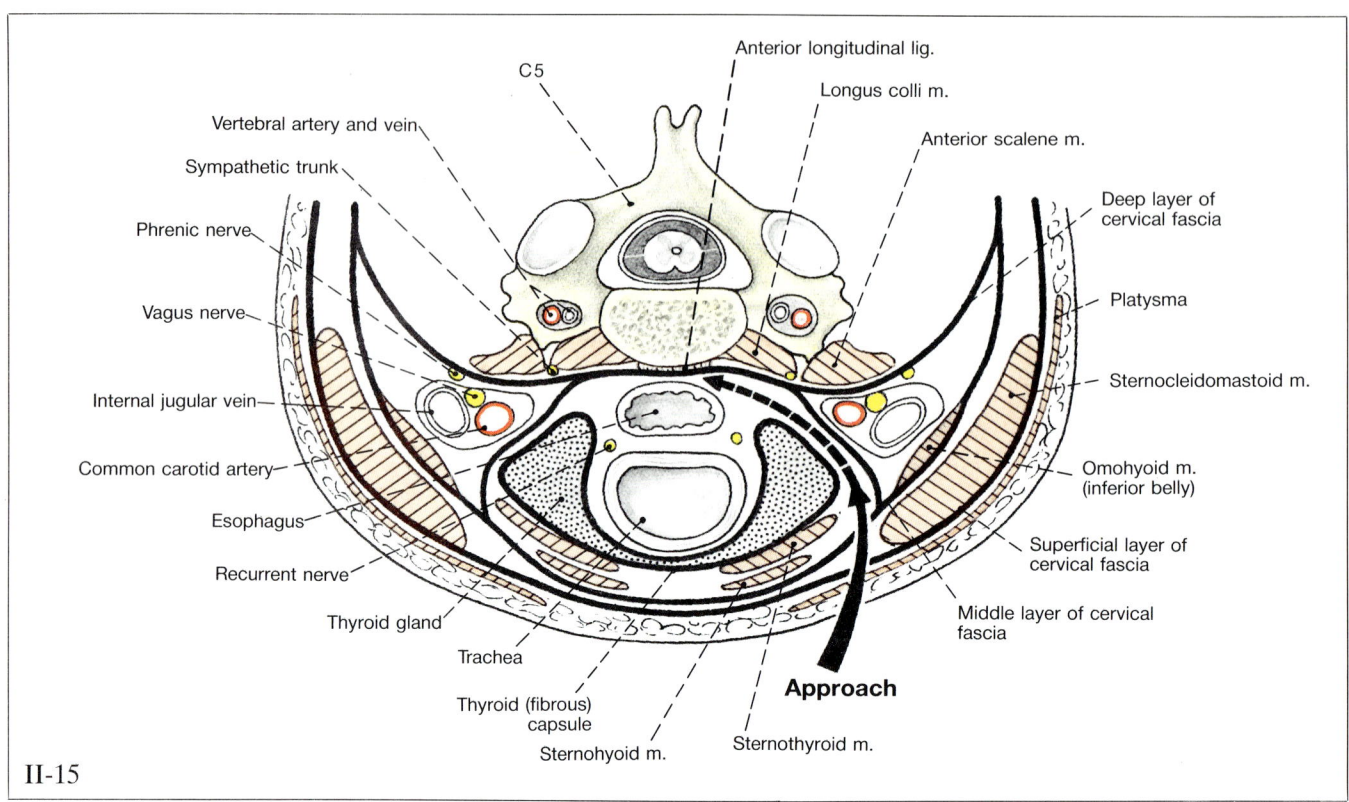

II-15

6. Divide the platysma in line with the skin incision. Enter into the deep neck medial to the sternocleidomastoid muscle (Fig. II-15).
7. Incise the pretracheal fascia longitudinally, adjacent to the lateral borders of the sternohyoid and sternothyroid muscles and medial to the neurovascular bundle. The latter, with the carotid artery, is readily palpated as is also the anterior aspect of the vertebral body. Deeper structures are developed by blunt dissection, with one finger palpating the carotid pulse and protecting the carotid sheath.
8. The recurrent nerve gives off a descending branch that accompanies the neurovascular bundle and an ascending branch that lies in the groove between the esophagus and the trachea.
9. Carefully displace the trachea, esophagus, and thyroid gland medially and reflect the neurovascular trunk laterally (Fig. II-16).
10. Palpate the vertebral body medial to the neurovascular trunk.
11. Split the prevertebral fascia with scissors in midline over the bodies of the vertebrae.
12. Incise the anterior longitudinal ligament with a scalpel. There is no muscular attachment to the vertebrae in the midline. Laterally, both the vertebral bodies and the transverse processes are covered by the longus colli muscle. The fibers of this muscle should not be disturbed because a network of sympathetic nerves (sympathetic trunk) is associated with them.
13. Lateral roentgenograms will identify the bodies of the vertebrae. The cricoid cartilage is usually at the level of C6.

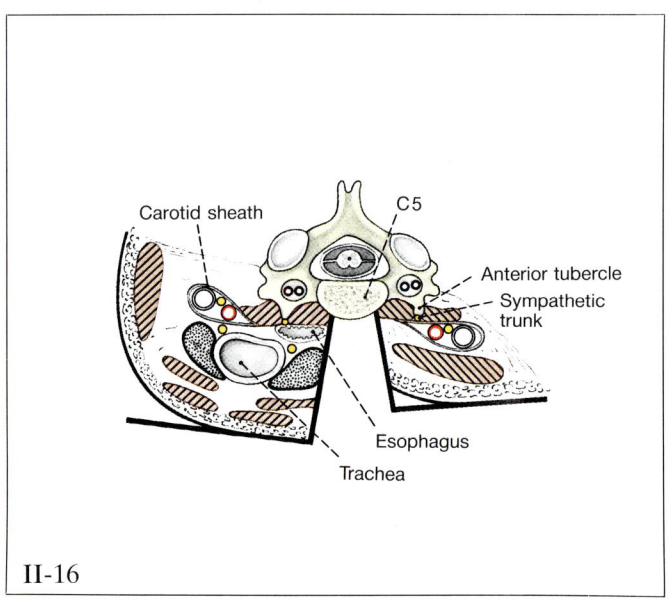

II-16

Notes

1. The level of the transverse skin incision can be determined as follows:

   Incision in the upper third of the neck for C3-C4,
   Incision in the middle third of the neck for C5-C6,
   Incision in the lower third of the neck for C7-T1.

2. Position of the patient: A small pillow placed transversely under the shoulders displays the neck better. The head end of the table is slightly elevated. This improves venous drainage and reduces hemorrhage.

3. The vertical longitudinal incision (skin incision B in Fig. II-14) is primarily used for an approach to multiple levels.

4. A better cosmetic result is achieved by incising the platysma along its fiber direction.

5. If necessary, the omohyoid muscle can be divided between two stay sutures. The latter facilitates reapproximation later. Dysphagia may ensue if the ends are not reunited.

6. The middle thyroid vein or veins must frequently be ligated (Fig. II-17). The course of the inferior thyroid vein is inconstant.

7. In the lower neck the inferior thyroid artery can be mobilized and retracted, or, if necessary, it may be doubly ligated. In the upper third of the neck, it is occasionally necessary to ligate branches of the external carotid, the superior thyroid, and the lingual arteries (in some cases also the facial artery). However, this usually should be avoided. The pattern of arteries and veins on the right side is indicated in Fig. II-17.

8. The most important step in the anteromedial procedure is the medial approach to the sternocleidomastoid muscle, i.e., the medial margin of the muscle should be clearly identified.

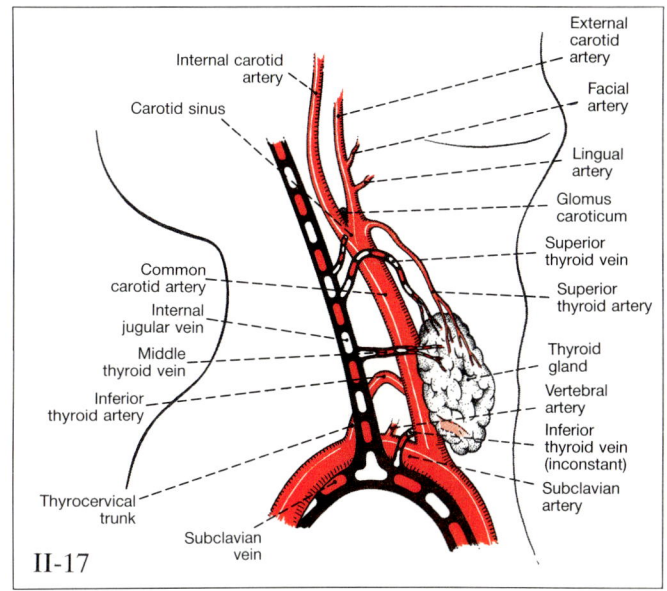

II-17

Variation for the Vertebral Artery – Spinal Nerve Root

Indications

1. Decompression of vertebral artery
2. Exploration of spinal nerve root

Operative Steps

1. Make the incision as in the anteromedial exposure, medial to the sternocleidomastoid muscle. The deep dissection is somewhat more lateral.
2. Dissect in the direction of the anterior tubercle of the transverse process (Fig. II-16).
3. The usually very prominent anterior tubercle of C6 (carotid tubercle) serves as a good landmark for determining the proper level in the lower neck region.
4. To gain access to the vertebral artery, perform a resection of the anterior part of the transverse process (transversotomy and partial transversectomy of Jung and Kehr, Fig. II-18a). Occasionally the anterior portion of the uncus must also be resected (Fig. II-18a).
5. Expose the nerve root completely from the front by performing an uncoforaminotomy (of *Verbiest*) with resection of the uncinate process (Fig. II-18b).

II-18a and b

Notes

1. The sympathetic trunk lies in front of the transverse process, either in the posterior wall of the carotid sheath or between the sheath and the longus colli muscle (Fig. II-15). The sympathetic trunk and the longitudinally oriented fibers of the longus colli muscle are retracted medially. The oblique portion of the muscle is detached from the anterior tubercle.
2. The anterior scalene muscle is separated from the anterior tubercle of C5 and C6.
3. Hemorrhage from the plexus of veins accompanying the vertebral artery is controlled by compression and packing.

Superficial Cervical Lymph Nodes
Lateral Triangle of the Neck

Transverse Exposure

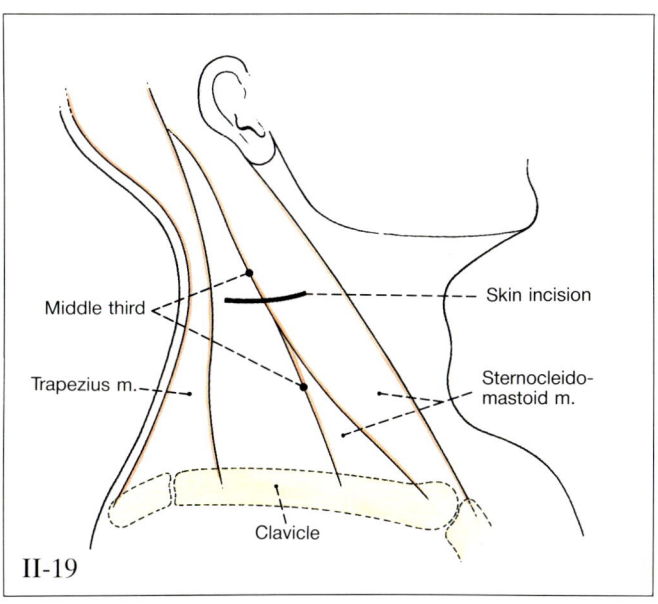

Indications

1. Biopsy of lymph nodes
2. Exploration of accessory nerve.

Operative Steps

1. Make a short, barely 5-cm-long transverse skin incision beginning immediately under the junction of the upper and middle thirds of the posterior margin of the sternocleidomastoid muscle and continuing posteriorly (Fig. II-19).
2. Carefully dissect and visualize the lymph nodes, using meticulous hemostasis (Fig. II-20).

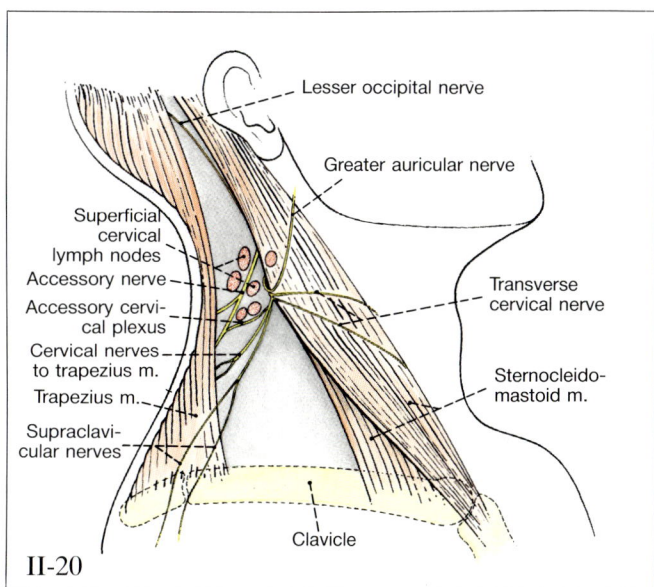

Notes

1. In the vicinity of the internal jugular vein, the accessory nerve runs caudally in the carotid triangle and contributes branches to the deep side of the sternocleidomastoid muscle. Although variable in its course, the nerve enters the posterior triangle close to the junction of the upper and middle third of the muscle and is intimately associated with a group of superficial cervical lymph nodes. The nerve then descends obliquely to the deep surface of the trapezius muscle (Fig. II-20).
2. Variable branches of the cervical nerves (C2-C4) supply the trapezius muscle (Fig. II-20) after contributing communicating rami to the accessory of the superficial cervical lymph nodes in the lateral neck region can easily cause complications involving lesions of the accessory nerve and/or the delicate motor branches of the cervical nerves, all of which contribute to the innervation of the trapezius muscle.
4. A lesion of the accessory nerve in the carotid triangle causes paresis of the sternocleidomastoid muscle and paralysis of the trapezius muscle. Injury to the accessory nerve and possibly also the cervical nerves in the posterior triangle causes varying degrees of paralysis of the trapezius muscle. This is observed clinically as inability or reduced ability to elevate or abduct the arm above the horizontal plane.
5. Occasionally the accessory nerve terminates in the sternocleidomastoid muscle.

Cervical Rib

Anterior Exposure

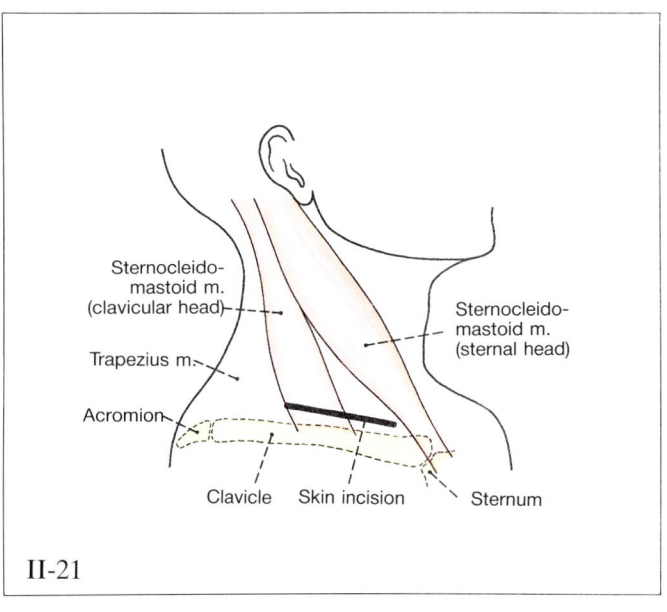

II-21

Indications

1. Excision of a cervical rib
2. Scalene syndrome

Operative Steps

1. Begin the skin incision in the supraclavicular fossa at the anterior border of the trapezius muscle; continue it to the sternal attachment of the sternocleidomastoid muscle. The incision roughly follows the skin crease of the neck (Fig. II-21).
2. After reflecting the skin, divide platysma at a slightly lower level but in the same direction as the skin incision. Retract the platysma to bring into view the underlying muscles, nerves, and vessels.
3. Cut the lateral half of the clavicular portion of the sternocleidomastoid muscle between two clamps (Fig. II-22). This facilitates hemostasis.
4. Retract the muscle medially to expose the tendon of the omohyoid muscle as well as the tendinous attachment of the anterior scalene muscle (Fig. II-23).
5. The phrenic nerve crosses the anterior scalene muscle from lateral to medial.
6. To expose the anterior scalene muscle better, retract the omohyoid muscle cranially. Avoid injury to the phrenic nerve.
7. The pleura and the neurovascular bundle, as well as the vertebral artery, lie medial to the anterior scalene muscle.

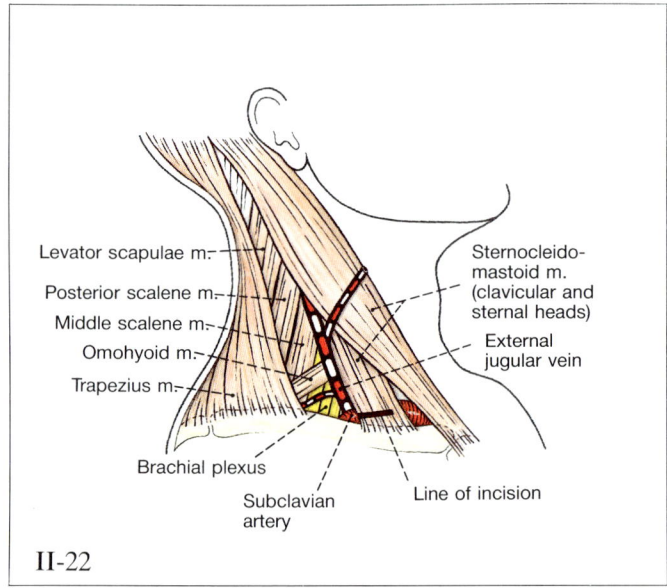

II-22

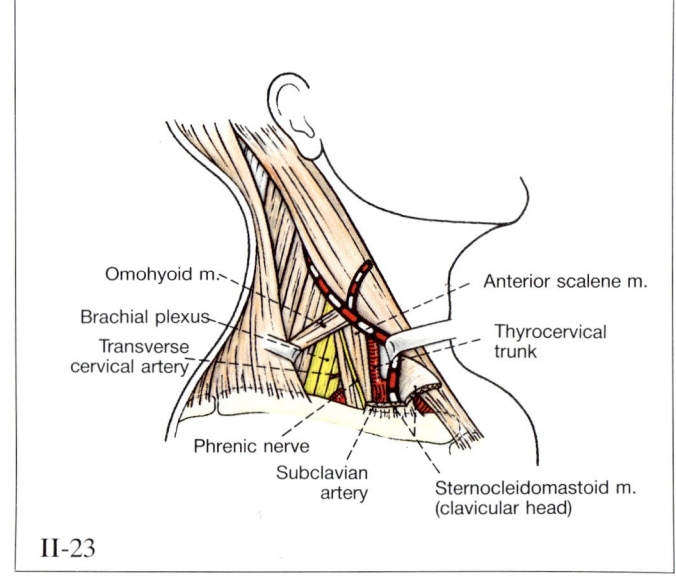

II-23

Cervical Rib — Anterior Exposure

8. Free the phrenic nerve completely before retracting it medially.
9. Divide the anterior scalene muscle between two clamps. Avoid the subclavian artery and the pleura, which lie in a deeper plane behind and medial to the scalene muscle (Fig. II-22, II-23, and II-24).
10. Cutting the anterior scalene muscle results in a somewhat anterior displacement (release) of the subclavian artery and the medial cord of the brachial plexus (Fig. II-26). This affords a view of the cervical rib.
11. This anterior approach to the cervical rib is preferred over the lateral or posterior approach because it is surgically simpler and less apt to cause injury to the brachial plexus.

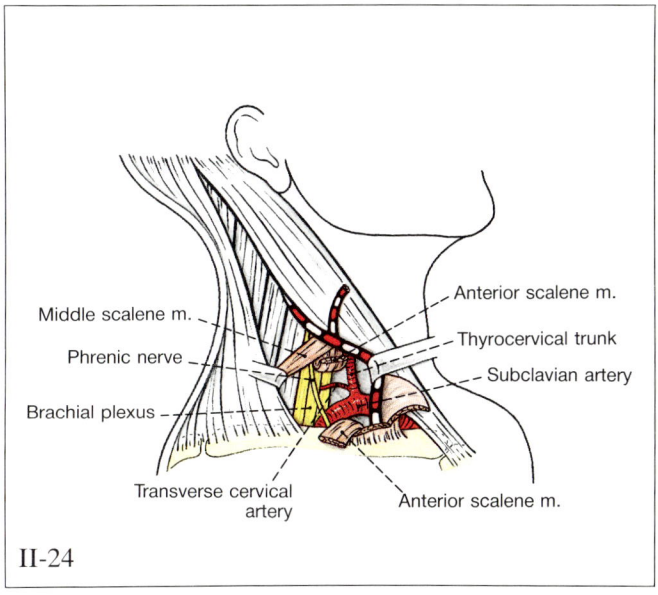

II-24

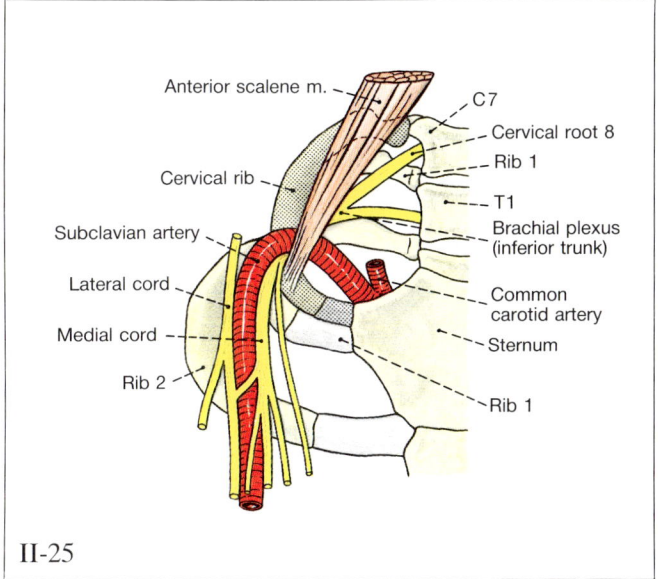

II-25

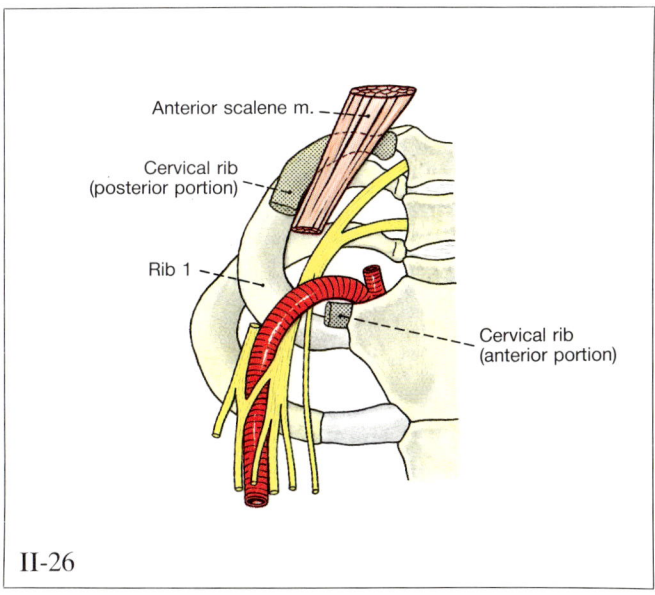

II-26

C. Thoracic Spine

Posteromedial Exposure

Dorsal Exposure

Indications

1. Fusion of the spine
2. Laminectomy
3. Infections in arches or spinous processes
4. Prolapsed thoracic disc

Operative Steps

1. Place the patient in a prone or lateral position (slightly inclined forward) or a stooped sitting position. The prone position is usually preferred.
2. Make a posterior longitudinal incision over the spinous processes of the desired segment of the spine from T1 to T12 (Fig. II-27, skin incision A). Usually only a part of the incision is adequate; subsections are indicated by broken lines in Fig. II-27.
3. The paraspinal longitudinal and curved incisions (Fig. II-27, skin incision B and C, respectively) are alternative approaches. Lateral extensions of the incision are possible by making short transverse cuts or a hinged flap.
4. Reflect the skin to expose the deep fascia over the spinous processes and split it down to the bone.
5. The musculature that attaches to the midline (Fig. II-28) is reflected off the spinous processes and the vertebral arches with the aid of a chisel or a rasp. It is helpful to finish the muscle detachment on one side before preparing the remaining side. This facilitates hemostasis.

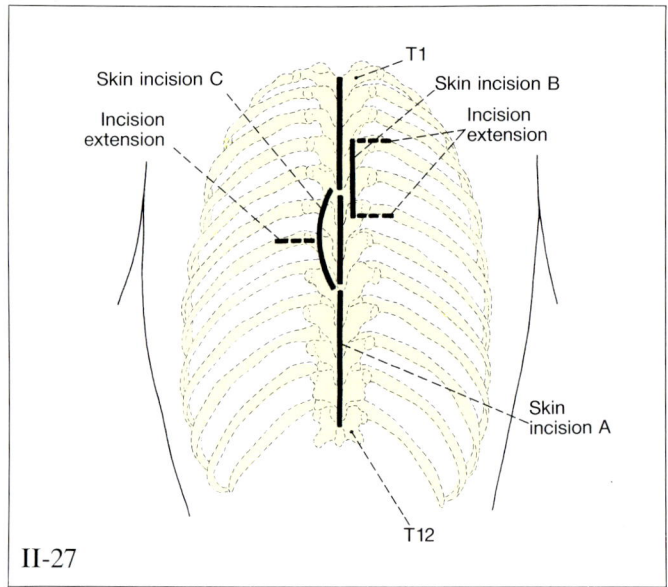

II-27

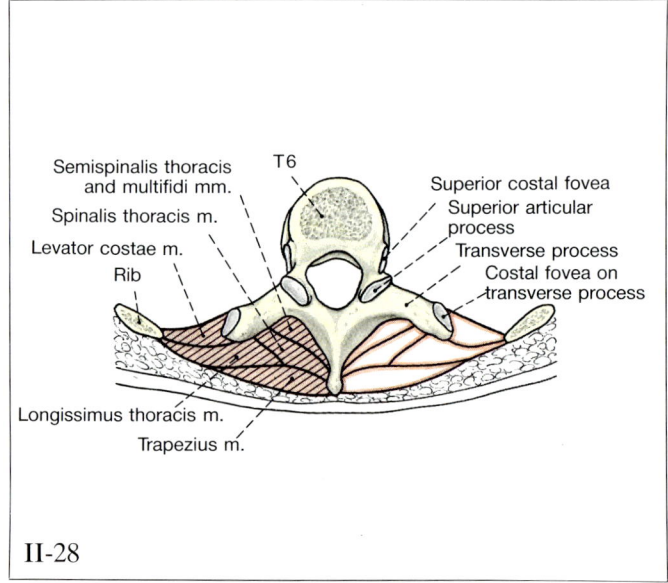

II-28

Thoracic Spine — Posteromedial Exposure

6. Reflect the paraspinal muscles to their respective sides (Fig. II-29).
7. Using the transverse extensions of the incision (see point 3), divide both fascia and musculature transversely.
8. For further augmentation of the field, resect the transverse process of the vertebra. Compare this with the posterolateral exposure.
9. To explore the intervertebral disc, remove the lamina on one side and, if necessary, its root.
10. The neurovascular bundle at the lower margin of the rib serves as a guide for the spinal nerve and the intervertebral disc. The intercostal nerve runs to the intervertebral foramen.

Notes

1. If the point of the chisel is too narrow or the rasp is too fine, the tip of the instrument can break off in the interlaminar space and cause a lesion of the spinal cord. A similar accident between the transverse processes can cause a hemothorax, in which case a larger operative field will be required for ligating the vessels.
2. The preoperative positioning of the patient is important to prevent compression of the abdomen and unnecessary hemorrhage.
3. The direct approach through the vertebral canal to the intervertebral disc in the thoracic region of the spine is more difficult than a similar procedure in the lumbar region because the spinal cord with the dura virtually fills the vertebral canal and is less mobile and very sensitive.
4. For extension of the field, see the details under the posterolateral exposure.

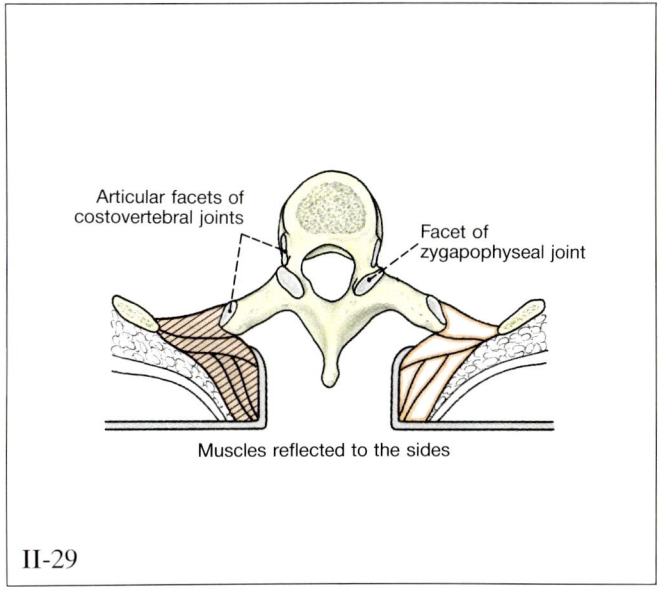

II-29

Posterolateral Exposure
Costotransversectomy

Indications

1. Exposure of the anterolateral aspect of the vertebral body – excision of a diseased part, exploration of the disc, biopsy
2. Opening and draining an abscess
3. Exploration and removal of a tumor

Operative Steps

1. Make a 12- to 15-cm paravertebral longitudinal incision adjacent to the spinous processes, 3–6 cm from the midline. The midpoint of the incision should be over the desired vertebra (Fig. II-30, skin incision A). It must be remembered that in the thoracic region the tip of a spinous process is approximately 5 cm below the level of the corresponding vertebral body.
2. Make a second incision from the midpoint of the first and continue it laterally over the rib, which should be partially resected.
3. Reflect the skin to reveal the deep fascia that encloses the erector spinae muscles.
4. Divide these muscles down to the rib in the direction of the skin incision.
5. When the muscle flaps are reflected, the vertebral arch, the transverse process, and the rib are seen.
6. Example for determining the proper level: If the T5-T6 intervertebral disc is to be explored, the fifth rib should be exposed.
7. After incising and removing the capsule of the costotransverse joint, detach the transverse process at its base with a chisel. Remove about 7–8 cm of the vertebral end of the rib subperiosteally.
8. Prior orientation to the course of the intercostal neurovascular bundle is helpful.
9. The head of the rib may also be mobilized and disarticulated (but not just turned and pulled out). In this case one must stay strictly in the subperiosteal plane to prevent unnecessary hemorrhage. The periosteum in front of (anterior to) the head of the rib with the intercostal muscles, as well as the endothoracic fascia and the parietal pleura are pushed out of the way, forward.

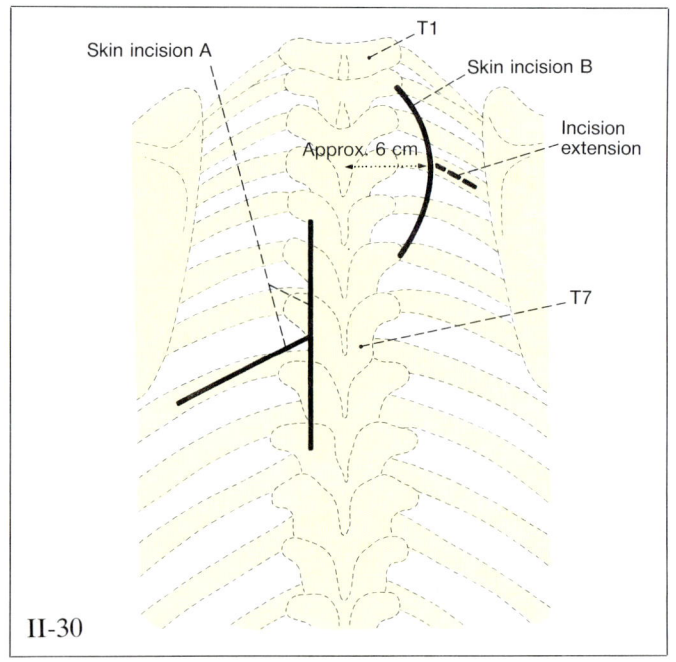

II-30

Thoracic Spine — Posterolateral Exposure

10. After removal of the transverse process and the approximately 10-cm-long portion of the vertebral end of the rib, the left side of the vertebral body, the lateral aspect of the disc, the aorta, and the slightly translucent parietal pleura are brought into view (Fig. II-31).
11. The lateral part of the arch and, if necessary, its pedicle can be resected for inspection of the posterior aspect of the disc (in prolapse of the disc).
12. Dissection of the neurovascular bundle that runs near the lower border of the rib and continues under the transverse process is useful for orientation. Tracing the intercostal nerve medially through the intervertebral foramen leads to the vertebral canal. After the rib is resected, the next higher intercostal neurovascular bundle is unexpectedly close.
13. Incision of the costal pleura for the purpose of expanding the field or accidental entry into the pleural cavity leads to collapse of the lung. In this case use a sponge-armed large hemostat to keep the lung out of the operative field. Prior to closure place a Bulau drain.
14. It is not absolutely necessary to suture the costal pleura in this region during wound closure.
15. An accidental small pleural lesion can be promptly closed while maintaining intrapulmonary pressure.
16. In any case take a postoperative x-ray on table to look for a pneumothorax.

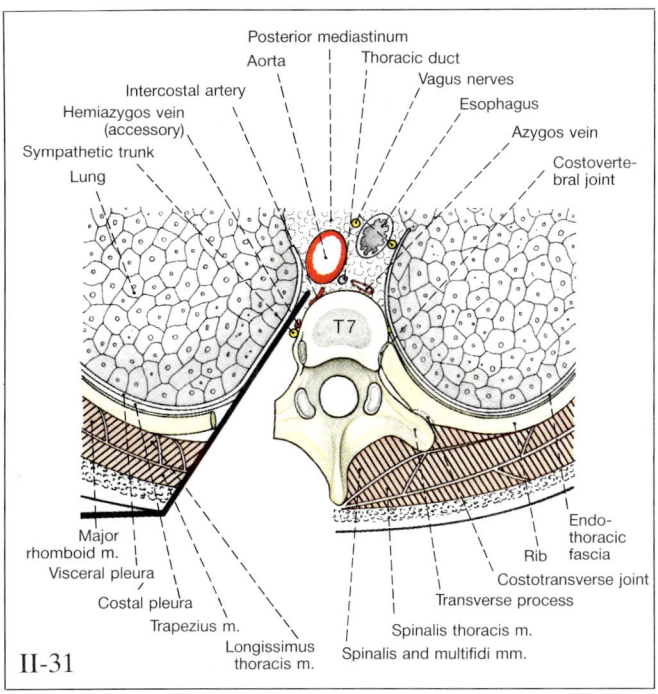

II-31

Alternative

1. Make a curved skin incision (Fig. II-30, skin incision B) whose lateral extension ends at the edge of the paraspinal musculature.
2. Detach the paraspinal musculature subperiosteally and displace it medially.
3. A transverse extension of the incision can be made if necessary.

Notes

1. A generous skin incision is important. For an augmented view, expose two or three ribs simultaneously.
2. In the upper and middle regions of the thoracic spine, the trapezius and part of the rhomboid muscle must be divided in the direction of the incision. At the middle and lower levels of the thoracic spine, the same holds true for the latissimus dorsi muscle. Fig. II-1 illustrates the fiber direction of the muscles.
3. In the upper half of the thoracic spine, it is helpful to elevate the periosteum of the ribs by starting medially and proceding laterally. In the lower half the opposite is preferred.
4. When needed, two (to three) vertebral ends of the ribs can be resected. The intercostal vessels are ligated. In the midthoracic area this cannot be done with impunity because the vessels may contribute to the blood supply of the spinal cord.
5. The intercostal nerves usually are preserved. If required, however, two (or a maximum of three) of the nerves can be surgically cut.
6. The left posterolateral approach is preferred because the aorta is more readily mobilized.
7. In case of postoperative lymph leakage, the thoracic duct or the cisterna chyli are ligated, the latter at the level of the diaphragm. Usually the wound closes by itself so that the drain can be removed after approximately 5 days; if not, a reexploration is required.
8. Technically, it is easier to perform a costotransversectomy in the upper half of the spine because of the less well developed paraspinal musculature.

D. Lumbar Region

Lumbar Spine

Posteromedial Exposure

Indications

1. Laminectomy – hemilaminectomy
2. Prolapsed disc – hemilaminotomy
3. Fusion of spine
4. Fractures

Positions

1. The operation is performed with the patient in the prone position. To prevent venous stasis in the operative field, the abdomen should be compression-free. Compare with position recommendations in Part II, section A.
2. To achieve this the anterior iliac crest and the thorax are supported by pillows. A firm ring-shaped pillow is also useful. Both hip joints are flexed to decrease the lordosis. The knees are supported by padding. The position is indicated in Fig. II-32. A small adjustable bench with bilateral supports can also be used to obtain the desired flattening of the lordosis.
3. The slightly inclined operating table – head low, buttocks high – will improve venous drainage.
4. The knee-chest position may at times be preferred (Fig. II-33). With a compression-free abdominal cavity, it has the advantage of affording maximal interlaminar separation (kyphosis).
5. The above position, however, has considerable disadvantages. The nerve root is stretched and therefore less movable and more readily injured. This position also affects the intervertebral spaces so that a prolapsed disc that has not yet ruptured may slide back and remain unnoticed during the operation. The unnatural position also makes it difficult to evaluate a possible lumbar stenosis (fornix and lateral recess

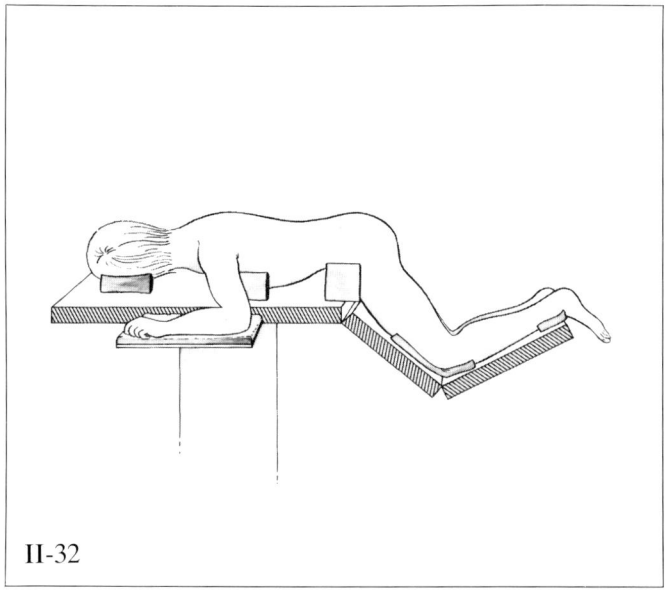

II-32

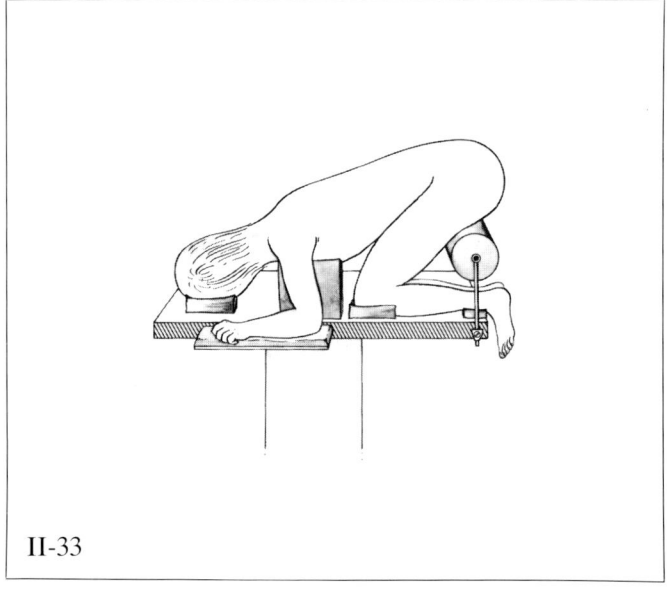

II-33

Lumbar Spine — Posteromedial Exposure

stenosis). The sharply angled knees can also contribute to congestion of the legs.

6. The simple prone position is preferred for fusion operations because it corresponds to the subsequently desired erect posture (Fig. II-34). The iliac crests and thorax are supported by pillows. The groin should be free from pressure.

7. A stable side position is effective for very obese patients. The desired flattening of the lumbar lordosis can be achieved by drawing the limbs up. A pillow supporting the flank or a corresponding elevation of the operating table makes possible the additional interlaminar separation on the side away from the table.

Operative Steps

1. Make a posterior longitudinal incision in the midline over the spinous processes of the vertebrae – in the present example, over L4–L5 (Fig. II-35).
2. Reflect the skin to reveal the posterior layer of the thoracolumbar fascia, which is split in the midline down to the spinous processes. The topographical relationships are indicated in Fig. II-36.
3. Alternatively, divide the fascia by two parallel paraspinal incisions.
4. Then detach the musculature from both sides of the vertebral arch with the aid of a wide chisel or a rasp, proceeding laterally along the spinous processes and the vertebral arches. It is helpful to first free the muscles on one side, where bleeding can be controlled with moist compresses during preparation of the opposite side. Remnants of the thoracolumbar fascia on the spinous processes facilitate reattachment later.

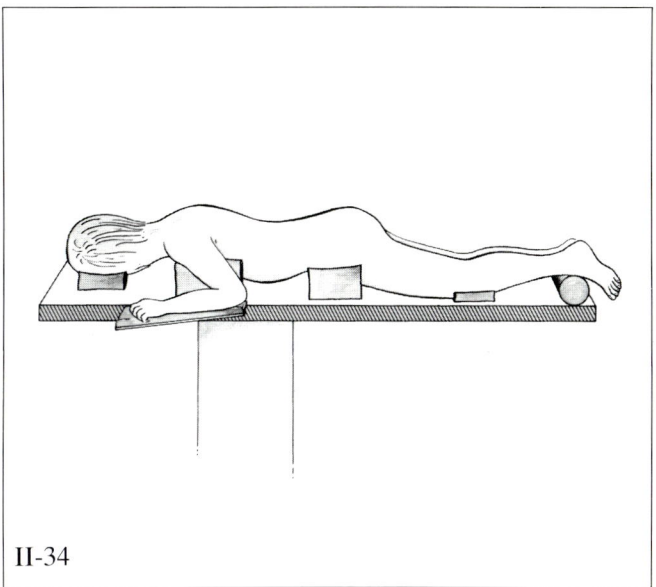

II-34

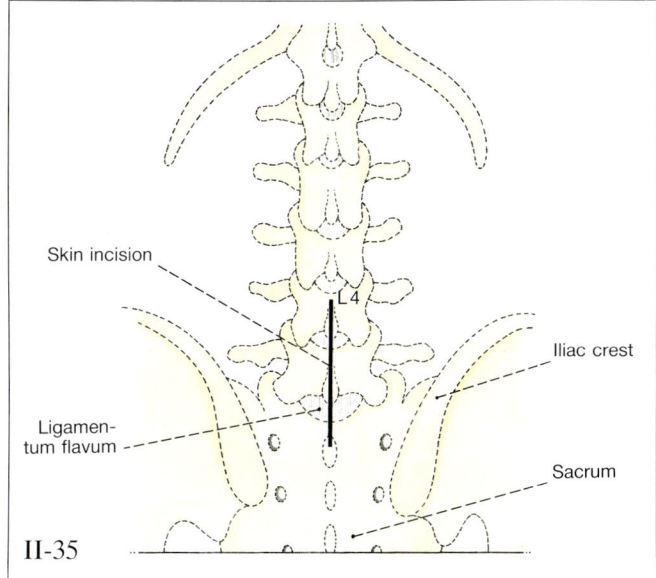

II-35

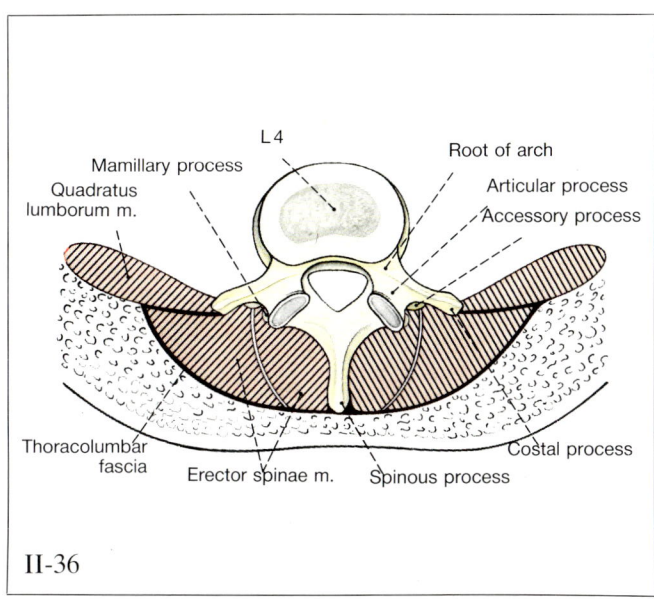

II-36

5. Firmly retract the paraspinal musculature to both sides, preferably by using a self-retaining retractor. The vertebral arch, the zygapophyseal joints, and the ligamentum flavum are now exposed (Figs. II-37 and II-38).
6. Create a unilateral fenestration into the vertebral canal by carefully incising the ligamentum flavum with a pointed scalpel at the lower margin of the arch of L 4 from medial to lateral along the course of the spinal nerve. The ligament is then elevated with a small clamp or a dural hook.
7. Pass a small right-angled dissector under the ligamentum flavum to carefully loosen the dura from the ligament.
8. Resect the ligament piecemeal with a small punch, or complete the incision of the ligament along the upper edge of the arch of L 5 and then remove the ligament.
9. At the level of L 4-L 5 and higher lumbar segments, it is frequently necessary to enlarge the window. This can be done by removing the lower edge of the arch of L 4 and the medial part of the zygapophyseal joint with a punch (or by using a chisel, gripping it firmly). The upper edge of the arch of L 5 may also be resected (laminotomy).
10. Displace the epidural adipose tissue to bring into view, through the window, the dura and the L 5 nerve root with its dural sleeve (Fig. II-39). After careful neurolysis a prolapsed disc may be revealed over the shoulder or in the axilla of the nerve root.
11. To expose the nerve root in the lateral recess of the vertebral canal, it might be necessary to perform a foraminotomy for a lateral enlargement of the window.
12. To obtain a limited view of the intervertebral disc, displace the spinal nerve root medially and incise crosswise the posterior longitudinal ligament over the disc space.

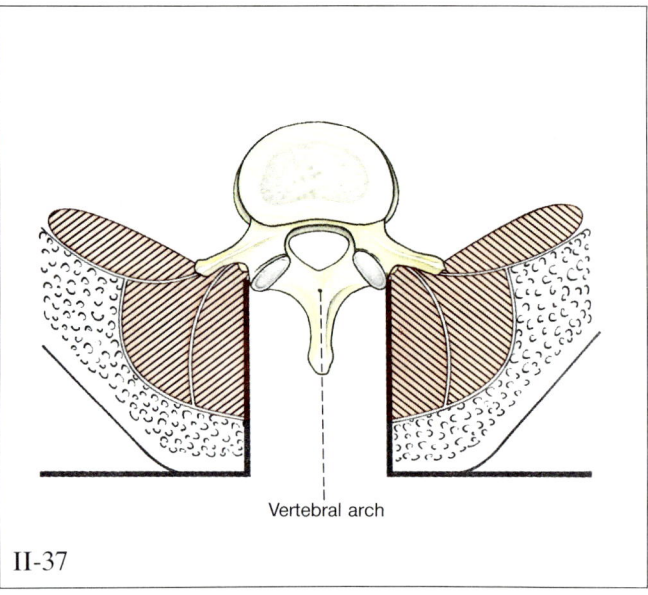

II-37

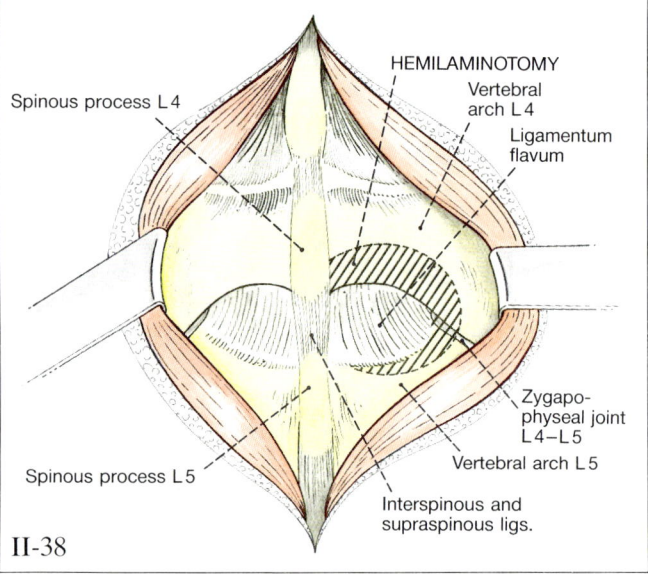

II-38

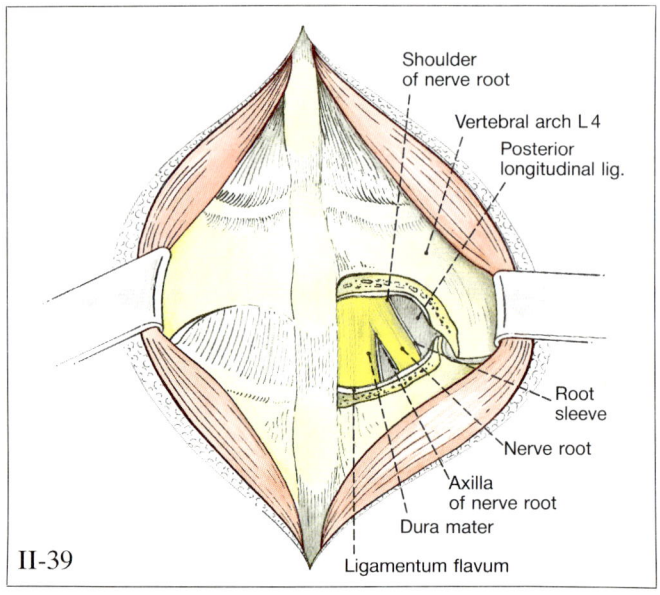

II-39

Lumbar Spine — Posteromedial Exposure

13. Anatomical relationships are illustrated in Figs. II-40 and II-41.

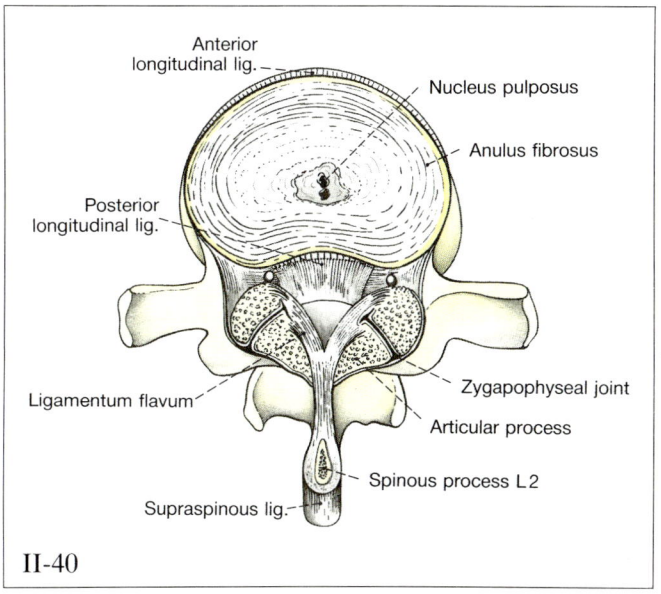

II-40

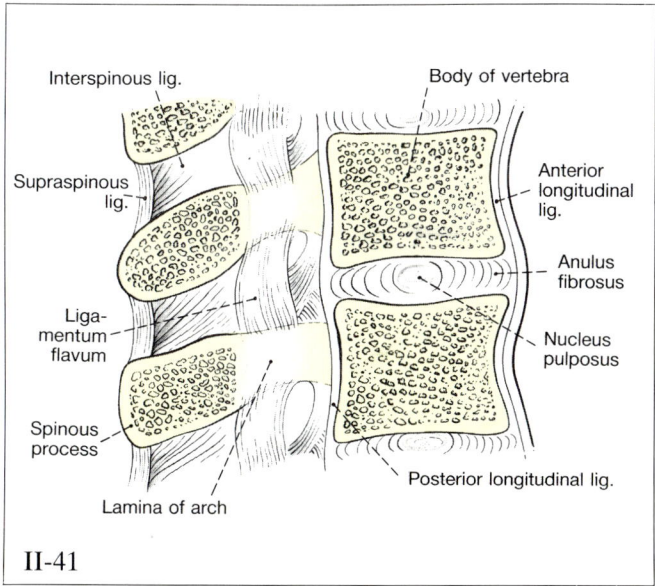

II-41

Alternative

1. Occasionally there is pronounced overlapping of the vertebral arches (particularly in older persons), or scar tissue is present from a previous operation, or a more substantial exposure is deemed necessary. Access to the ligamentum flavum can then be facilitated by removing midline wedges of bone with segments of the corresponding spinous processes from which the interspinous ligaments have been removed.
2. The expansive exposure of the ligamentum flavum affords the opportunity to incise the ligament so as to create a flap, which is later used to cover the window (method of Cloward) (Fig. II-42).

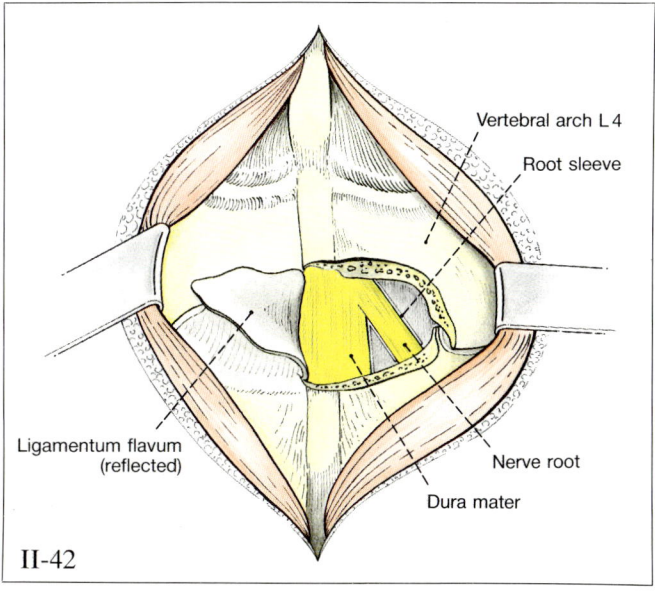

II-42

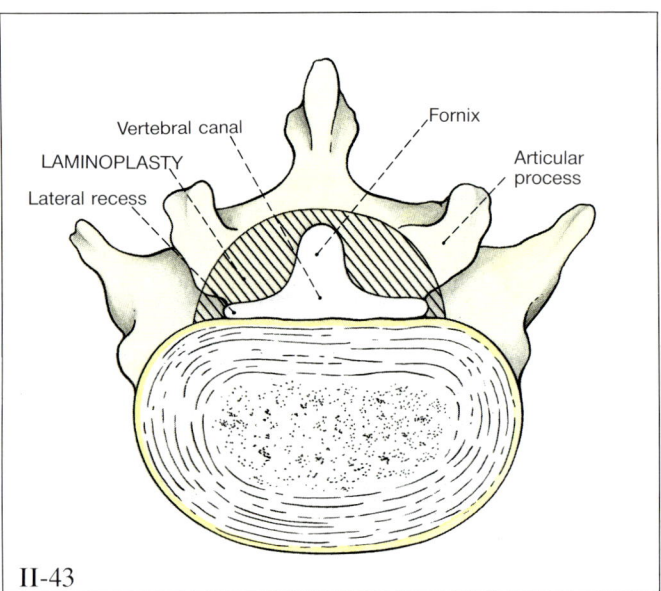

II-43

Laminoplasty

1. In the case of lumbar stenosis, it is often impossible to obtain an adequate view of the spinal nerve without resecting portions of the vertebral arch by performing a hemilaminectomy, laminectomy, and/or a foraminotomy with partial facetectomy.
2. In many cases the alternative is to remove the inner portion of the vertebral arch. This ensures continuity of the arches and stability of the spine (Fig. II-43). Sometimes this can be done unilaterally (hemilaminoplasty). The craniocaudal width of the arch also can be decreased using this method. Overlapping projections of the cranial margin of the vertebral arch, as seen in hyperlordosis, can be effectively removed with a wide resection to relieve the bilateral stenosing effect.
3. Tunneling under the vertebral arch and decompressing the nerve root are achieved by using a right-angled drill, a curved small chisel, a punch rongeur, and a curved fine rasp.

Notes

1. Identification of the last vertebral arch of the lumbar spine serves as a guide for establishing the proper segmental level. On palpation the arch feels like a rough transverse elevation that clearly differs from the sacrum. The latter has a smooth posterior surface.
2. By elevating and rocking the presacral spinous process, slight movements can be elicited in the vertebral arch and the zygapophyseal joints. Of course, the spinous process of S1 is immovable.
3. To locate the proper level, it is necessary to use roentgenograms for comparisons because of the not infrequent fusions in the lumbosacral joint.
4. When errors do occur in identification, it is almost always the next higher level that is selected.
5. The paraspinal musculature is supplied by the dorsal primary rami of the spinal nerves, which enter the muscles from their lateral aspect. Therefore, there is no danger of interrupting the innervation by displacing the muscles as far as the zygapophyseal joints.
6. At the lumbosacral level (L5-S1), it is usually possible to prepare a wide area of the ligamentum flavum for fenestration without partial resection of the vertebral arch.
7. Bleeding from epidural veins is controlled with cautery (bipolator). Temporary compression with application of fibrin foam is frequently adequate.
8. Hemorrhage, which prevents safe exposure of the nerve root, can be controlled with moist felt packs (tagged with a string) above and below the field.
9. An accidental nick in the dura should be sutured or covered with Gelfoam. If the dural edges can not be approximated, a small muscle flap from the paraspinal musculature should be placed over the lesion. A drain is not recommended in this case.

Lumbar Transversectomy
Posterolateral Exposure

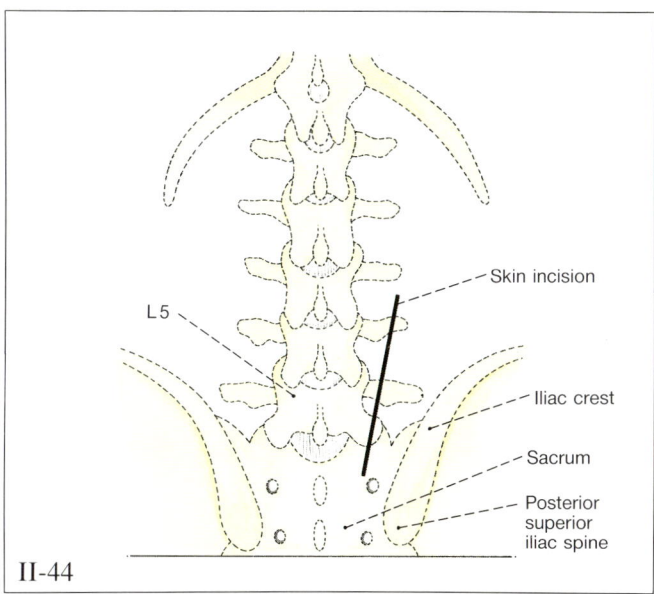

II-44

Indications

1. Tumors associated with the vertebral body
2. Inflammatory processes
3. Biopsies
4. Posterolateral fusion of vertebrae

Operative Steps

1. Make a 10-cm longitudinal incision beginning approximately 4 cm lateral to the spinous process and directed caudally and slightly toward the midline. The midpoint of the incision should be over the desired body of the vertebra. It ends just medial to the posterior superior iliac spine.
2. Reflect the skin and split the posterior layer of the thoracolumbar fascia over the iliocostalis and longissimus thoracis muscles.
3. Incise these muscles in a longitudinal direction down to the transverse processes.
4. Detach the transverse processes at their bases with a sharp chisel.
5. The psoas major muscle is now seen. This muscle and the transverse process with its muscle attachments are carefully displaced laterally.
6. The inferior vena cava and the aorta lie directly in front of the psoas major muscle on the right and left sides, respectively.
7. At this stage in the operation, the lumbar vessels and nerves are brought into view. These structures run diagonally through the operative field and are retracted.
8. The side of the body of the lumbar vertebra is now exposed. Deep angular retractors are employed for a good view of the field.

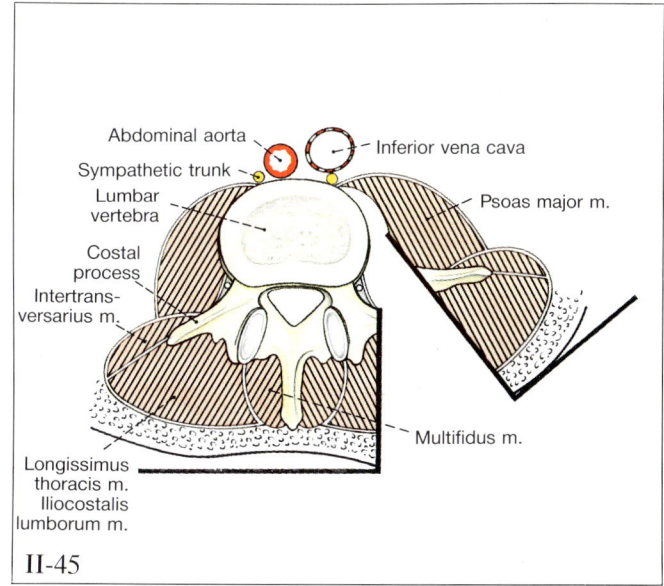

II-45

Notes

1. This line of incision has an advantage over the posteromedial approach in that the vertebra can be reached without opening the vertebral canal. However, it does cut across the long extensor muscles.
2. The view of the vertebral body is somewhat limited. There is also the danger of injury to the abdominal aorta and the inferior vena cava. The posterior branches of the vena cava are particularly troublesome.
3. The paraspinal approach may be used for a posterolateral fusion. Bilateral parallel incisions are then required.
4. The ipsilateral zygapophyseal joint can also be reached with an identical incision. Even the intervertebral foramen and the exit of the spinal nerve can be exposed.

Lumbosacral Junction

Anterior Exposure

Transperitoneal Exposure

Indications

1. Inflammatory processes and tumors of L4-S1
2. Reduction of spondylolisthesis at L5-S1
3. Lumbosacral instability
4. Fusion of L5-S1

Operative Steps

1. Make an anterior abdominal midline incision from a point about 2 cm above the umbilicus to the pubic bone (Fig. II-46, skin incision A).
2. Reflect the skin to expose the linea alba.
3. Incise the linea alba and the underlying peritoneum in the midline beginning immediately under the umbilicus.
4. Lower the head end of the table so that the small intestine can be displaced cranially with moist compresses.
5. The promontory is now brought into view (Fig. II-47).
6. The bifurcation of the aorta and the left common iliac vein must be protected.
7. Incise the peritoneum over the lumbosacral joint. Avoid injury to the somewhat laterally situated nerves, vessels, and sympathetic trunk.
8. Retract the peritoneum and the presacral nerve to expose the lumbosacral union. Ligate the median sacral artery and vein to prevent unnecessary bleeding.
9. A Steinmann pin is driven into the body of the vertebra to keep the ilecal vessels out of the way.

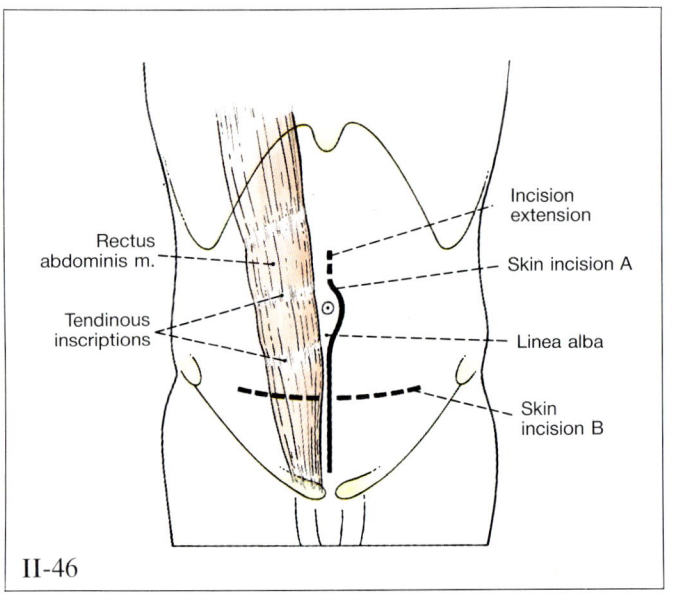

II-46

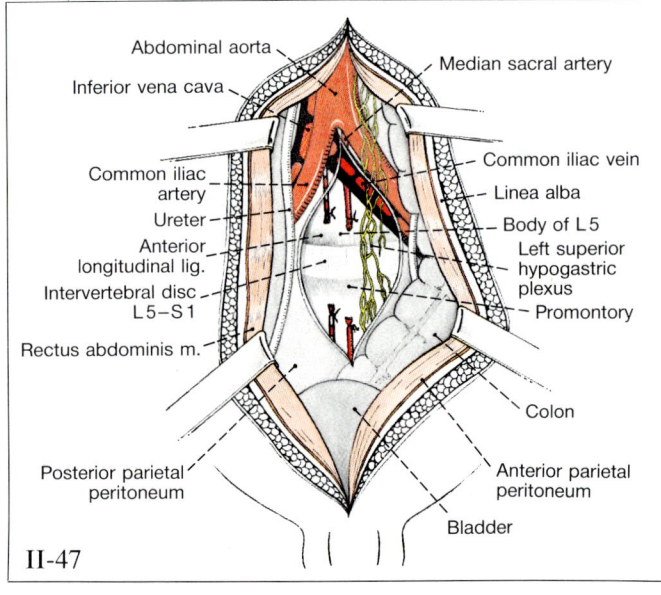

II-47

Alternative Transverse Incision

1. Make the transverse incision at the level of a line connecting the anterior superior iliac spines (Fig. II-46, skin incision B). This line of incision may also be placed lower, i.e., corresponding to Pfannenstiel's incision.
2. Retract the rectus abdominis muscle on both sides.
3. The transverse incision affords a wider exposure and is cosmetically more desirable than the longitudinal incision.

Notes

1. With the anterior approach it is easy to injure the superior hypogastric plexus (presacral nerve), particularly in front of the 5th lumbar vertebra and the presacral intervertebral disc. The plexus is connected with the lumbar sympathetics through a network of fibers.
2. To prevent lesions of the plexus, do not use cautery in the prevertebral and presacral regions. Retroperitoneal hemorrhage can be controlled by compression or, in some cases, by ligatures.
3. Lesions of the prevertebral plexus and ganglia lead to disturbances in sexual function and retrograde ejaculation.
4. The parietal peritoneum, which lies in intimate contact with the posterior lamina of the thin rectus sheath, should be guarded.
5. After carefully incising the peritoneum over the bifurcation of the aorta, identify the left common iliac vein. It frequently passes obliquely across the L5-S1 disc as an inconspicuous band.
6. Dissection of the vessels can be facilitated by prevertebral injection of physiological saline.
7. The left lateral approach to the body of L4 necessitates ligation of the segmental lumbar vein.
8. The bifurcation of the aorta and the pattern of branching of the inferior vena cava are quite variable with respect to level and morphology. From the common iliac vein there is frequently a segmental branch that runs dorsally and can be torn when the common iliac is retracted.

Sacroiliac Joint

Posterolateral Exposure

Indications

1. Inflammatory processes
2. Tumors
3. Irreducible fractures

Operative Steps

1. Make a curved skin incision along the outer lip of the posterior third of the iliac crest to the posterior superior iliac spine. Continue it caudally and laterally along the fiber direction of the gluteus maximus muscle (Fig. II-48).
2. Detach the thoracolumbar fascia from the iliac crest.
3. Release the sacrospinalis muscle and its aponeurosis subperiosteally and reflect them medially.
4. The posterior margin of the sacroiliac joint is now exposed.
5. Mobilize the gluteus maximus muscle as a hinged flap. Place the upper segment of the incision between the edges of the gluteus maximus and medius muscles and conduct it in the fiber direction of the gluteus maximus (Fig. II-49).
6. Reflect the gluteus maximus muscle laterally and downward. Now the posterior portion of the iliac bone can be seen.
7. Locate the lower limit of the sacroiliac joint by palpating the boundaries of the greater sciatic foramen.
8. In this region the piriformis muscle can be identified, with the superior gluteal artery above it and the sciatic nerve below it (Fig. II-50).
9. To open the sacroiliac joint, remove a 1 × 2-cm segment of the iliac bone. This window can be enlarged if necessary.

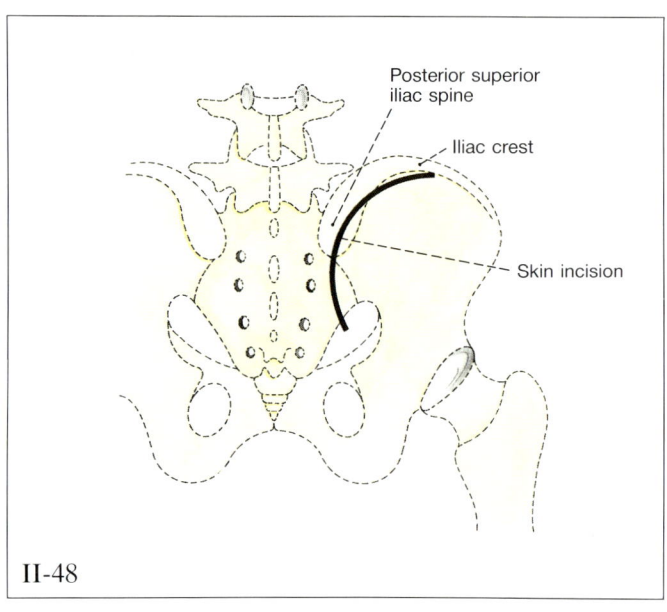

II-48

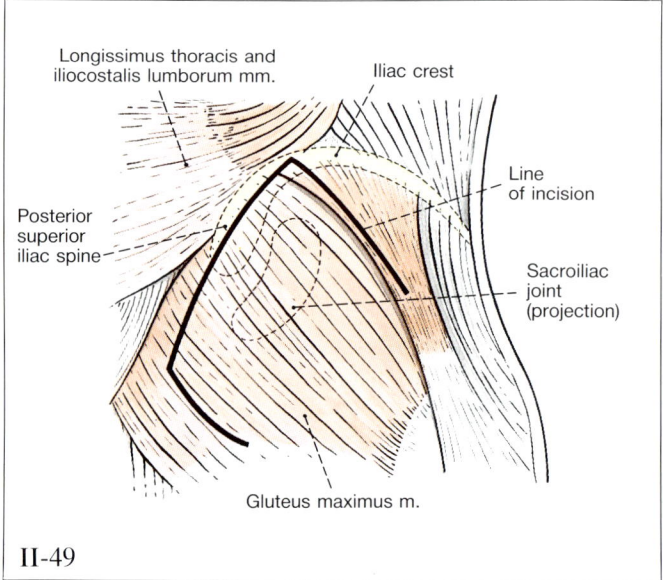

II-49

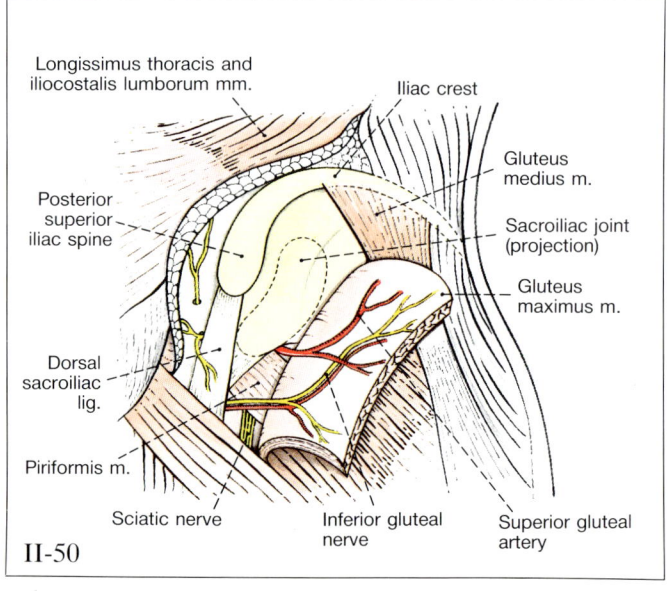

II-50

Zygapophyseal Joint/Sacroiliac Joint — Posterior Exposure

Lumbosacral Zygapophyseal Joint and Ipsilateral Sacroiliac Joint

Posterior Exposure

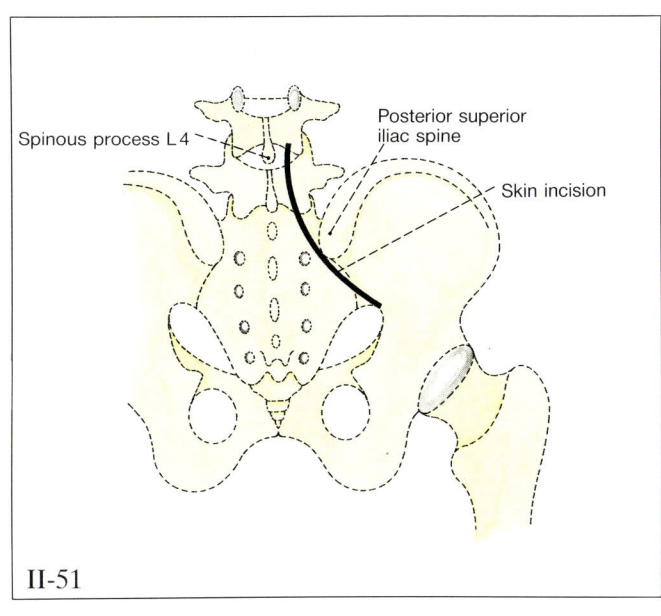

II-51

Indications

1. Instability of the zygapophyseal and sacroiliac joints
2. Inflammatory processes of the lumbosacral zygapophyseal and sacroiliac joints
3. Irreducible fractures of the lumbosacral zygapophyseal and sacroiliac joints

Operative Steps

1. Make a curved, approximately 12-cm skin incision beginning at the lateral side of the spinous process of L4 and continue it caudally and laterally under the posterior superior iliac spine (Fig. II-51).
2. Reflect the skin laterally and make two muscle incisions (Fig. II-52).
3. Place the first incision in the midline from the spinous process of L4 to the median sacral crest opposite S2 (Fig. II-52).
4. With a chisel or a wide rasp, detach the musculature from the side of the spinous processes and the vertebral arches.
5. Place the second incision along the line of origin of the gluteus maximus muscle, beginning at the level of S3 and continuing cranially and laterally along the dorsal margin of the iliac crest to the gluteus medius muscle. From this point the incision is angled caudally and laterally between the gluteus maximus and medius muscles (Fig. II-52).
6. The vertebral arch and the area of the iliac bone overlying the sacroiliac joint are now exposed (Fig. II-53).

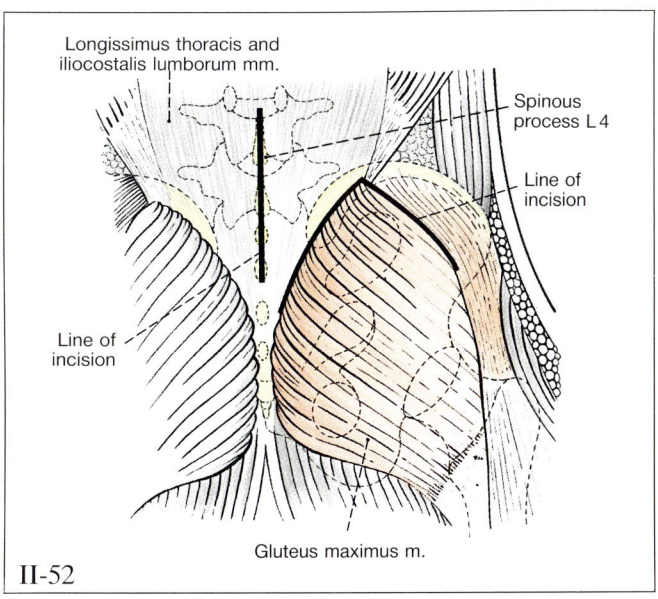

II-52

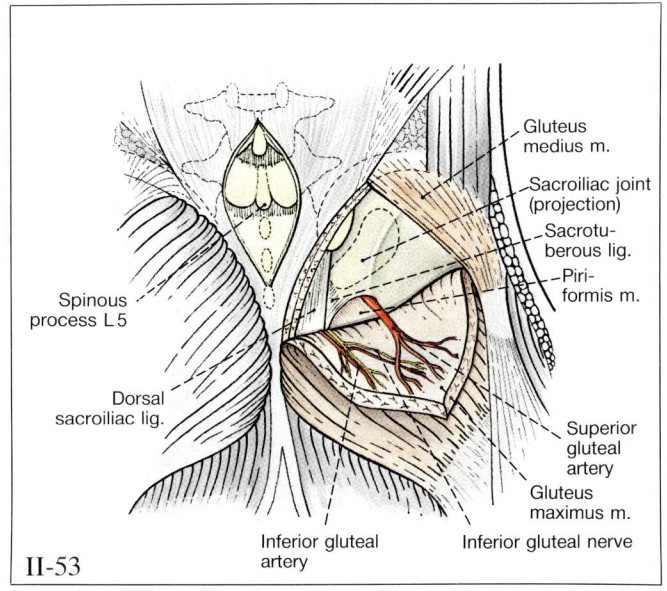

II-53

Bilateral Lumbosacral Zygopophyseal Joints and Both Sacroiliac Joints

Indications

1. Instability of the lumbosacral zygapophyseal and sacroiliac joints
2. Inflammatory processes in the region of the lumbosacral zygapophyseal and sacroiliac joints
3. Irreducible fractures of the lumbosacral zygapophyseal and sacroiliac joints

Operative Steps

1. Make an approximately 15-cm-long curved skin incision with the convexity facing caudally. Begin on the posterior surface of the iliac bone, cross the midline at the level of the posterior superior iliac spine, and end on the opposite iliac bone (Fig. II-54, skin incision A).
2. After reflecting the skin, make three incisions, as indicated in Fig. II-55:
   a) A longitudinal incision from the spinous process of L4 to the median sacral crest opposite S2 (Fig. II-55).
   b) An incision on the right side along the origin of the gluteus maximus muscle, beginning at the level of S3 and continuing along the posterior aspect of the iliac crest to the gluteus medius muscle. The line of the incision is then angled caudally and laterally between the gluteus maximus and medius (Fig. II-55).
   c) Repeat procedure b on the left side.
3. Reflect the muscles to expose the zygapophyseal joints and the areas over both sacroiliac joints (Fig. II-56).

Alternative

1. The skin incision can also be made longitudinally in the midline from L4 to S2 (Fig. II-54, skin incision B).
2. The dissection is then continued laterally in the subcutaneous plane.

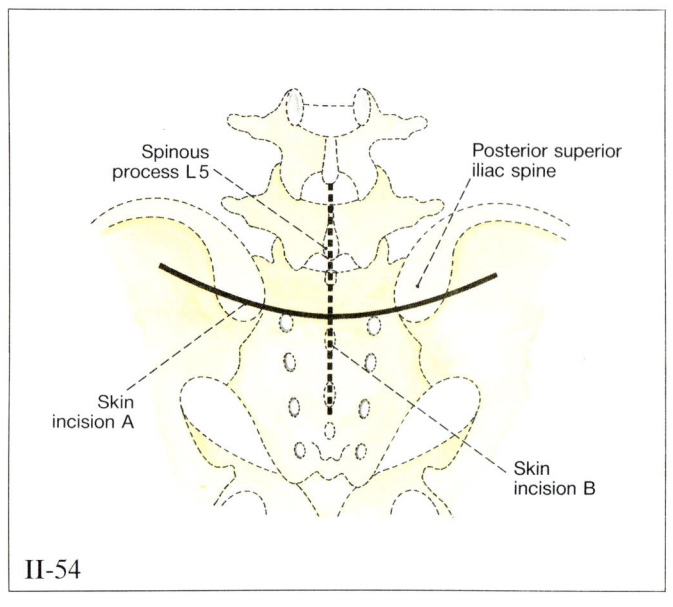

II-54

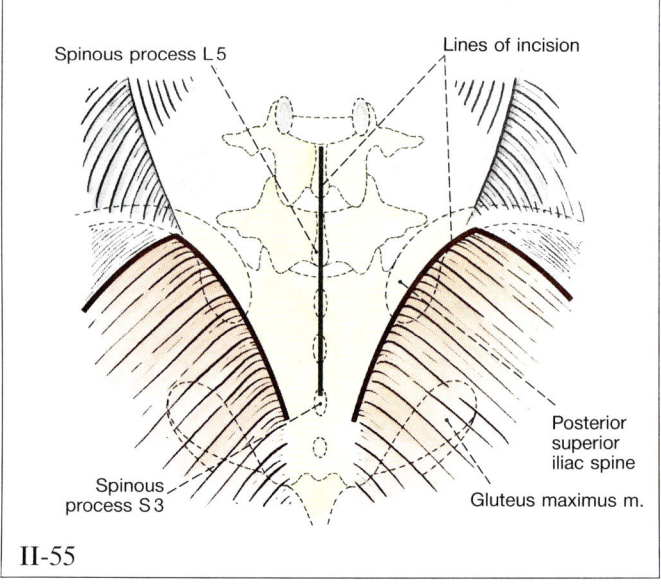

II-55

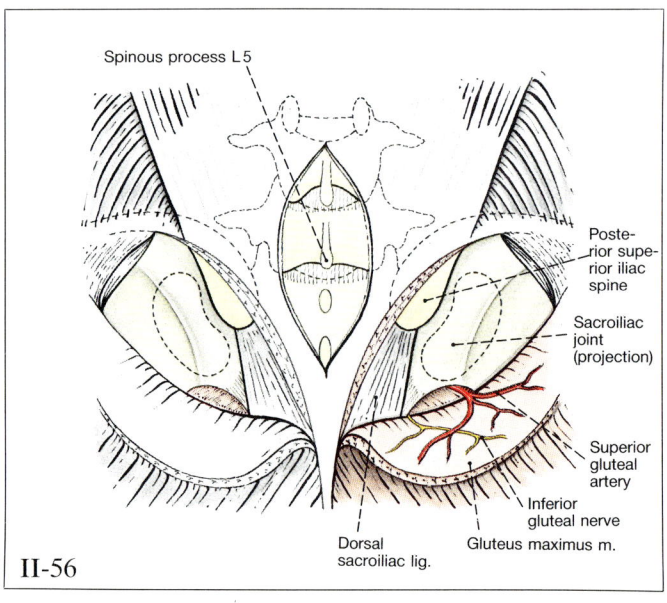

II-56

E. Pelvis

Ilium – External Surface

Lateral Exposure

Indications

1. Irreducible fractures
2. Tumors
3. Inflammatory processes

Operative Steps

1. Make a skin incision along the iliac crest from the posterior superior iliac spine to the anterior superior iliac spine (Fig. II-57).
2. Incise the superficial and deep fasciae and detach the muscles from the iliac crest close to the bone.
3. Reflect all musculature subperiosteally from the outside of the iliac bone.
4. Pack the intervening space between the muscles and the ilium to control bleeding from the nutrient vessels.
5. The outer surface of the ilium is now completely exposed (fig. II-58).

Notes

1. A narrow bony rim can be obtained with a chisel and included with the muscle origins to facilitate reattachment later.
2. In children the muscles are preferably detached with a narrow cartilaginous rim.

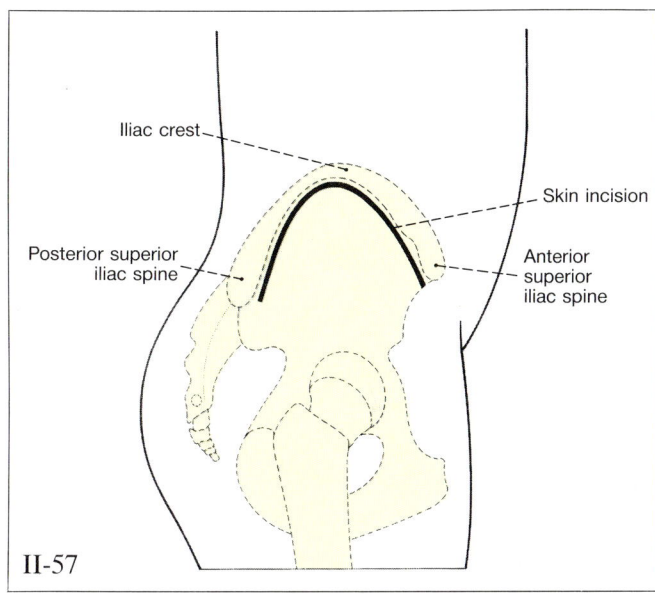

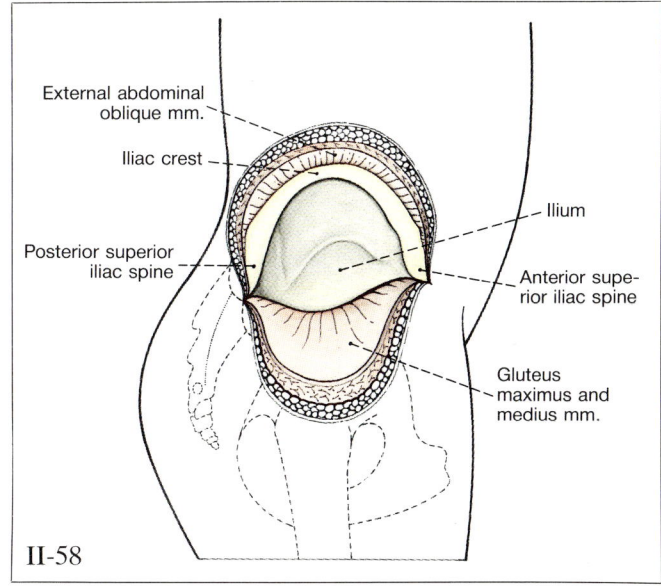

Iliac Fossa

Indications

1. Irreducible fractures of the ilium
2. Irreducible fractures of the superior part of the acetabulum
3. Tumors
4. Inflammatory processes

Operative Steps

1. Begin the skin incision approximately over the middle of the iliac crest, continuing over the anterior superior iliac spine and following the sartorius muscle distally and medially for about 3–5 cm (Fig. II-59).
2. Incise the abdominal wall musculature 1–2 cm from the origin on the crest (Fig. II-60). This facilitates reattachment.

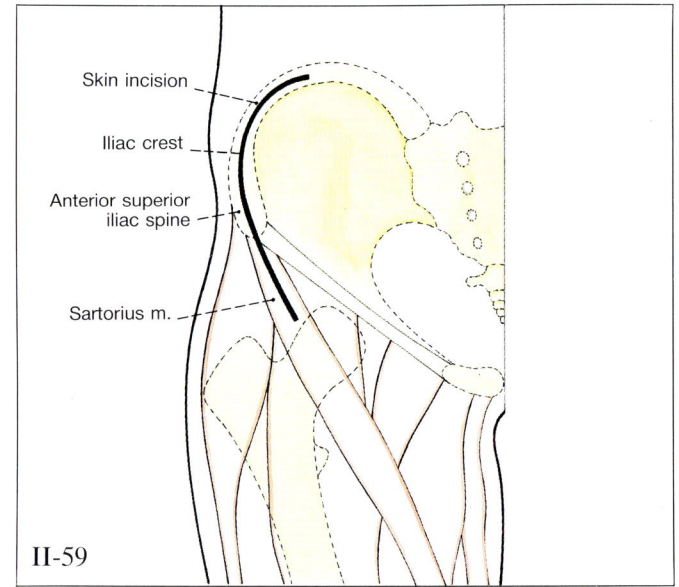

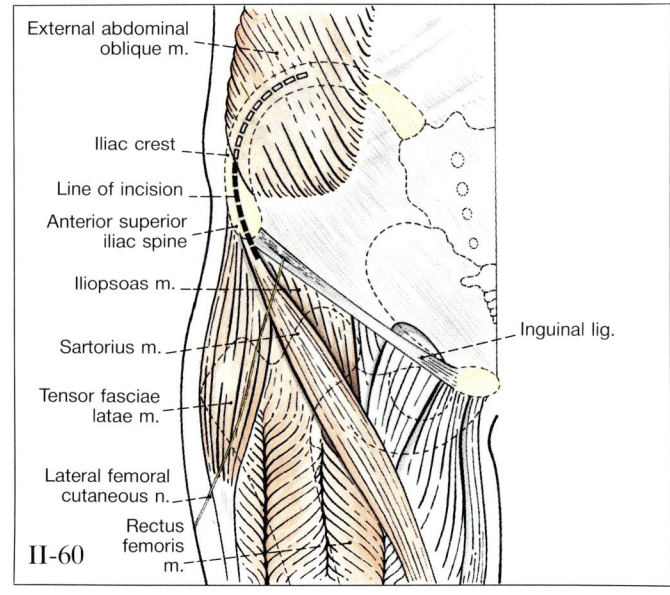

Iliac Fossa — Exposure

3. Reflect the abdominal musculature medially to expose the iliacus muscle (Fig. II-61).
4. Incise the iliacus muscle close to the iliac crest and reflect it from the ilium subperiosteally. The iliac fossa is now exposed (Fig. II-62).
5. Release the inguinal ligament from the anterior superior iliac spine and reflect it with the abdominal musculature (Fig. II-62).
6. Firm medial retraction of the psoas muscle gives a better overview of the upper part of the acetabulum and the capsule of the hip joint.

Notes

1. If a less extensive exposure is adequate, the abdominal muscles and the iliacus muscle can be detached as one unit.
2. When making the incision over the sartorius muscle, avoid injuring the lateral femoral cutaneous nerve.

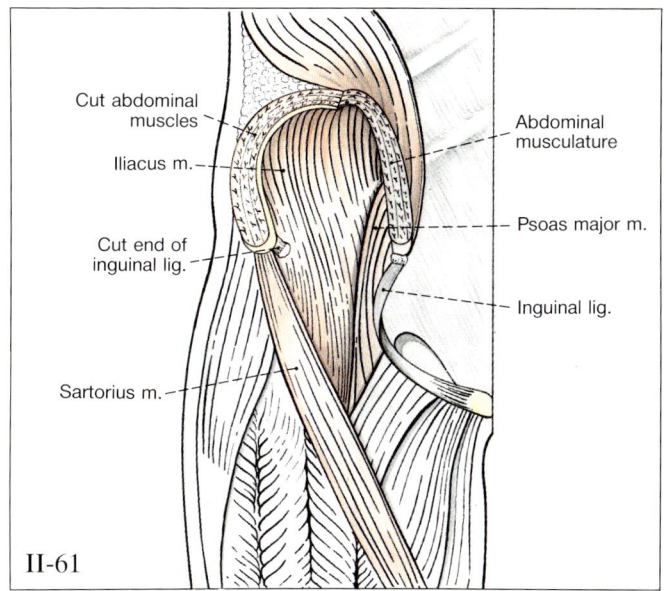

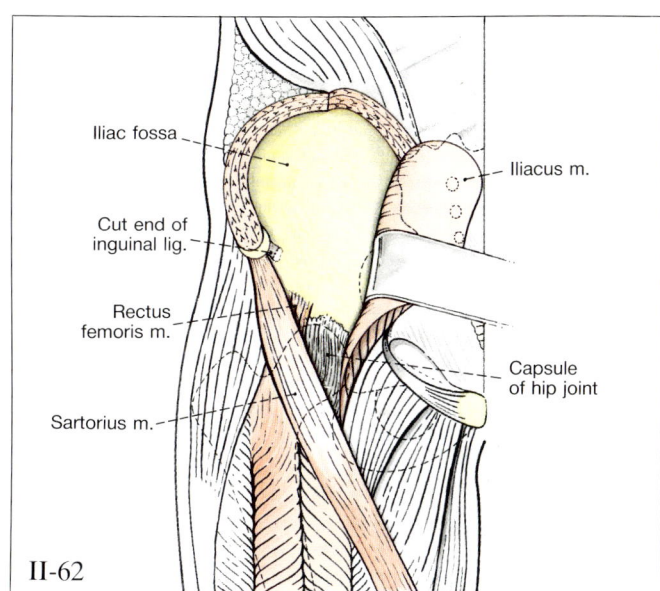

Iliac Crest

Anterolateral Exposure

Indication

Removal of chips from the iliac crest

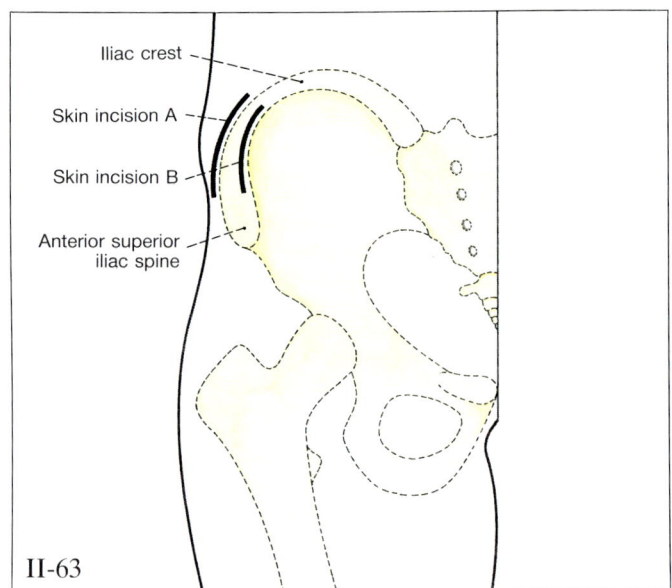

II-63

Operative Steps

1. Make a medial skin incision over the internal lip of the iliac crest or 2 cm lateral (along the outer lip) (Fig. II-63). The length of the incision (5–10 cm) depends on the desired exposure.
2. The line of incision along the iliac crest should pass through the tendinous origin of the muscles and include the periosteum on the medial or lateral sides.
3. Detach the muscles and drive a pointed Hohmann retractor into the depth (inside) of the pelvic wall to keep the musculature out of the way.

Notes

1. The line of incision is anterolateral along the iliac crest and should terminate at a safe distance from the anterior superior iliac spine. If there is extensive removal of chips, the spine may break off. Furthermore, the lateral femoral nerve can be injured.
2. It is usually preferable to remove the chips from the inside of the ilium (iliac fossa). Cosmetically undesirable depressions may ensue after removal from the outside.

Posterior Exposure

Indication

Removal of bone chips and spongiosa with the patient in the prone position

Operative Steps

1. Make a slightly curved skin incision along the iliac crest, beginning at the posterior superior iliac spine (Fig. II-64, skin incision A).
2. Detach the gluteal musculature from the outer lip of the iliac crest. With a wide rasp reflect the muscle mass from the outside of the ala, downward and laterally.
3. Reattachment of the musculature later is facilitated if a narrow rim of bone is removed with the gluteal muscles.
4. After driving two pointed Hohmann retractors deep into the ala, expose the site for obtaining chips.
5. From a cosmetic standpoint, better results are obtained with a transverse incision (of Louis) beginning at the posterior superior iliac spine (Fig. II-64, skin incision B).

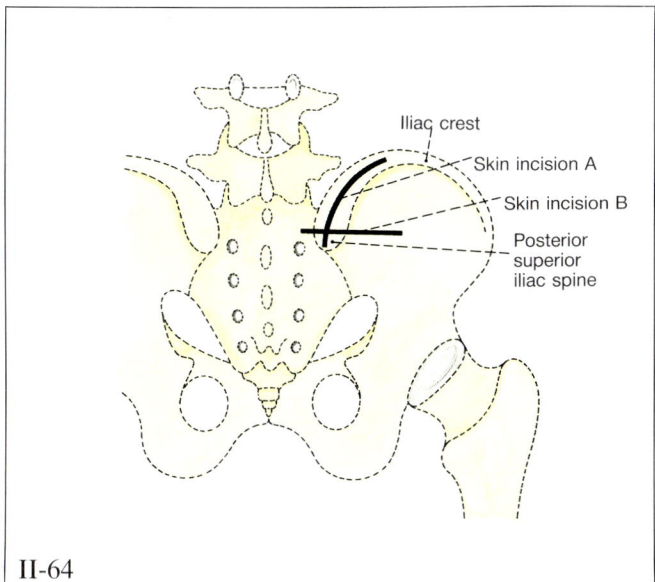

II-64

Alternative Exposure of Louis

1. Make an approximately 8-cm-long oblique incision from medial to lateral, crossing the iliac crest 2–3 cm above the posterior superior iliac spine and terminating about 5 cm to the side of the latter (Fig. II-65).
2. Reflect the soft tissues medially and laterally (or forward and backward).

Notes

1. From experience it seems that the conventional line of incision along the iliac crest causes considerable and prolonged postoperative pain. Occasionally there is also a deepening of the scar because of detached muscle insertions.
2. The oblique line of incision avoids severing the cutaneous nerves (superior clunial nerves). By this approach the gluteal musculature is not divided transversely through its bony attachment so that the continuity with the lumbodorsal fascia is retained.
3. Use Gelfoam and bone wax to maintain meticulous hemostasis of the area from which bone is removed. This is mandatory because hematomas are readily induced and the danger of secondary infections is increased.
4. A drain should not be placed in immediate contact with the bleeding surface because the negative pressure will interfere with hemostasis. Frequent changes of the drain bottle may even cause severe hemorrhages. In some cases the drain is kept open for only short periods of time (measured in minutes).

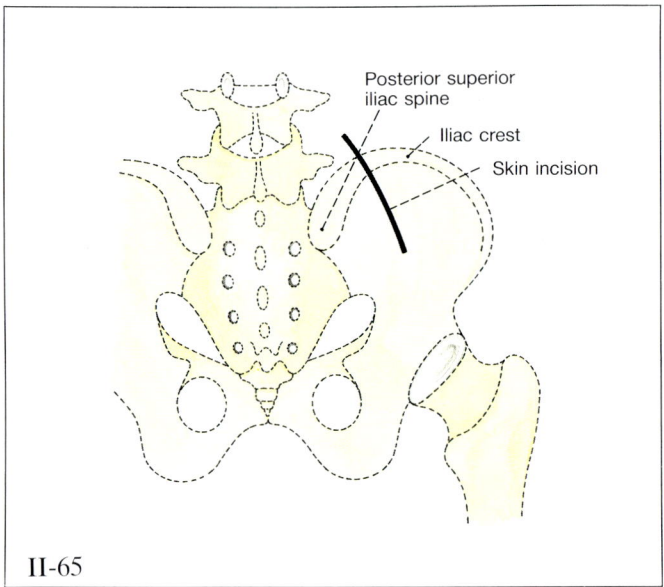

II-65

Ischium

Indications

1. Inflammatory processes
2. Tumors
3. Irreducible fractures

Operative Steps

1. With the patient in the lithotomy position, elevate the pelvis with pillows or towels.
2. Palpate the ischial tuberosity and the inferior ramus of the pubis.
3. Place the incision along the ramus of the ischium. Continue it posteriorly for 8–10 cm over the gluteus maximus muscle (Fig. II-66).
4. Identify the lower margin of the gluteus maximus muscle and elevate it with a finger so that the fibers that pass over the ischial tuberosity can be cut. This will expose the ischial tuberosity with the attached musculature and the sacrotuberous ligament on its medial margin (Fig. II-67).

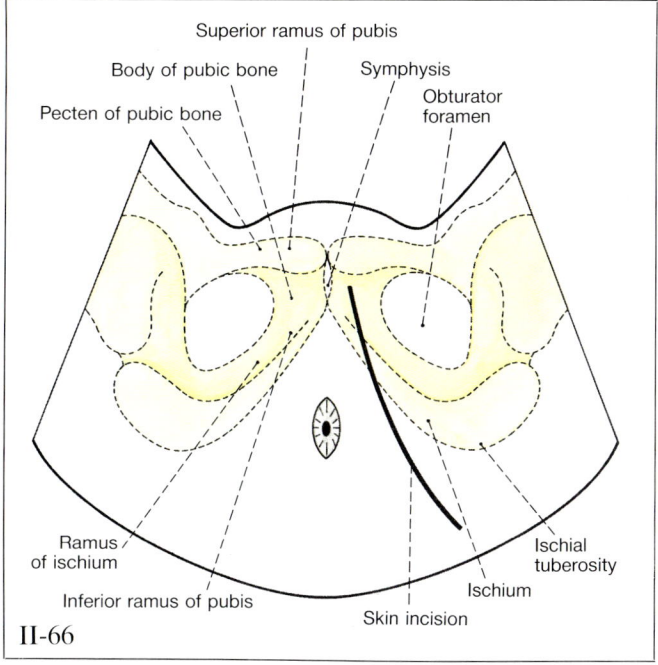

II-66

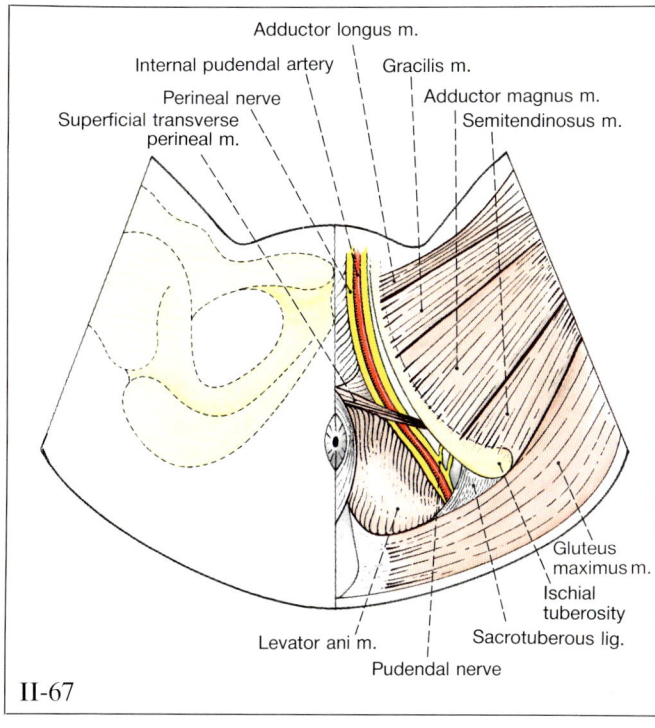

II-67

5. Incise the periosteum over the free bony edge of the tuberosity. Detach the muscle origins subperiosteally and reflect them laterally (Fig. II-68).
6. The periosteal incision is continued anteriorly along the ramus of the ischium and the inferior ramus of the pubic bone between the adductor muscles laterally and the perineal musculature medially.
7. Detach the adductor magnus muscle and reflect it laterally to get a better view of the lateral border of the bone.
8. Detach the adductor brevis, adductor longus, quadriceps femoris, and, finally, the external obturator muscle and reflect them laterally with the sciatic nerve. The lower border of the obturator foramen is now brought into view. Structures of importance are not encountered during this dissection, and there is no danger of serious hemorrhage.
9. Exposure of the medial border of the ischial ramus and the tuberosity is somewhat more perilous because of the course of the internal pudendal artery and vein. If the detachment of the ischiocavernosus and the transverse perineal muscles is done strictly subperiosteally, it is possible, deep in the operative field, to displace the pudendal nerve with the vessels and the obturator internus muscle. In the posterior portion of the field, the sacrotuberous ligament is released from the ischial tuberosity, bringing into view the lesser sciatic foramen (Fig. II-68).
10. There is now a good overview of the ischium.
11. The surgeon is again reminded to stay very close to the bone.

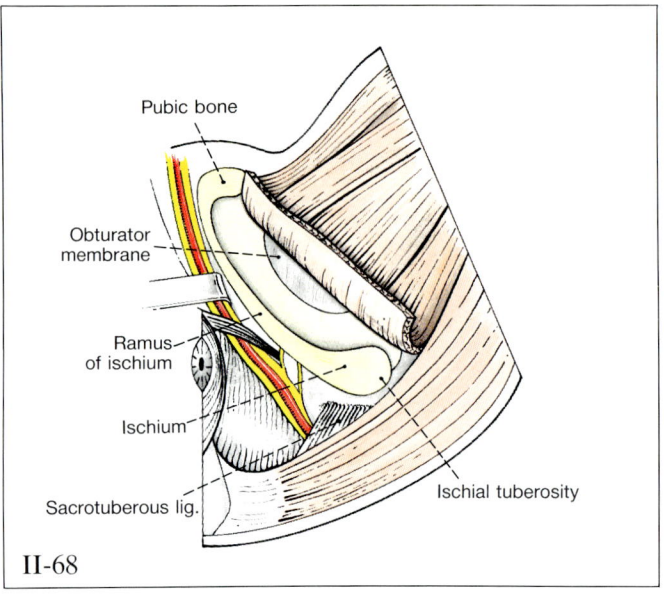

II-68

Note

The ischial tuberosity can also be reached with the patient in the prone position. This requires right-angle flexion at the hip joint and almost 90 degrees flexion of the knee joints.

Part III
Lower Limb

Contents Part III

Lower Limb

A. Hip Region 152
    Hip Joint 152
        Anterior Exposure 152
        Iliofemoral Exposure
        of *Smith-Petersen* 154
        Lateral Exposure
        of *Watson-Jones* 156
        Lateral Cup Incision
        of *Lexer-Murphy* 159
        Anterolateral Exposure 160
        Posterior Exposure 162
        Posterolateral Exposure
        of *Marcy* and *Fletcher* 164
    Intertrochanteric Neck of Femur 167
        Lateral Exposure 167
    Lesser Trochanter 169
        Exposure of *Nicola* 169

B. Thigh 170
    Shaft of the Femur 170
        Anterior Exposure 170
        Lateral Exposure 173
        Medial Exposure 175
        Posterior Exposure 176
    Distal Shaft of the Femur 178
        Posterior Exposure 178

C. Knee Region 179
    Knee Joint 179
        Applied Anatomy 179
        Arteries of the Knee Joint 180
        Anteromedial Exposure 181
        Medial Curved Incision 183
        Medial S-Incision 184
        Posteromedial Exposure (1) 185

        Anteromedial Exposure
        (Short or Long Medial *Payr* Incision) . . . 186
        Medial and Lateral
        Parapatellar Exposure 187
        Anteromedial Exposure
        of *Coonse-Adams* 188
        Anterior Curved *(Textor)* Incision 189
        Anterolateral Exposure 190
        Lateral Exposure 192
        Posterolateral Exposure 193
        Anteroposterior Exposure
        from Lateral Side 194
        Posteromedial Exposure (2) 194
        Posterocentral Exposure 196
        Safe Zone of the Distal Femur 196
    Head of Tibia with Knee Joint 197
        Anterior Exposure 197
    Head of Tibia 198
        Anterior Exposure 198

D. Leg 199
    Tibia 199
        Anterolateral Exposure 199
        Medial Exposure 201
        Posteromedial Exposure 203
    Fibula 204
        Lateral Exposure 204
        Alternative Exposures 205
    Fibula and Tibia 206
        Lateral Exposure 206
    Leg Compartments 207
        Anterolateral and
        Posteromedial Exposure 207
    Plantaris Tendon 208
        Posteromedial Exposure 208

Lower Limb — Contents Part III

- Sural Nerve ... 209
  - Posterolateral Exposure ... 209
- Achilles Tendon ... 209
  - Posteromedial or Posterior Exposure ... 209

E. Malleolar Region ... 210

- Talocrural Joint (1) ... 210
  - Anterior Exposure ... 210
  - Anterolateral Exposure ... 212
- Talocrural and Subtalar Joint (1) ... 213
  - Para-achillar Exposures ... 213
  - Posterolateral Exposure ... 214
  - Applied Anatomy ... 215
- Ankle Joints – Lateral Malleolus ... 216
  - Lateral Exposure (*Kocher* Incision) ... 216
  - Alternative Lateral Exposures ... 217
- Talocrural Joint (2) ... 218
  - Posterolateral Exposure of *Patrick* ... 218
- Subtalar Joint ... 219
  - Lateral Exposure ... 219
- Talocrural and Subtalar Joint (2) ... 220
  - Applied Anatomy ... 220
- Subtalar Joint ... 220
  - Medial Exposure ... 220
- Talocrural Joint – Medial Malleolus ... 222
  - Medial Exposures ... 222
- Tarsal Tunnel ... 223
  - Exposure ... 223

F. Foot ... 224

- Calcaneus ... 224
  - Lateral Exposures ... 224
  - Lateral Plantar Exposure ... 225
  - Medial Plantar Exposure ... 225
  - Mediolateral Exposure ... 226
  - Plantar Exposure ... 227
- Tarsus ... 229
  - Medial Exposure ... 229
  - Anterior Exposure ... 229
- Tarsus – Metatarsal Bone V ... 230
  - Lateral Exposure ... 230
- Metatarsal Bones ... 230
  - Anterior Exposures ... 230
- Sole of the Foot ... 231
  - Median Longitudinal Incision ... 231
  - Applied Anatomy ... 231
- Plantar Aspect of Forefoot ... 232
  - Plantar Exposure ... 232

G. Toes ... 233

- Metatarsophalangeal Joint of the Big Toe ... 233
  - Medial Exposure ... 233
  - Anteromedial Exposure ... 234
- Toes ... 235
  - Applied Anatomy ... 235
- Metatarsophalangeal Joints ... 236
  - Anterior Exposure ... 236
- Metatarsophalangeal Joints II–V ... 237
  - Plantar Exposure of *Gocht* ... 237
- Proximal Interphalangeal Joint ... 239
  - Anterior Exposure ... 239

A. Hip Region

Hip Joint

Anterior Exposure

Indications

1. Biopsy, Arthrotomy
2. Bone tumors
3. Removal of loose joint bodies
4. Open reduction of congenital hip dislocation
5. Open reduction of traumatic anterior dislocation
6. Resection of head and neck of femur
7. Synovectomy

Operative Steps

1. Make an approximately 12-cm-long skin incision from the anterior superior iliac spine distally and medially along the fiber direction of the sartorius muscle (Fig. III-1).
2. Split the superficial and deep fasciae to expose the proximal fourth of the sartorius and rectus femoris muscles. The lateral femoral cutaneous nerve, which runs about 2.5 cm distal to the anterior superior iliac spine, should be avoided during this step (Fig. III-2). The superficial circumflex iliac artery, which is also in this area, can be clamped, ligated, and cut.

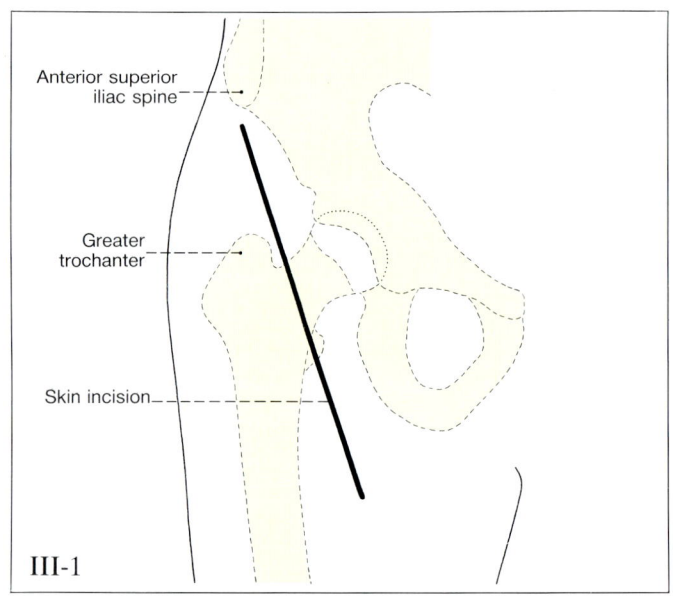

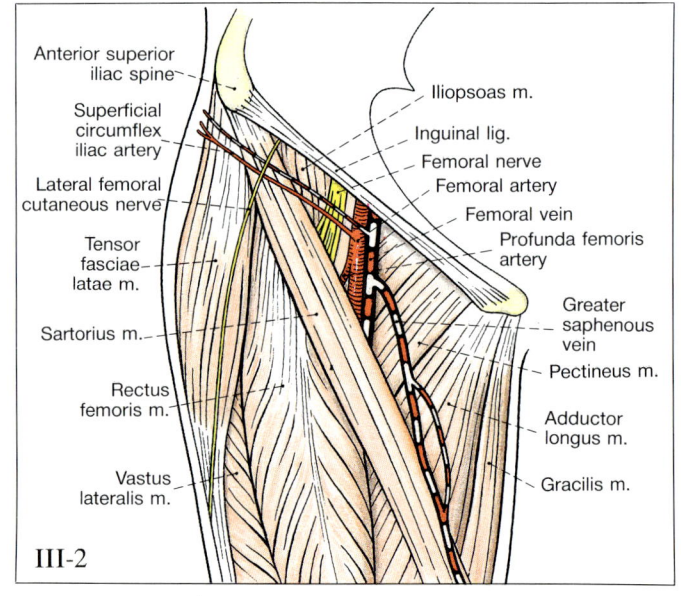

Hip Joint — Anterior Exposure

3. Retract the sartorius and iliopsoas muscles medially and displace the rectus femoris muscle laterally. The anterior portion of the joint capsule is now seen (Fig. III-3). The field can be augmented by dividing the rectus tendon 1.5 cm from its origin. The remaining tendinous stump facilitates reattachment later.
4. Retract the femoral nerve medially with great care.
5. Open the joint capsule with an inverted U-incision (Fig. III-4).

Notes

1. The rectus femoris muscle retracts rapidly after its division. To facilitate retrieval of the ends later, it is recommended that sutures be attached to both ends of the rectus tendon.
2. For a wider view of the hip joint, a Hohmann retractor can be tunneled forward between the iliopsoas muscle and the bone and hooked to the superior ramus of the pubis. The iliopsoas muscle and the vessels and nerves are thus displaced medially.
3. If necessary, the sartorius muscle can also be retracted laterally. This gives excellent exposure of the femoral nerve with its branches as well as the femoral artery and vein (but also makes these structures more vulnerable to injury).
4. In muscular individuals this exposure will not always permit luxation of the femoral head. In that case the line of incision can be directed cranially and continued over the iliac crest for the purpose of detaching the tensor fasciae latae muscle and the anterior portion of the gluteus medius muscle (see "Iliofemoral Exposure of *Smith-Petersen*").
5. In special cases it may be necessary to cut the iliopsoas muscle above the lesser trochanter. This should be done with a Z-shaped cut to facilitate reapproximation later. It is recommended that the ends of the tendon be tagged prior to cutting it.

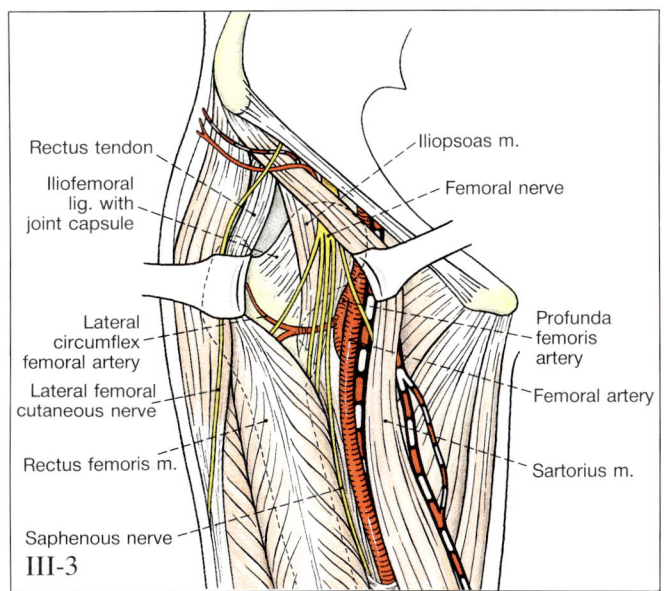

III-3

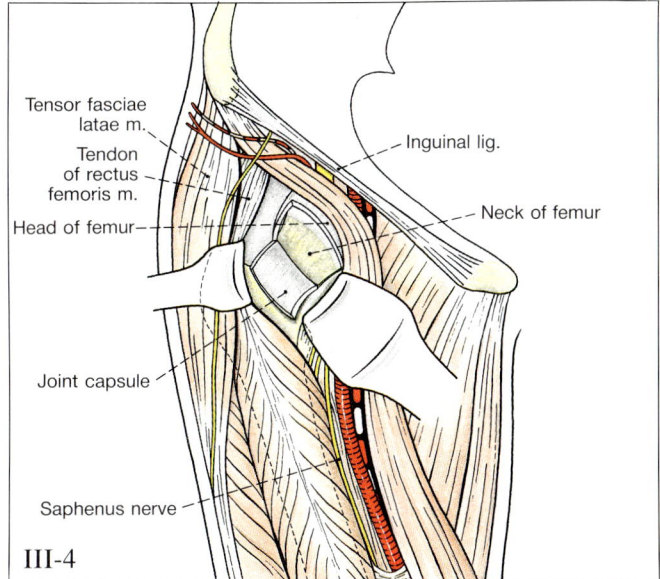

III-4

Iliofemoral Exposure of *Smith-Petersen*

Indications

1. Arthroplasty of hip joint, total replacement, partial replacement
2. Arthrodesis of hip joint
3. Acetabular osteoplasty
4. Certain cases of traumatic hip dislocation
5. Certain acetabular fractures
6. Certain fractures of the ilium
7. Tumors of the anterior aspects of the alae
8. Synovectomy

Operative Steps

Before making the incision, mark the skin at the level of the anterior superior iliac spine in two or three places at right angles to the line of incision. This provides for good registration of the skin edges during wound closure.

1. Make a skin incision from the middle of the iliac crest to the anterior superior iliac spine and extend it distally and slightly laterally for about 10–12 cm (Fig. III-5).
2. Cut through the superficial and deep faciae.
3. Detach the gluteus medius and tensor fasciae latae muscles with a chisel and include a narrow strip of bone from the iliac crest (cartilage in children) with the attached fascia (Fig. III-6). This procedure facilitates reattachment later.

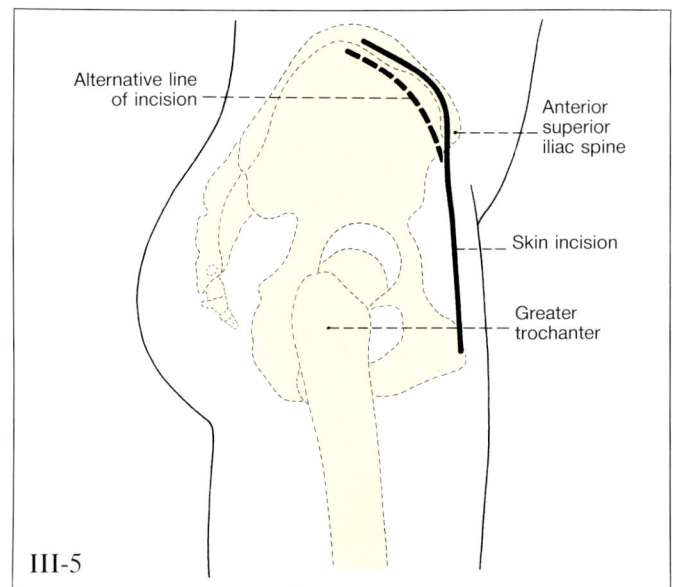

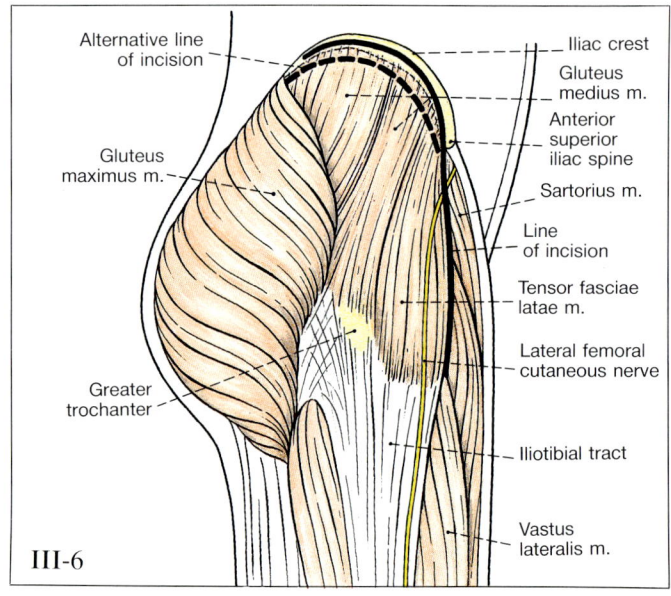

Hip Joint — Iliofemoral Exposure

4. Alternative: Cut through the gluteus medius and tensor fasciae latae muscles approximately 1½ cm below the iliac crest (Fig. III-7). This approach also makes later reattachment easier.
5. Detach the muscle mass from the external aspect of the ilium subperiosteally, and reflect it dorsally and downward (Fig. III-7). Pack the developed space to decrease hemorrhage from the nutrient arteries.
6. Displace the lateral femoral cutaneous nerve medially. It lies approximately 2.5 cm below the anterior superior iliac spine and runs over the sartorius muscle. The ascending branch of the superficial circumflex iliac artery also enters this area. If necessary, it can be clamped, ligated, and cut.
7. Continue the dissection through the deep fascia of the thigh between the tensor fasciae latae laterally and the sartorius and rectus muscles on the medial side.
8. Open the hip joint with an inverted U incision of the capsule (Fig. III-7). This brings into view the head and neck of the femur.
9. If a more complete exposure of the hip joint is required, the ligament of the femoral head must be cut with curved scissors so that the head of the femur can be dislocated by external rotation of the thigh.
10. At the time of closure, suture the capsule, reposition the periosteum with the gluteus medius muscle against the ilium, and attach the reflected musculature carefully to the iliac crest. This procedure prevents a cosmetically undesirable pitting of the cutaneous scar.
11. When suturing the skin, carefully observe the cutaneous markings that were made preoperatively at the level of the anterior superior iliac spine.

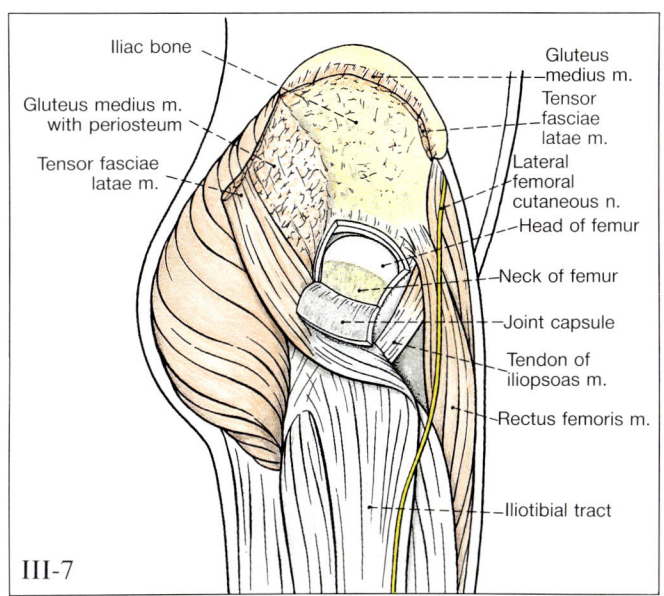

III-7

Notes

1. There is usually no danger of injury to nerves or vessels with this approach (except for a branch of the lateral femoral cutaneous nerve).
2. This exposure can be augmented by detachment of the capsular origin of the rectus femoris muscle and division of its tendon (after preparatory applications of tags).
3. A better overview is also obtained by passing a Hohmann retractor between the iliopsoas muscle and the bone and anchoring it behind the superior pubic ramus.

Lateral Exposure of *Watson-Jones*

Indications

1. Total replacement
2. Fractures
3. Dislocations
4. Inflammatory processes (synovectomy)
5. Replacement of prosthesis

Operative Steps

1. Place the patient in a supine position.
2. Make a lateral longitudinal incision beginning 2–6 cm above the tip of the trochanter and ending one hand's breadth below the greater trochanter (Fig. III-8). The incision can be extended in the direction of the anterior superior iliac spine. In this case a slightly curved line of incision is preferred, similar to that in the anterolateral approach.
3. Alternative lines of incision are directed posteriorly, i.e., dorsally (Fig. III-9). Skin incision A (Fig. III-9) corresponds to the Charnley modification. Skin incision B ends just short of the posterior superior iliac spine. In these approaches, a corresponding incision is made in the gluteus maximus muscle along its fiber direction. Further development of this exposure may later involve removal of a slice of the trochanter (see step 7).

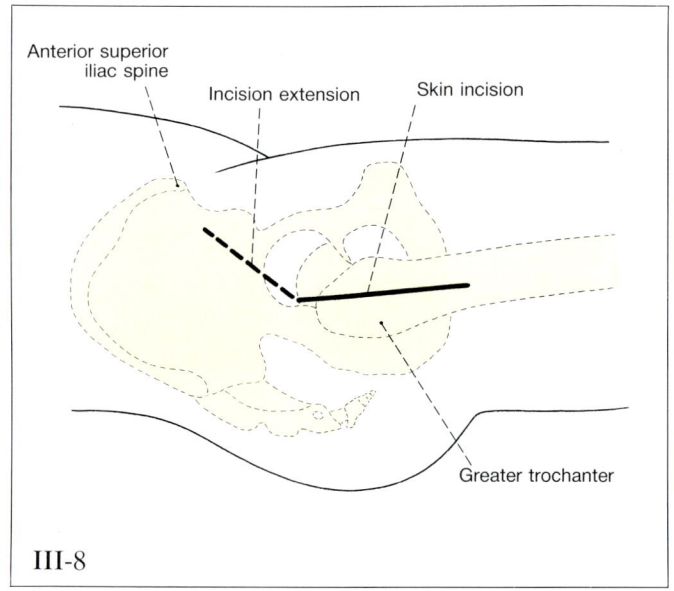

III-8

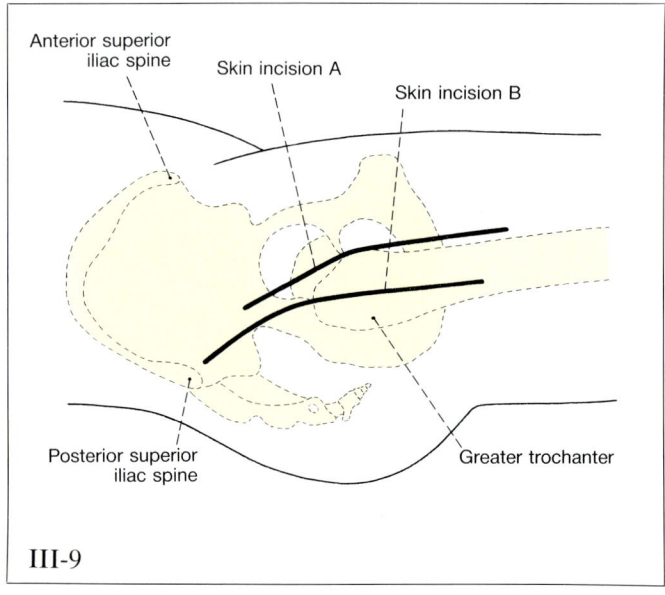

III-9

4. Locate the plane between the gluteus medius and tensor fasciae latae muscles. A Hohmann retractor behind the head of the femur will retain the soft tissues toward the medial side (Fig. III-10).
5. Detach the anterior fibers of the gluteus medius muscles from the trochanter so as to obtain a better view of the lateral and anterior aspects of the femoral head.
6. If an augmented exposure is desired (for total replacement), the greater trochanter is chipped off from the front in such a way that it can be hinged back on the posterior intact margin (Fig. III-11).
7. As an alternative, a slice of the trochanter can be obtained with a chisel applied to its distal margin. The piece of the greater trochanter with the attached muscle can then be elevated and kept out of the way with a Steinmann nail driven into the bone above the acetabulum (Fig. III-12).
8. Incise the capsule along the anterior aspect of the neck of the femur.
9. Release the capsule along the intertrochanteric line.
10. Reflect it forward and backward.
11. Retract the vastus lateralis muscle distally or split it lengthwise so that the base of the greater trochanter and the proximal part of the femoral shaft are exposed (Fig. III-11).

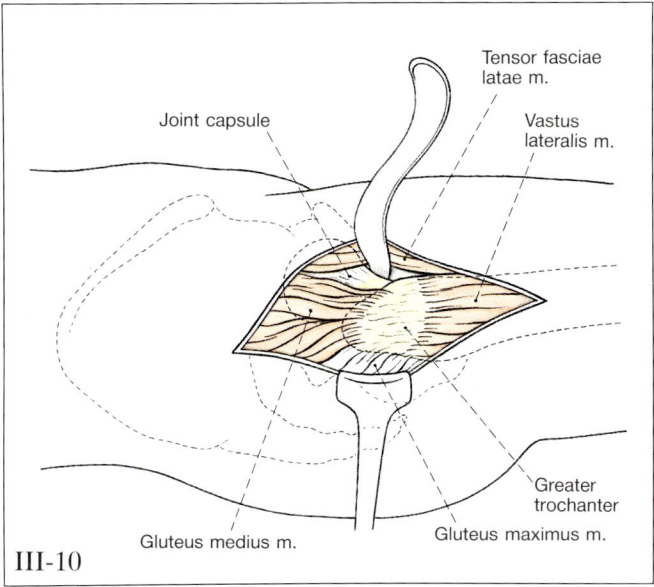

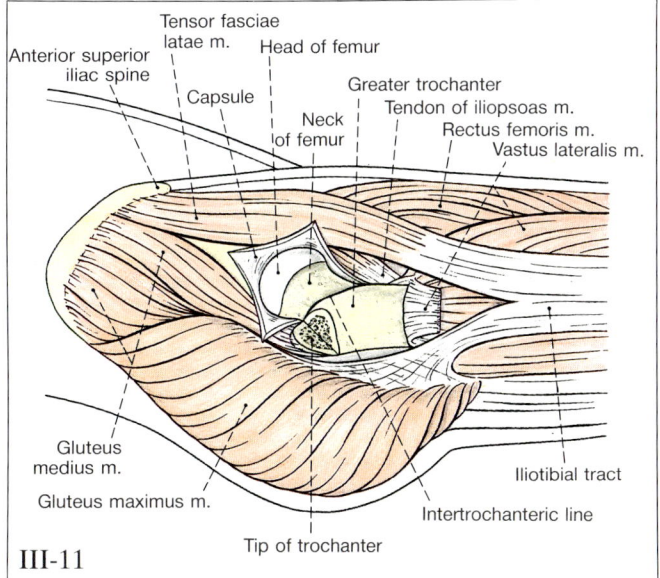

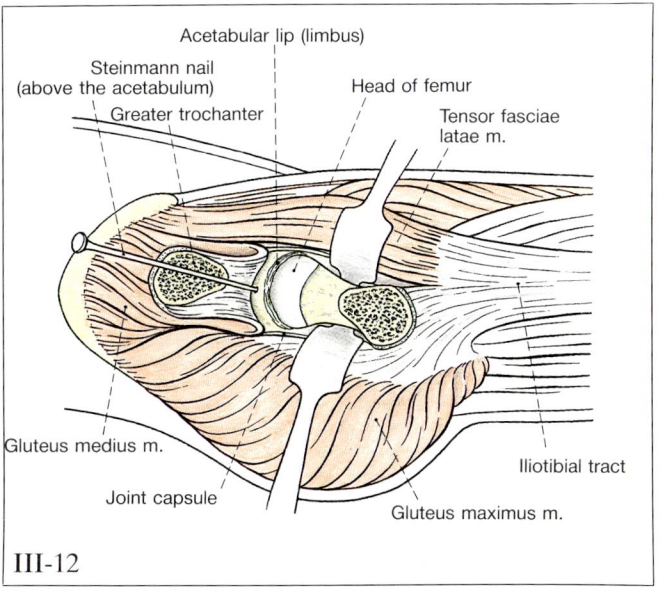

12. Disarticulate the head of the femur from the acetabular fossa by external rotation and adduction of the limb (Fig. III-13).
13. Reattach the trochanter slice by applying a figure-of-eight wire with a proximal loop behind the trochanter musculature and a distal loop through a drilled canal in the femur (Fig. III-14a).
14. An alternative method for reattachment using two wire loops is indicated in Fig. III-14b.

Notes

1. The line of incision is standard for total hip replacement or open reduction and fixation of a femoral head fracture.
2. Severe hemorrhage is rarely encountered.
3. Additional transverse relaxing incisions of the anterior and posterior edges of the fascia lata afford a better overview.
4a. Removal of the trochanter by the *R. Schneider* method is a useful variation in which a saddle-shaped osteotomy is performed (at an angle of about 135 degrees) with the oscillating saw.
4b. To reattach the trochanter, two canals are drilled in a longitudinal direction so that the wire coming from the neck of the femur can be passed over the tip of the trochanter through the attached musculature. The ends of the wires are tied at the base of the trochanter.
5. The supine patient should be positioned near the edge of the operating table. In this way the soft tissues of the buttocks project slightly beyond the table and do not interfere with the operative field.
6. The trochanter region is best exposed by flexing and adducting the limb over the opposite knee.
7. Tension on the joint capsule before it is incised is achieved by lateral rotation.

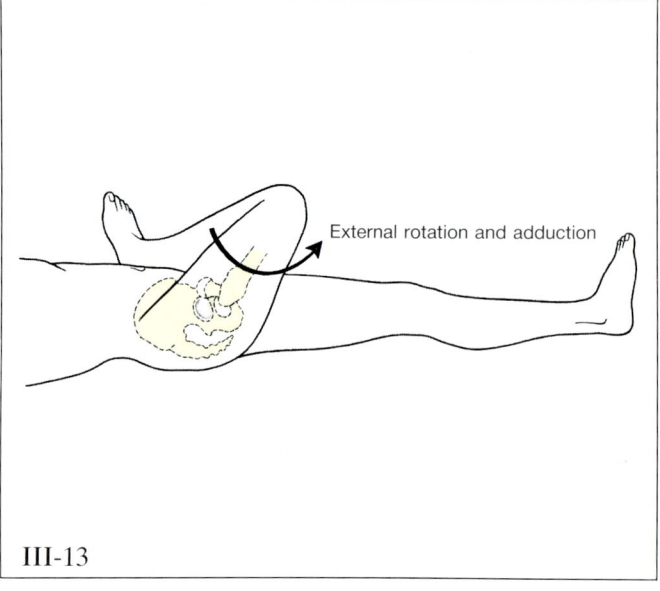

III-13

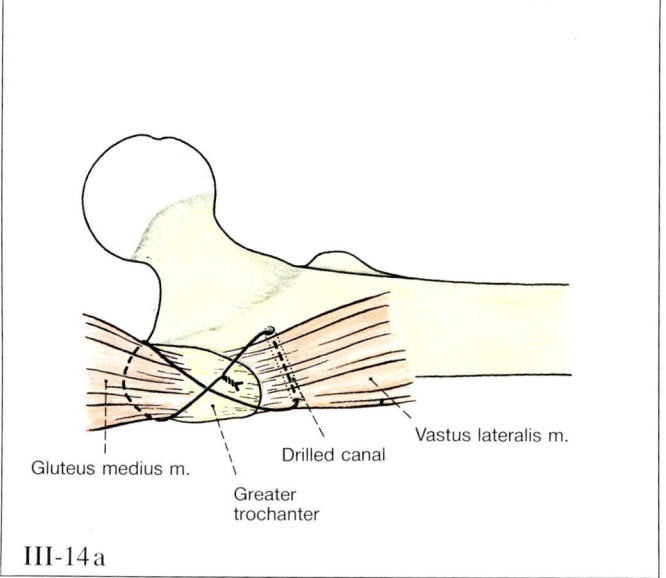

III-14a

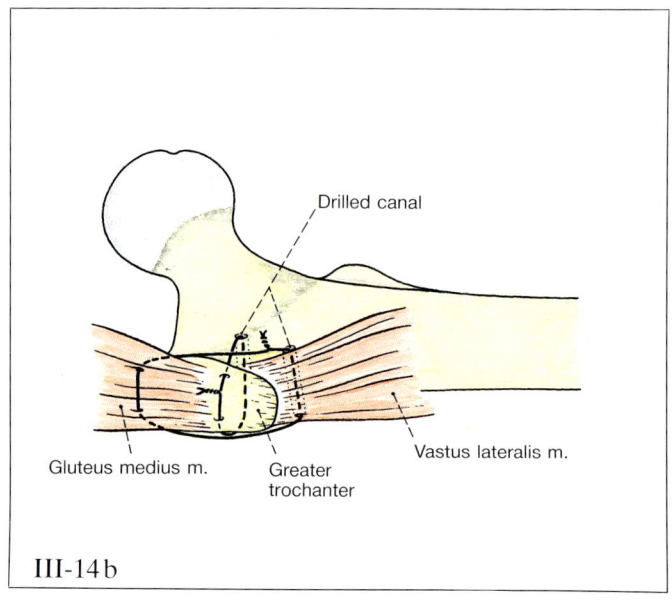

III-14b

Lateral Cup Incision
of *Lexer-Murphy*

Indications
1. Hip arthroplasty
2. Total hip replacement
3. Arthrodesis of hip joint

Operative Steps
1. Begin the skin incision under the anterior superior iliac spine. Continue it distally in a U-shaped fashion under and behind the greater trochanter to a point a hand's breadth below the posterior superior iliac spine (Fig. III-15).
2. Separate the pelvitrochanteric musculature forward and backward, forward toward the tensor fasciae latae.
3. With a chisel remove a thick slice of the greater trochanter and elevate the slice with the attached pelvitrochanteric muscles (Fig. III-16).
4. Develop the field dorsally by splitting the gluteus maximus muscle along the line of the incision.
5. The proximal aspect of the joint capsule is exposed by retracting the greater trochanter.
6. Incise the capsule longitudinally along the upper limits of the neck of the femur to expose the head and the neck.
7. When closing the wound, reattach the greater trochanter with wires (see Figs. III-14a and III-14b). Furthermore, attach the fascia of the vastus lateralis muscle to the trochanter slice with interrupted sutures.

Notes
1. Although this line of incision provides a good view of the head and neck of the femur, it has become obsolete.
2. The *Lexer-Murphy* approach is improved by adding a distal longitudinal incision from the center of the "U" (Fig. III-15).

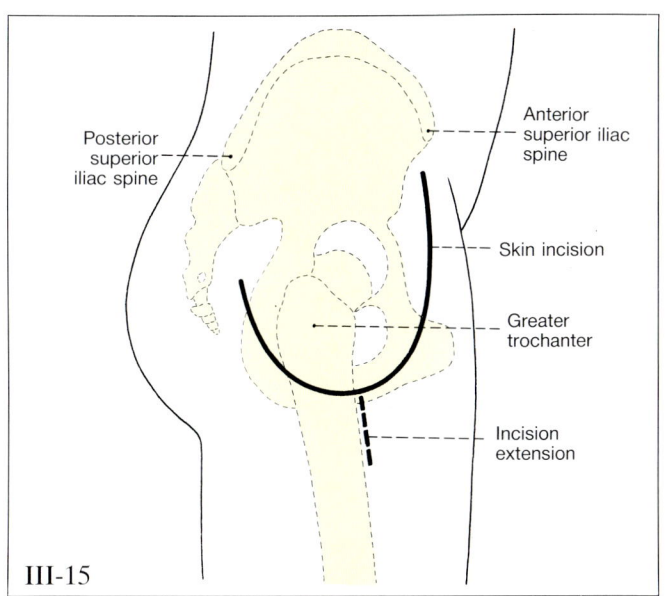

III-15

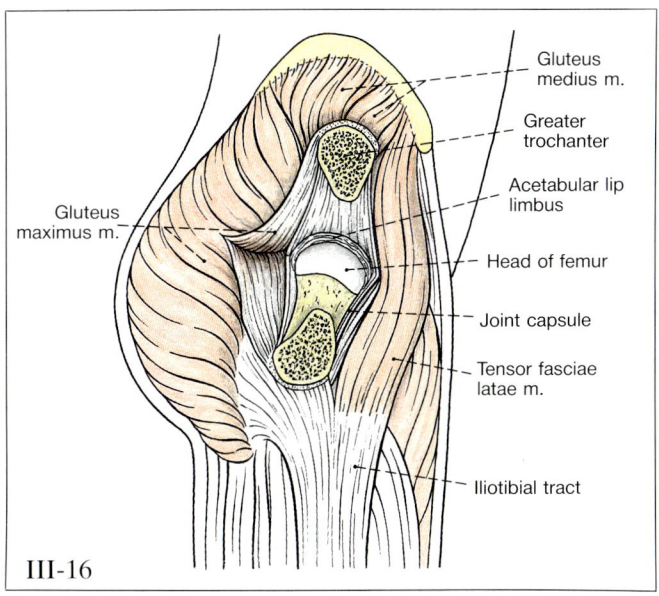

III-16

Hip Joint — Anterolateral Exposure

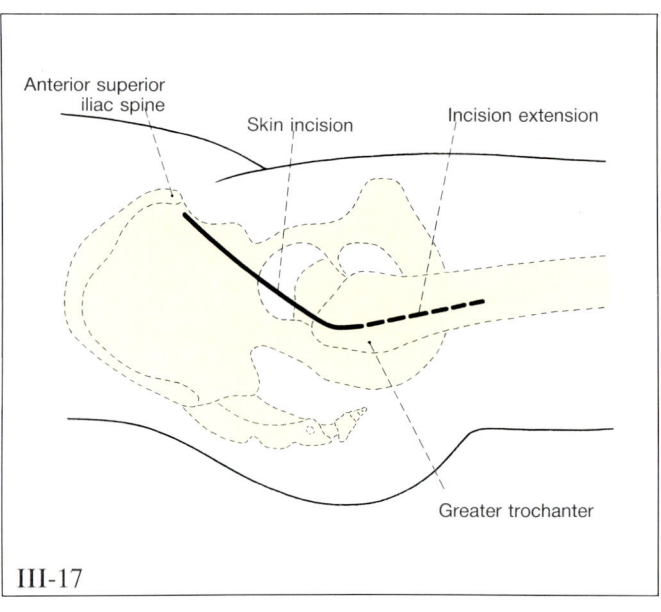

III-17

Anterolateral Exposure

Indications

1. Total replacement
2. Fractures and dislocations
3. Epiphysiolysis of the femoral head
4. Inflammatory processes
5. Synovectomy

Operative Steps

1. Place the patient in a supine position.
2. Begin the skin incision immediately under the anterior superior iliac spine and continue it obliquely across the hip toward the tip of the greater trochanter. At this point curve the incision to follow the long axis of the femur for about 3 cm (Fig. III-17). A distal extension is possible.
3. Split the fascia and, if necessary, excise the trochanteric bursa.
4. Locate the plane between the tensor fasciae latae and the anterior border of the gluteus medius muscle (Fig. III-18). Ligate the transversely running blood vessels. Bluntly separate the muscles from the deep structures and reflect them forward and backward.
5. Expose the joint capsule by passing a Hohmann elevator behind the femoral neck above and below, i.e., in the front and in the back (Fig. III-19).

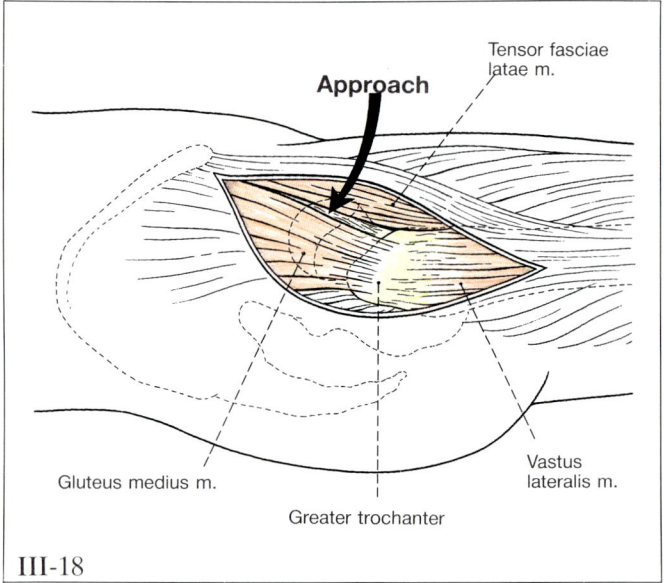

III-18

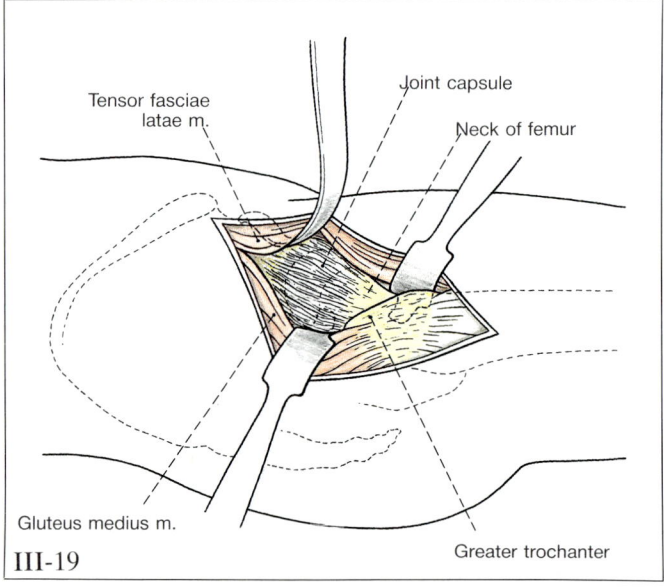

III-19

Hip Joint — Anterolateral Exposure

6. Pass another Hohmann retractor under the ventral musculature and stay close to the bone at the medial rim of the acetabulum so that the retractor can be hooked behind the superior ramus of the pubis. Retract the tensor fasciae latae and the rectus femoris muscles medially with the femoral nerve and vessels (Fig. III-20).
7. Incise the joint capsule lengthwise and detach it from the intertrochanteric line in such a way that it can be hinged back.
8. The head of the femur can now be resected, while the surrounding soft tissue is protected by the Hohmann retractors (Fig. III-21).

Notes

1. The exposure is well suited for a total hip replacement operation. It does not require separation of the greater trochanter.
2. With careful dissection the exposure is not associated with any great risks. Traction on the Hohmann retractor behind the superior pubic ramus should be moderate to prevent injury to the femoral nerve.
3. If the operative field is crowded, it is possible to cut the anterior attachment of the gluteus medius muscle on the greater trochanter.
4. Proximally, it is frequently difficult to locate the fascial plane between the tensor fasciae latae and the gluteus medius muscles. The separation of the two muscles is therefore best begun half way down, as seen in Fig. III-18.
5. Separation of the tensor fasciae latae and gluteus medius muscles in the proximal third of the incision can endanger the deeply running nerve supply to the tensor fasciae latae muscle.
6. The tensor fasciae latae muscle is supplied by a terminal branch of the superior gluteal nerve, which runs in the adipose layer between the gluteus medius and minimus muscles. In the proximal third of the incision, the motor nerve branch crosses the fascial plane and enters the tensor fasciae latae muscle. The nerve also can be dissected free and thus remain protected from accidental injury.
7. The most important point is that the proper fascial plane is entered between the tensor fasciae latae and the gluteus medius muscles.

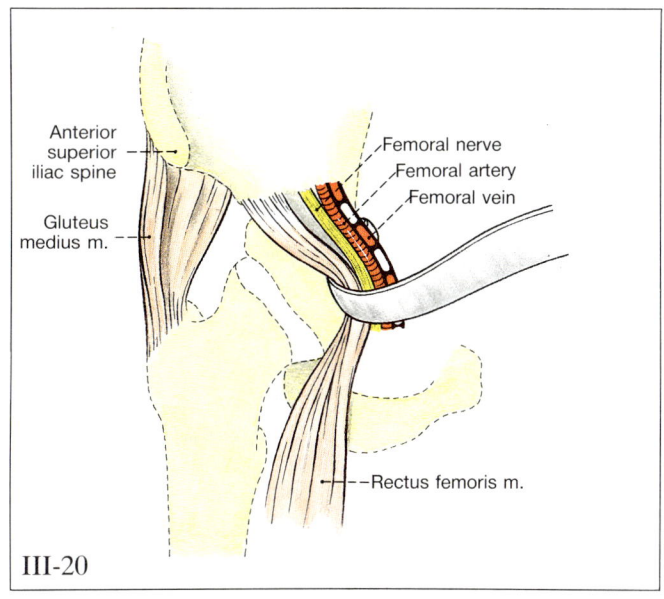

III-20

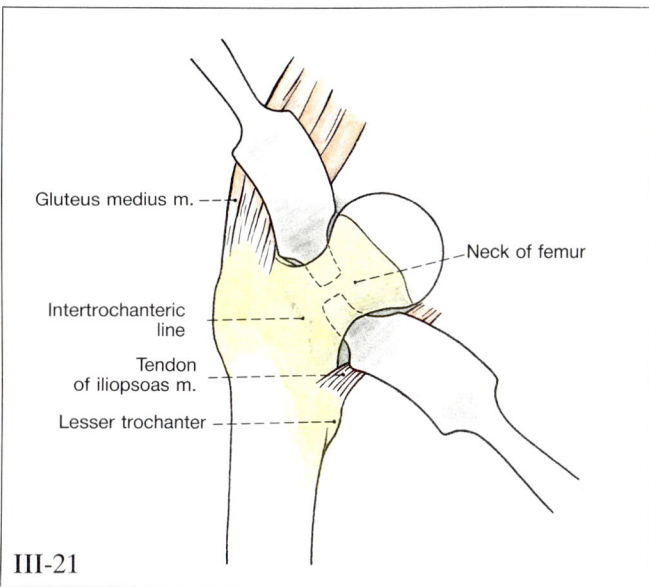

III-21

Posterior Exposure
Posterior Curved Exposure

Indications

1. Hip joint arthroplasty
2. Total hip replacement
3. Irreducible fractures of the posterior part of the acetabulum
4. Exploration of the sciatic nerve
5. Tumors in the gluteal region

Operative Steps

1. Position the patient face down or on the side, depending on the chosen procedure (see Notes).
2. Begin the angled skin incision approximately 2–3 cm below the posterior superior iliac spine. Continue the incision across the base of the greater trochanter to a point 2–3 cm beyond the latter (Fig. III-22). The angle of the incision should be near the tip of the trochanter.
3. An alternative incision with a caudally convex curve is illustrated in Fig. III-23.
4. Cut through the superficial and deep fasciae. Split the gluteus maximus muscle along its fiber direction to a point distal to the posterior superior iliac spine. The length of this split depends on the desired exposure (Fig. III-24). For didactic reasons, the gluteus maximus muscle has been split wide open in Fig. III-25 to illustrate the topographical relationships.

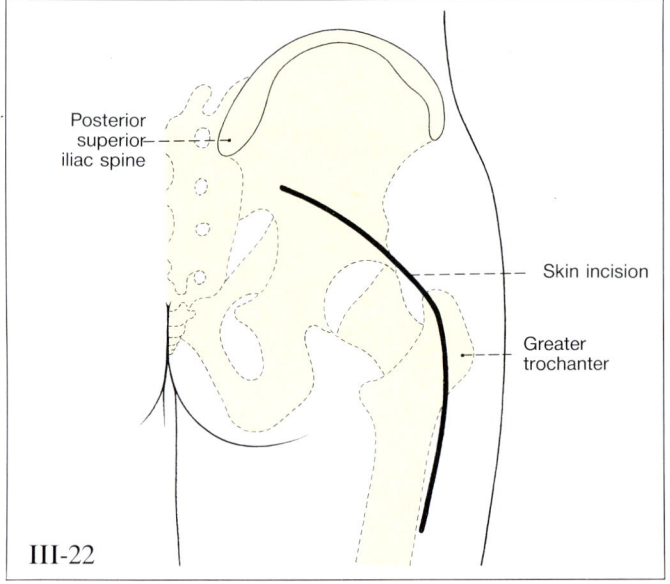

III-22

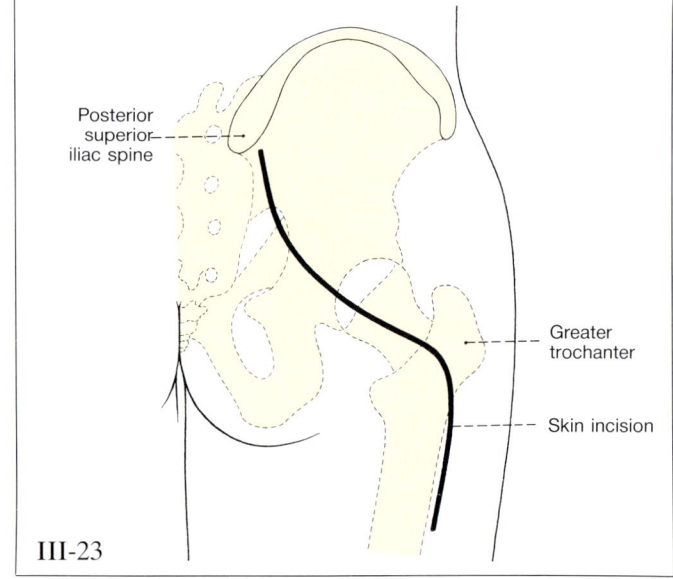

III-23

Hip Joint — Posterior Exposure

5. Extend the incision distally through the posterior aspect of the iliotibial tract.
6. Cut the taut aponeurosis of the gluteus maximus muscle which attaches to the outer surface of the greater trochanter (Fig. III-25).
7. Retract the split gluteus maximus muscle forward and backward to expose the sciatic nerve and the lateral rotators (Fig. III-25).
8. Rotate the femur medially and cut the tendons of the piriformis, superior gemellus, internal obturator, and inferior gemellus approximately 1.5 cm from their insertions (Fig. III-25). This will facilitate later reapproximation, which, however, is not essential.
9. Retract the muscles medially and the posterior aspect of the joint capsule is exposed (Fig. III-26).
10. Incise the joint capsule lengthwise and transversely to bring into view the posterior portions of the head and neck of the femur.

Notes

1. This posterior curved incision is also conveniently referred to as the "southern exposure."
2. If disarticulation of the femoral head is planned, the lateral patient position is preferred.
3. The lateral rotators can be separated from the trochanter with an electric knife to prevent hemorrhage.
4. Particular care should be taken to prevent injury to the superior gluteal artery and the inferior gluteal nerve when splitting the gluteus maximus.
5. Many useful modifications of this exposure have been added during the years (see "Posterolateral Approach of *Marcy* and *Fletcher*"), in which splitting of the gluteus maximus muscle is unnecessary.
6. Cutting of the quadratus femoris is optional (risk of hemorrhage from the lateral femoral circumflex artery).
7. Injury to the superior gluteal artery is dangerous because it retracts rapidly into the pelvic cavity. A retroperitoneal approach may be indicated to stop the hemorrhage.

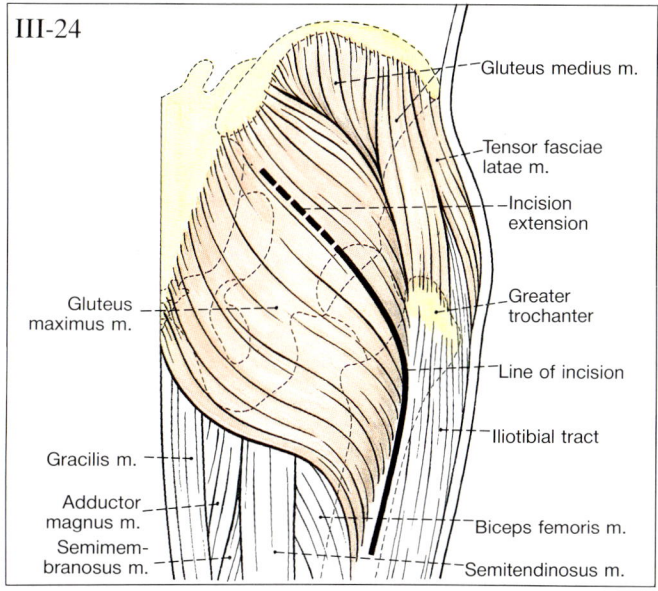

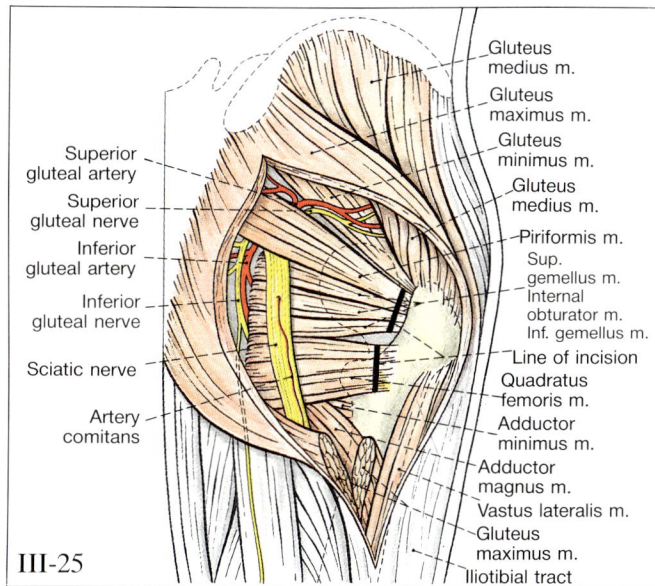

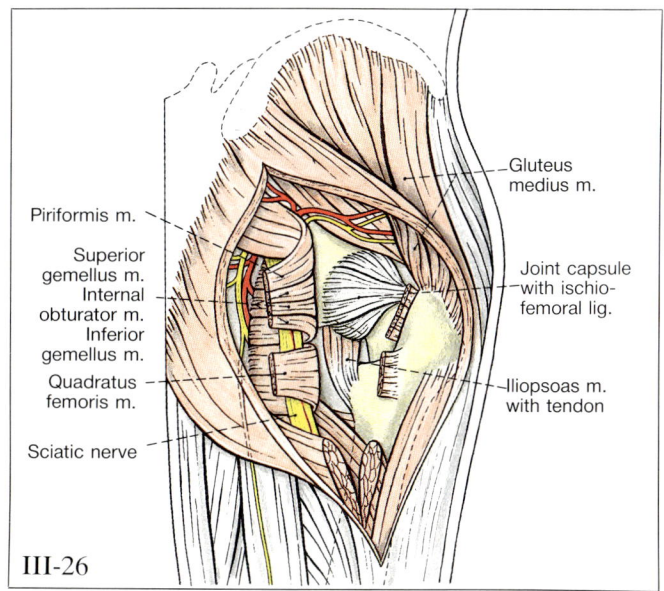

Posterolateral Exposure of *Marcy* and *Fletcher*

Indications

1. Arthroplasty
2. Total replacement
3. Irreducible fractures of the posterior part of the acetabulum

Operative Steps

1. Position the patient on the healthy side. Secure the position with lateral supports and sand bags (Fig. III-27). The limb to be operated on should be draped free for mobility.
2. Begin the skin incision approximately 5 cm in front of the posterior superior iliac spine. Continue the incision distally and anteriorly over the greater trochanter and along the thigh for approximately 7–8 cm (Fig. III-28).

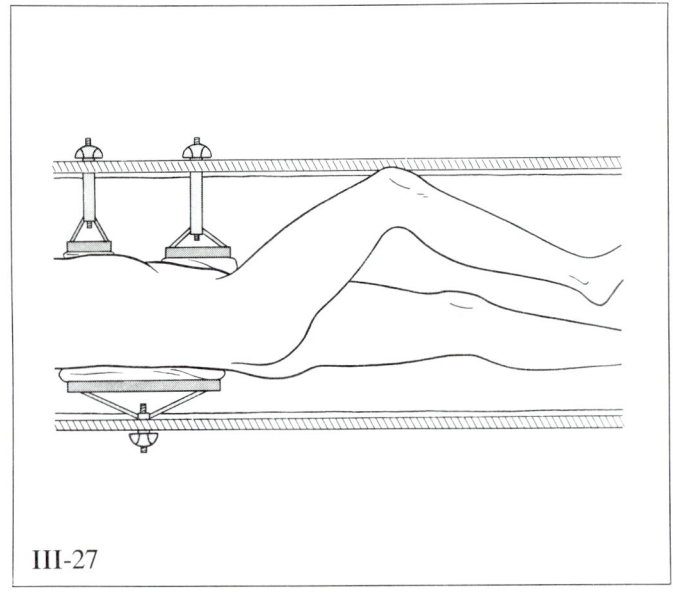

III-27

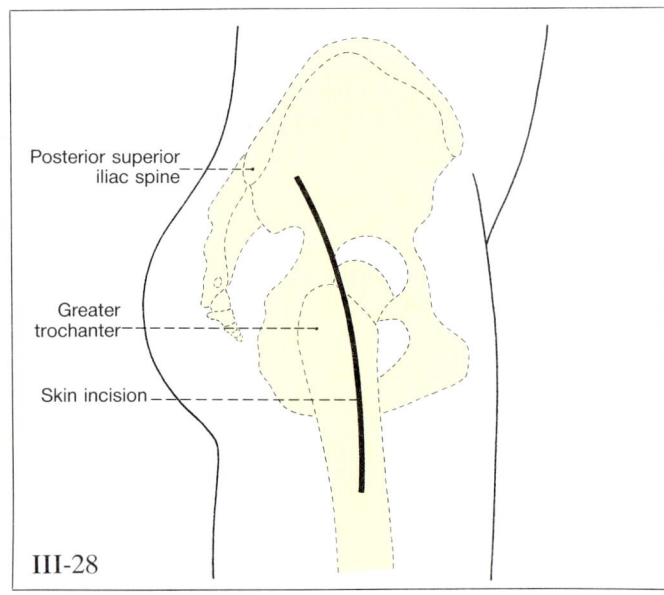

III-28

Hip Joint — Posterolateral Exposure

3. Incise the gluteal fascia along the anterior margin of the gluteus maximus muscle (Fig. III-29, incision A).
4. Split the iliotibial tract starting from below. This will open the trochanteric bursa. Excise the bursa. By extending the incision proximally between the gluteus maximus and the tensor fasciae latae muscles, it is possible to retract the gluteus maximus muscle with the posterior portion of the iliotibial tract toward the back. This exposes the lateral rotators and the greater trochanter (Fig. III-30).
5. As an alternative, incision B in Fig. III-29 may be elected.
6. Divide the piriformis, the gemelli, the internal obturator, and the quadratus femoris muscles (Fig. III-31), leaving a stump of each muscle for ease of reapproximation later. Use an electric knife to control hemorrhage.
7. Retract the lateral rotators and the pelvitrochanteric musculature to expose the posterior aspect of the joint capsule (Fig. III-31).

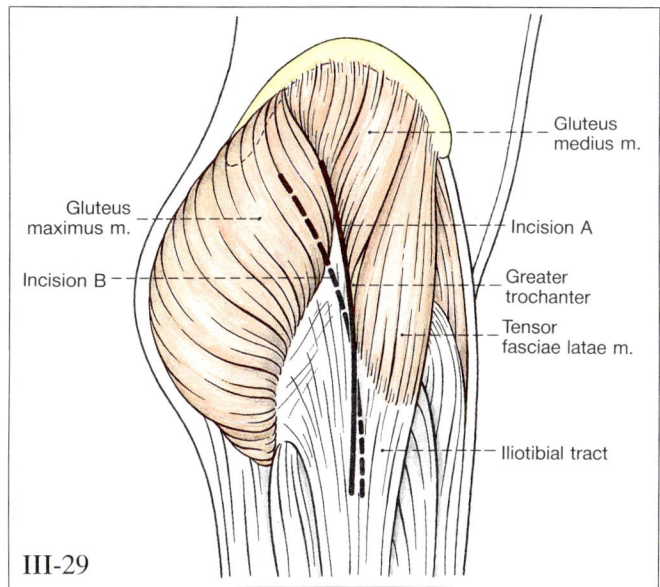

III-29

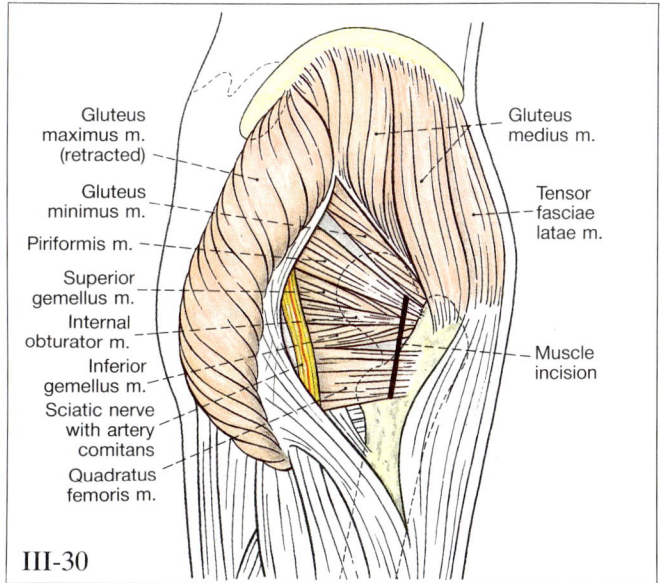

III-30

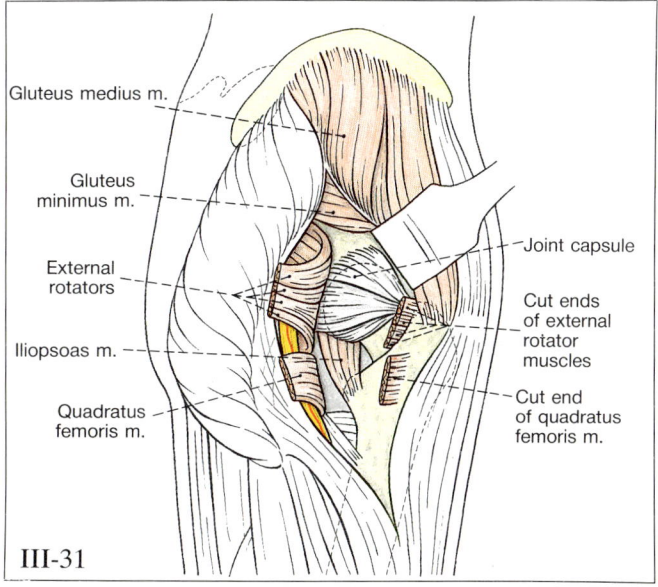

III-31

Hip Joint — Posterolateral Exposure

8. After the capsule is incised (Figs. III-32 and III-33), the hip joint can be disarticulated by flexion, adduction, and medial rotation of the femur (Fig. III-34).

Notes

1. This is a standard and uncomplicated exposure, and the blood loss is mild.
2. With this approach there is no need to split the gluteal musculature (incision A).
3. The length of the incision in the direction of the posterior superior iliac spine is determined by the required exposure. It is frequently sufficient to only reflect the piriformis muscle a short distance to prevent injury to the superior gluteal artery and nerve. Regardless of the approach, these particular structures should always be guarded (see Fig. III-25).
4. The reattachment of the lateral rotators is not essential. Neglecting to do this does not cause an apparent functional loss.
5. It is not necessary in every case to detach the external obturator and the quadratus femoris muscles in order to obtain a good overview.
6. Compare the notes on the Posterior Exposure.

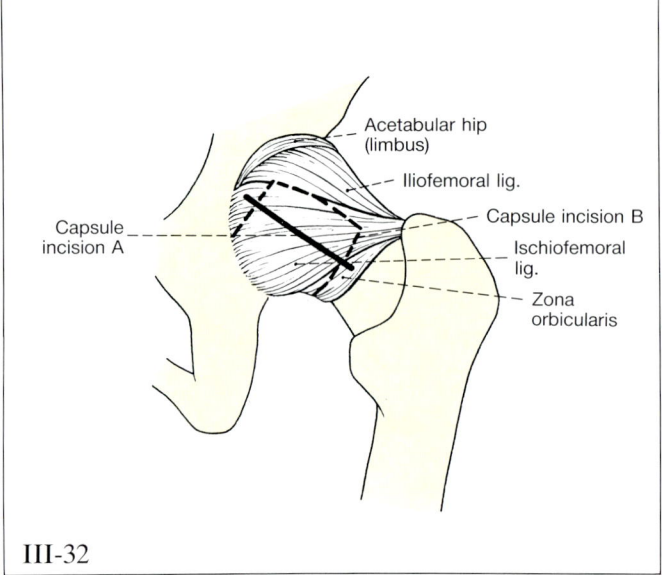

III-32

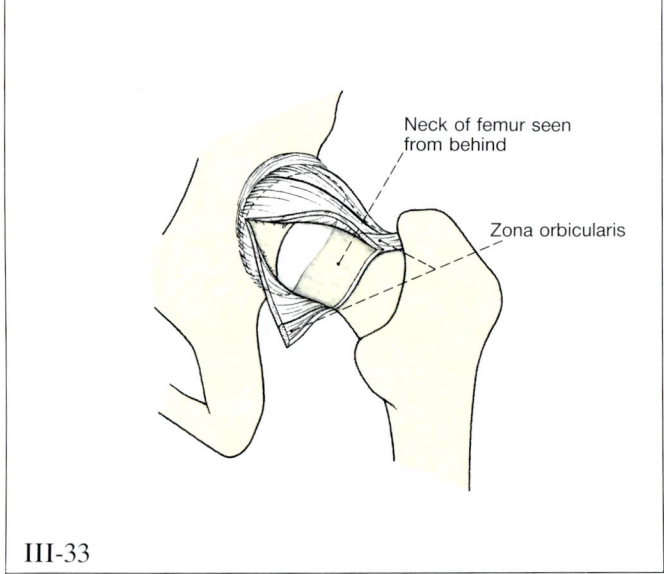

III-33

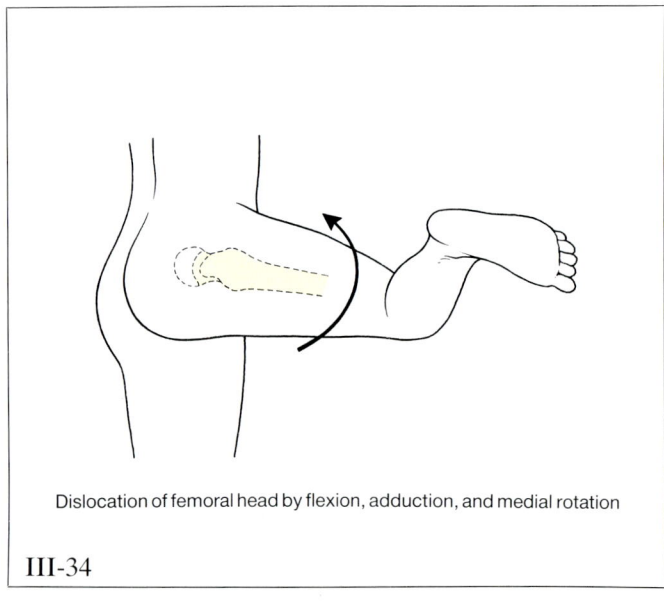

Dislocation of femoral head by flexion, adduction, and medial rotation

III-34

Intertrochanteric Neck of Femur

Lateral Exposure

Indications

1. Osteotomy
2. Tumors or inflammatory processes

Operative Steps

1. Place the patient in the supine position with the limb rotated medially.
2. Begin a straight incision one or two fingers' breadth below the tip of the trochanter, and continue it for 12–14 cm below the base of the trochanter (Fig. III-35) in case a subsequent plate fixation is planned.
3. Incise the fascia lata longitudinally (Fig. III-36).
4. Find the origin of the vastus lateralis muscle at the base of the trochanter.

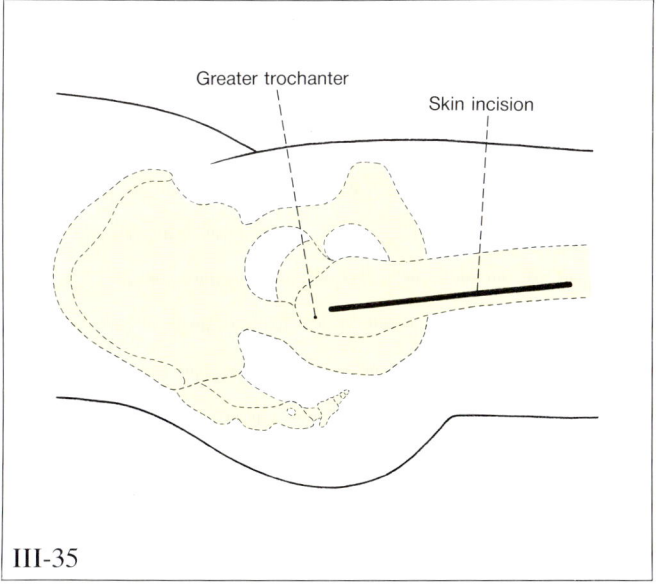

III-35

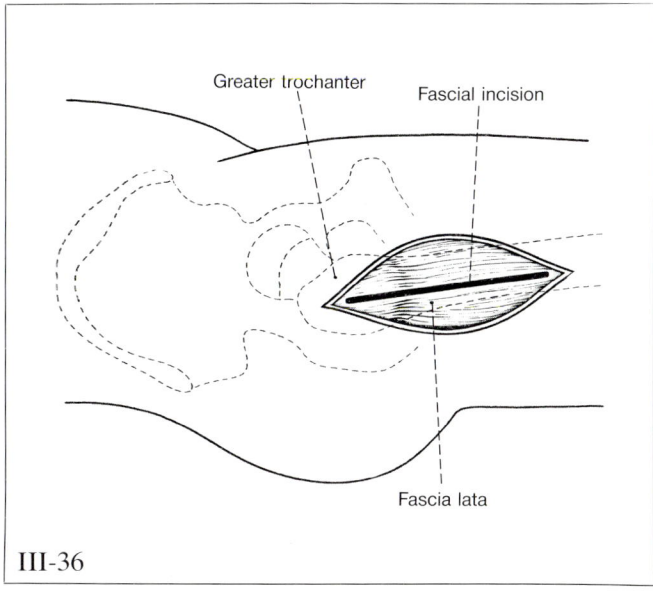

III-36

5. Cut across the origin of the vastus lateralis muscle, leaving a stump of muscle and associated fascia for later reattachment (Fig. III-37). Angle the incision and continue along the lateral margin of the muscle.
6. Detach the vastus lateralis muscle from the lateral intermuscular septum and the lateral aspect of the shaft of the femur by sharp dissection and the use of a rasp.
7. Elevate the periosteum in the intertrochanteric region with a rasp.
8. Pass Hohmann retractors under the intertrochanteric neck of the femur from the medial and lateral sides. This will displace the soft tissues (Fig. III-38).

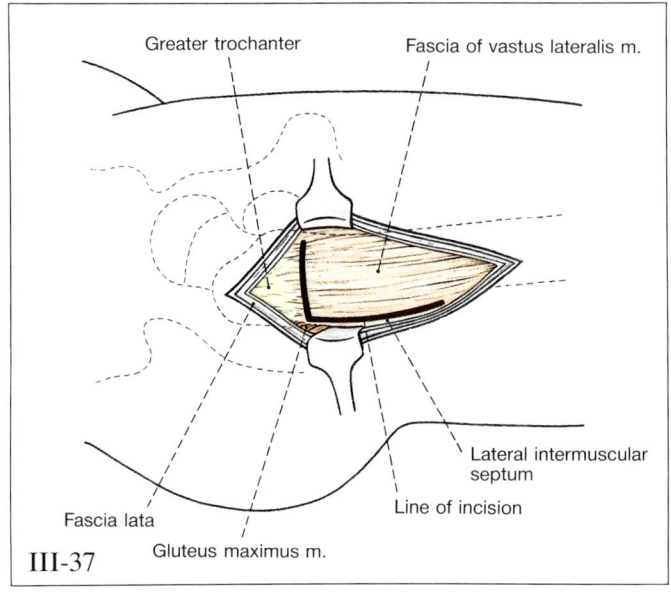

III-37

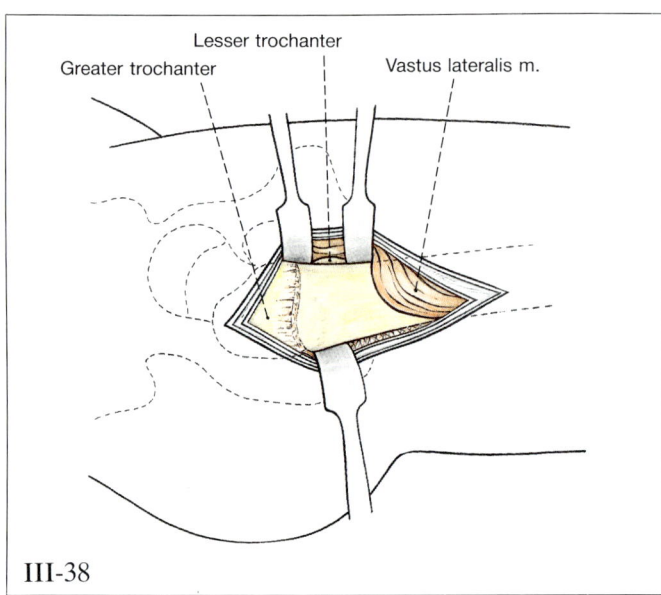

III-38

Lesser Trochanter

Exposure of *Nicola*

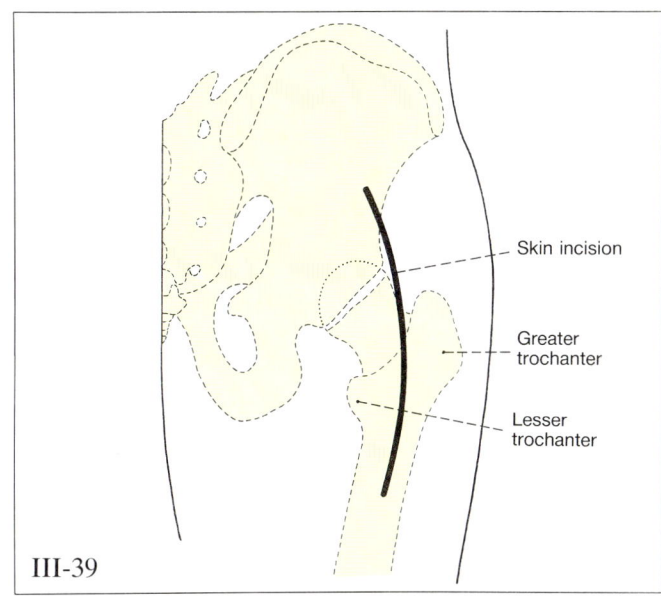

Indications

1. Tumors
2. Biopsy

Operative Steps

1. Place the patient in the prone position.
2. Begin an approximately 10-cm-long curved dorsal incision about 3–4 cm above the tip of the trochanter at the midsacral level, and extend it distally for another 5–6 cm (Fig. III-39).
3. Retract the skin and subcutaneous fat medially and laterally to expose the deep fascia over the gluteus maximus muscle.
4. Incise the strong aponeurosis of the gluteus maximus muscle for about 10 cm, beginning distally (Fig. III-40).
5. Detach the lower part of the quadratus femoris muscle and retract it proximally; carefully displace the sciatic nerve medially (Fig. III-41).
6. Detach the iliopsoas muscle from the lesser trochanter with a rasp. The part of the tendon that inserts on the femoral shaft below the lesser trochanter should be left intact. The lesser trochanter is now exposed (Fig. III-41).

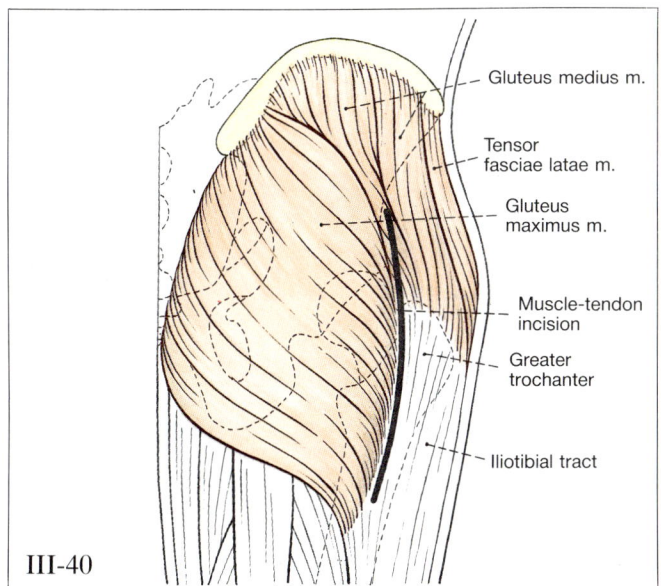

Notes

1. To prevent unnecessary hemorrhage, the sciatic nerve should not be further exposed.
2. Compare with the notes on the posterior exposure of the hip joint.

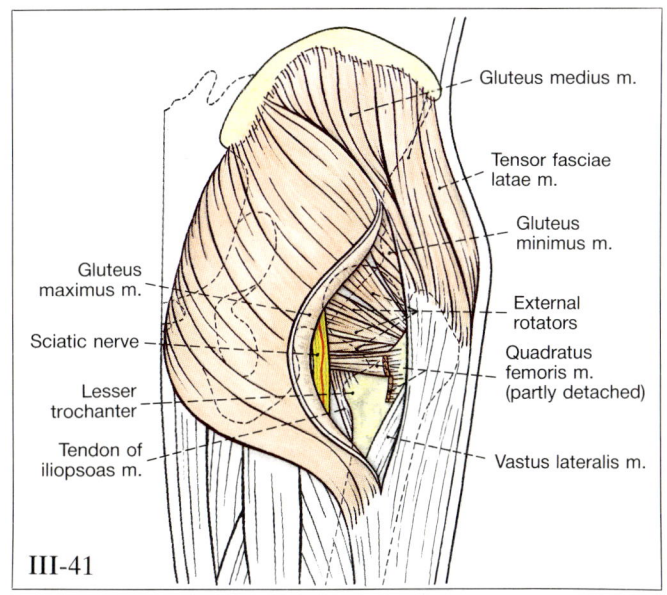

B. Thigh

Shaft of the Femur

Anterior Exposure

Indications

1. Fractures of the femoral shaft
2. Bone tumors
3. Inflammatory processes

Operative Steps

1. Make a skin incision over the shaft of the femur along a line connecting the anterior superior iliac spine and the lateral margin of the patella (Fig. III-42).
2. Enter the space between the rectus femoris and the vastus lateralis muscles (Fig. III-43). The point of entry is about one hand's breadth below the greater trochanter.

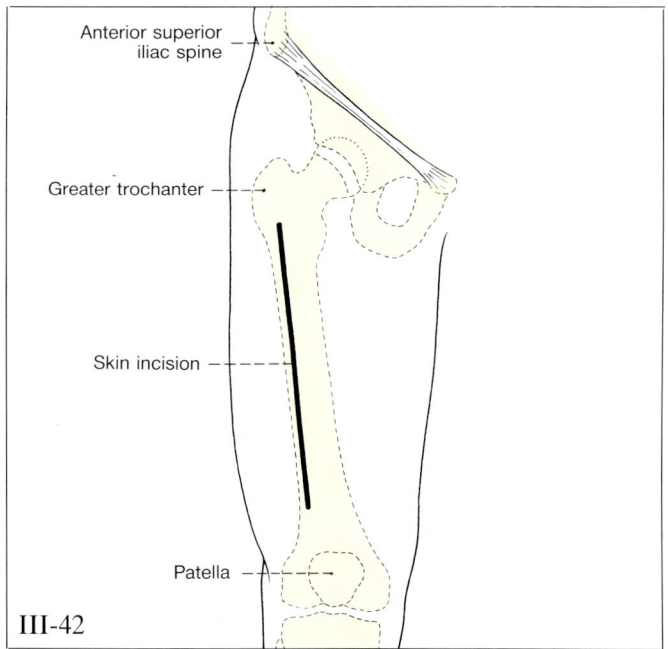

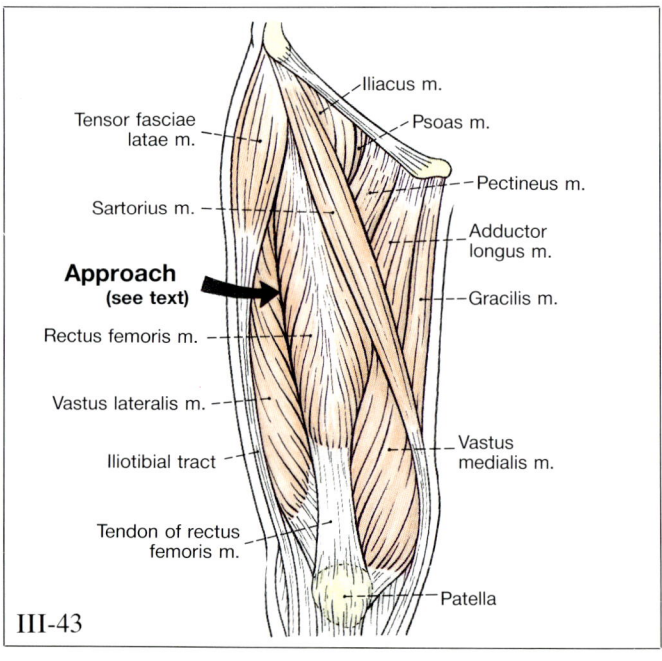

Shaft of the Femur — Anterior Exposure

3. Retract the rectus femoris muscle medially (Fig. III-44).
4. Dissect through the vastus intermedius muscle along its fiber direction down to the femur. Elevate the muscle subperiosteally to expose the anterior and lateral aspects of the femur (Fig. III-45).
5. The nerve branches to the vastus lateralis muscle and the lateral femoral circumflex artery are seen in the upper part of the operative field. These structures must be retracted before the upper portion of the vastus intermedius is incised (Fig. III-45). The neurovascular bundle can be freed by blunt dissection with the fingers.

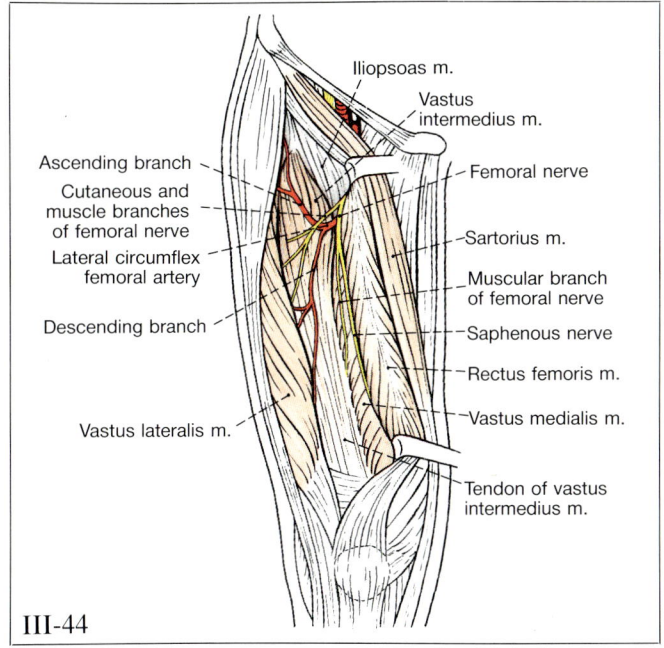

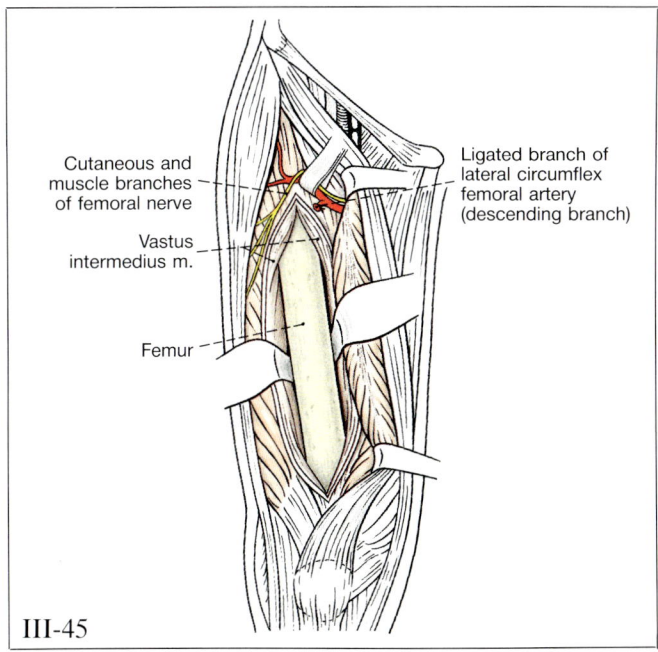

Shaft of the Femur — Anterior Exposure

6. The topographical anatomy and the approach are illustrated in a cross section of the thigh (Fig. III-46).
7. The operative field may be augmented by extending the incision proximally to the anterior superior iliac spine and distally, past the patella, to the lateral margin of the tibial tuberosity (Fig. III-47). This makes possible a simultaneous exposure of the femoral shaft and the hip and knee joints. The extension that reaches the hip joint corresponds to the approach by *Smith-Petersen*.

Notes

1. In the upper third of the field, the safety of the lateral femoral circumflex artery and vein as well as branches of the femoral nerve must be ascertained. This is particularly important in the proximal extension of the field (Fig. III-47).
2. If necessary, the vastus lateralis muscle can be widely mobilized toward the back.
3. During the postoperative healing process, adhesions may develop involving the vastus intermedius, thus limiting flexion at the knee joint. For this reason it is important that exercises be initiated as soon as possible.
4. Total replacement of the femur is an indication for the incision extension presented under step 7.
5. A proximal or distal part of the exposure is frequently adequate.

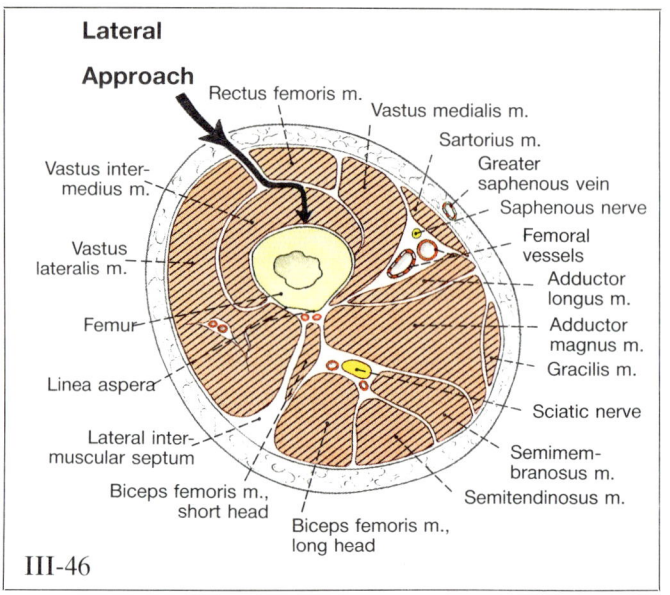

III-46

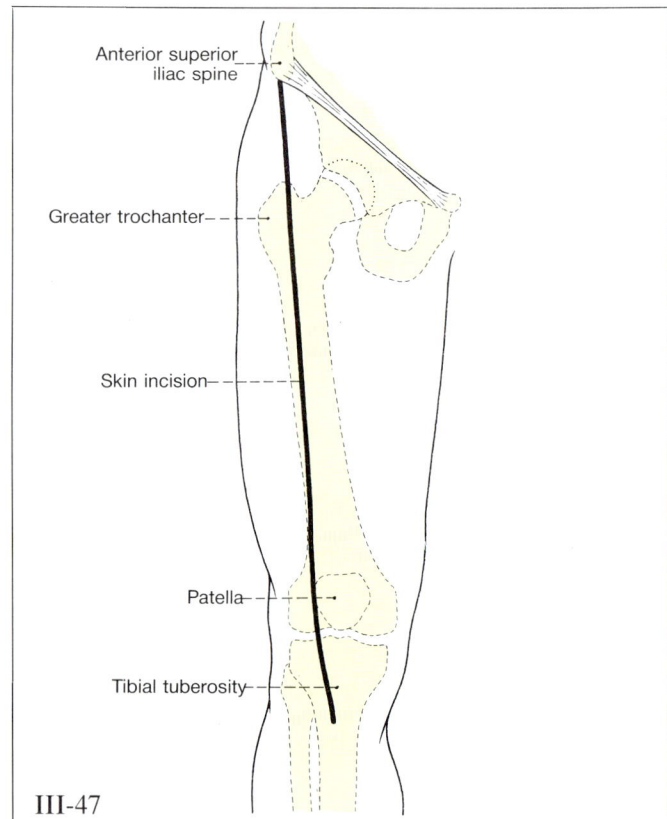

III-47

Shaft of the Femur — Lateral Exposure

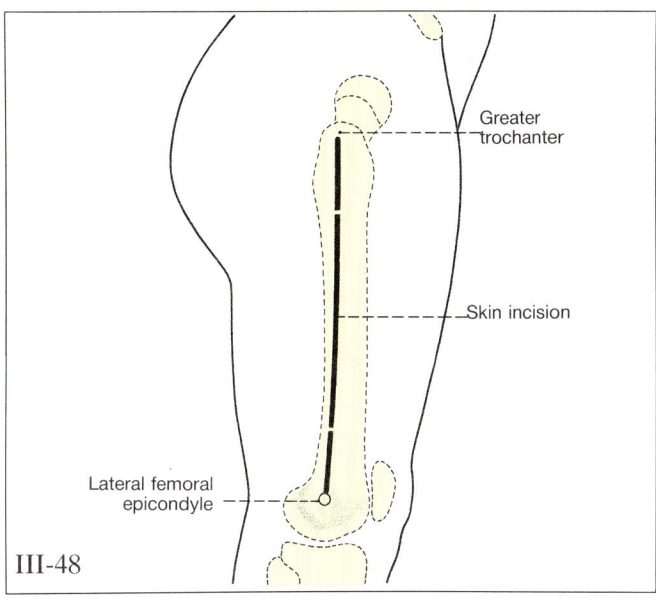

III-48

Lateral Exposure

Indications

1. Complicated fractures of the femoral shaft
2. Bone tumors
3. Inflammatory processes
4. Application of a plate

Operative Steps

1. Make a longitudinal incision from the tip of the greater trochanter to the lateral epicondyle of the femur or a subsection of this incision as deemed appropriate for the procedure (Fig. III-48).
2. Split the fascia lengthwise (Fig. III-49). Lift the vastus lateralis muscle. Locate the posterior margin of the vastus lateralis muscle at the lateral intermuscular septum (Fig. III-49). Split the muscle fascia along the posterior border.
3. Expose and ligate the transversely running perforating arteries. Incise the periosteum lengthwise and displace it forward and backward with a rasp (Fig. III-50).
4. Place Hohmann retractors under the shaft of the femur and the exposure is completed.

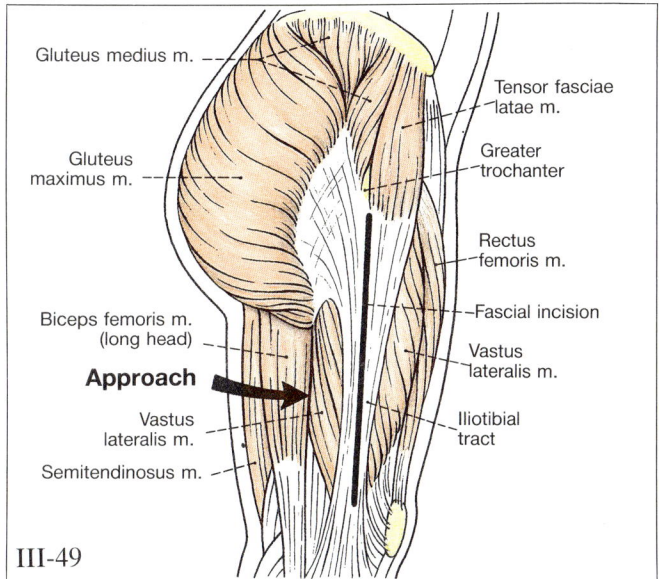

III-49

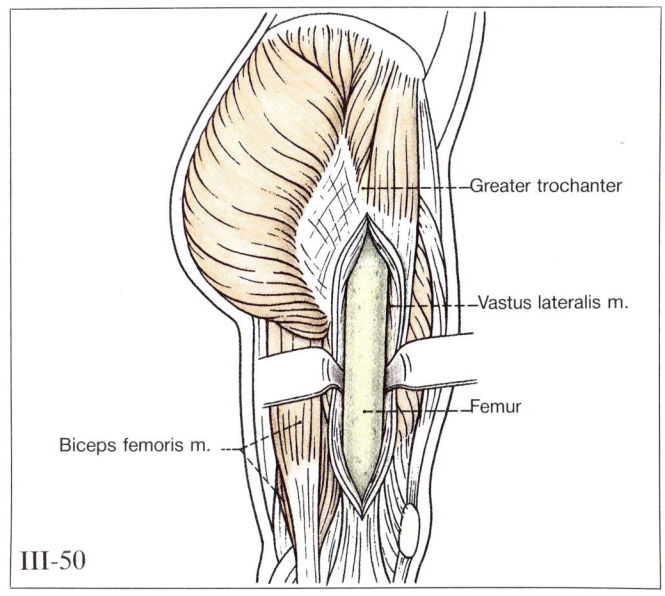

III-50

Shaft of the Femur — Lateral Exposure

5. The topographical anatomy and the approach are illustrated in a cross section of the thigh (Fig. III-51). This shows that the vastus lateralis muscle must be separated from the lateral muscular septum (bluntly).
6. Extension of the incision distally to the lateral margin of the tibial tuberosity is indicated in Fig. III-52.

Notes

1. This exposure is also referred to as a mailbox approach because the soft tissues (vastus lateralis muscle) are flipped forward like a lid.
2. Basically, a direct lateral approach is also possible. This involves splitting the iliotibial tract and the vastus lateralis and intermedius muscles in the direction of their fibers. The indirect lateral approach, however, is preferred because the muscles are left intact. Adhesions and interference with the innervation are therefore prevented.

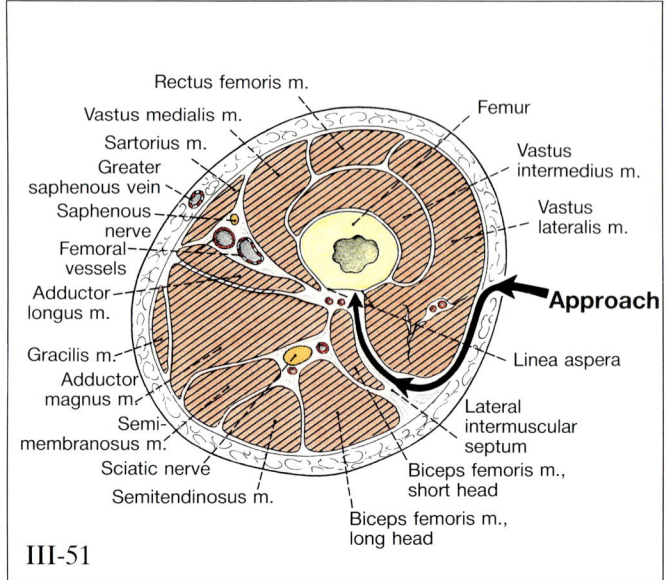

III-51

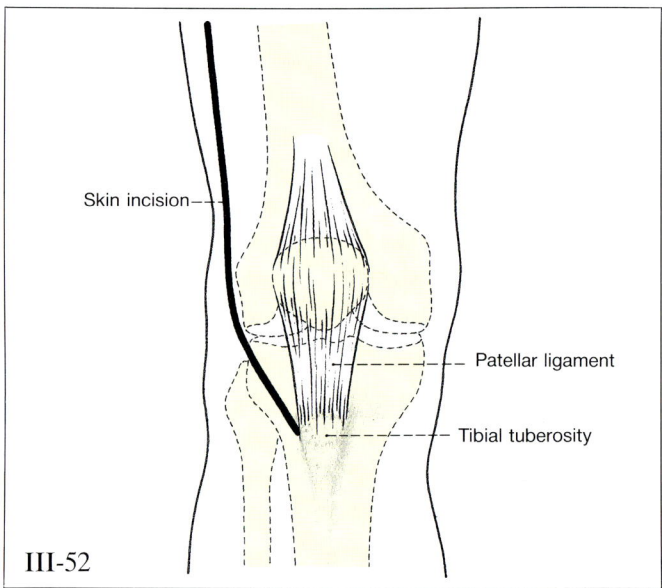

III-52

Shaft of the Femur — Medial Exposure

Medial Exposure

Indications

1. Bone tumors of the medial femoral condyle
2. Fracture of the condyle
3. Medial supracondylar osteotomy
4. Angular plate osteosynthesis
5. Exploration of the adductor canal

Operative Steps

1. Make a 15- to 20-cm skin incision from the medial femoral epicondyle upward in front of the adductors (Fig. III-53).
2. Expose the deep fascia over the adductor muscles down to the medial epicondyle, which is devoid of muscular attachments. The deep fascia lies behind the vastus medialis muscle (Fig. III-54).
3. The synovial cavity of the knee joint should not be opened. Retract the sartorius muscle posteriorly (or ventrally – see Notes) to expose the tendon of the adductor magnus muscle (Fig. III-55).
4. The saphenus nerve, which runs deep to the sartorius muscle, must be protected.
5. With blunt dissection, expose the femur in the popliteal region.
6. Retract the large vessels and nerves dorsally.
7. A clear view of the medial aspect of the femur is obtained by also retracting the adductor magnus tendon toward the back and the vastus medialis muscle forward.

Notes

1. No muscle is cut with this exposure.
2. Wound closure involves merely returning the muscles to their original sites.
3. The sartorius muscle is retracted ventrally when the middle third of the femur is exposed and dorsally with distal exposure.
4. If a more comprehensive exposure of the femoral shaft is desired, the adductor muscles can be detached and reflected posteriorly after cutting the vastoadductor membrane.

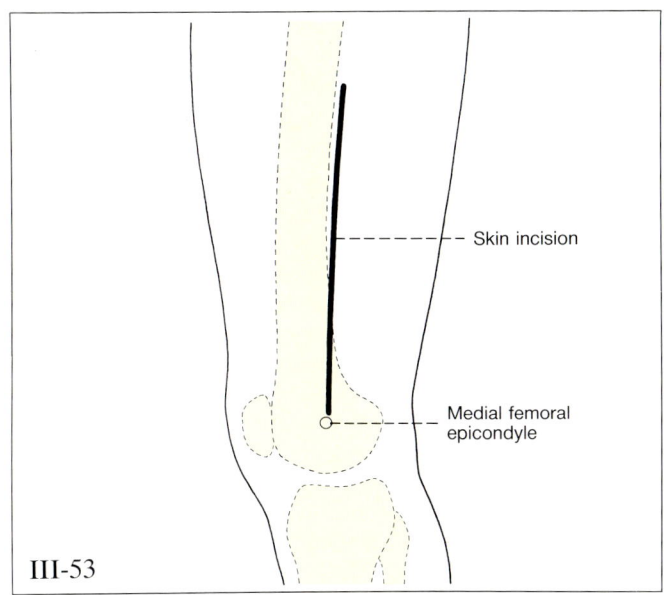

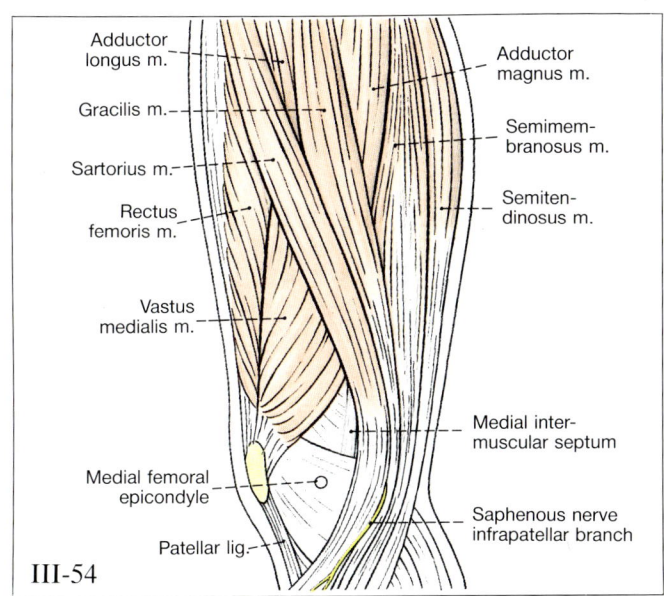

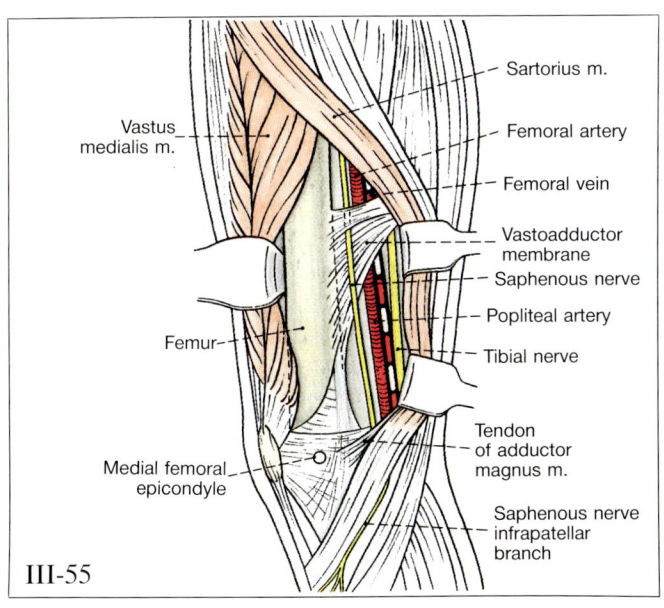

Shaft of the Femur — Posterior Exposure

Posterior Exposure

Indications

1. Tumors
2. Fractures of the femoral shaft
3. Exploration of the sciatic nerve

Operative Steps

1. Place the patient in the prone position.
2. Make a longitudinal incision on the back side of the thigh, beginning at the junction of the upper and middle third and ending just short of the popliteal fossa (Fig. III-56).
3. Retract the long head of the biceps muscle and the posterior femoral cutaneous nerve to the lateral side, and the semimembranosus and semitendinosus muscles to the medial side (Figs. III-57 and III-58). This exposes the popliteal artery and vein and the sciatic nerve, which runs on the short head of the biceps muscle (Fig. III-58).

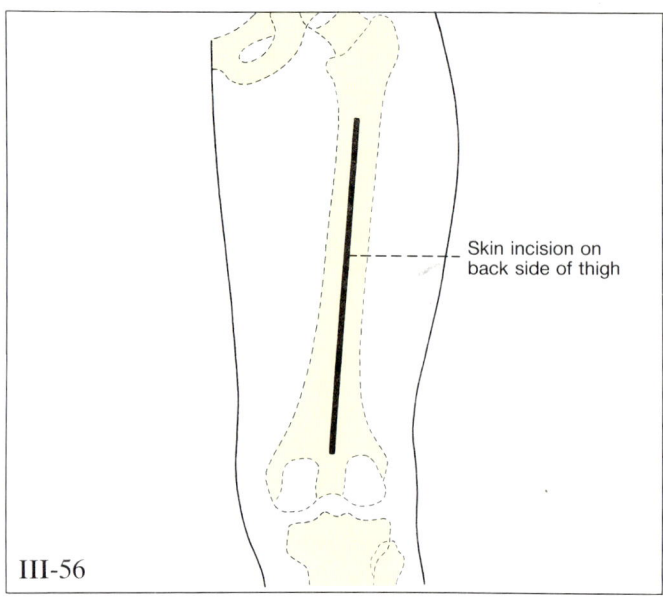

III-56

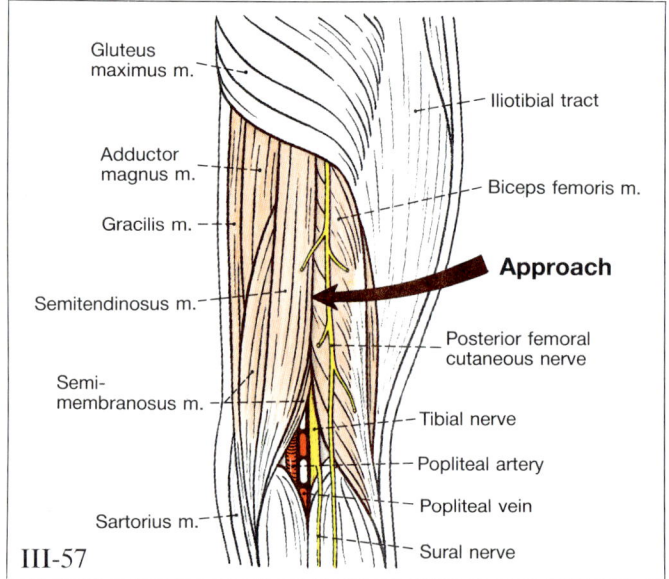

III-57

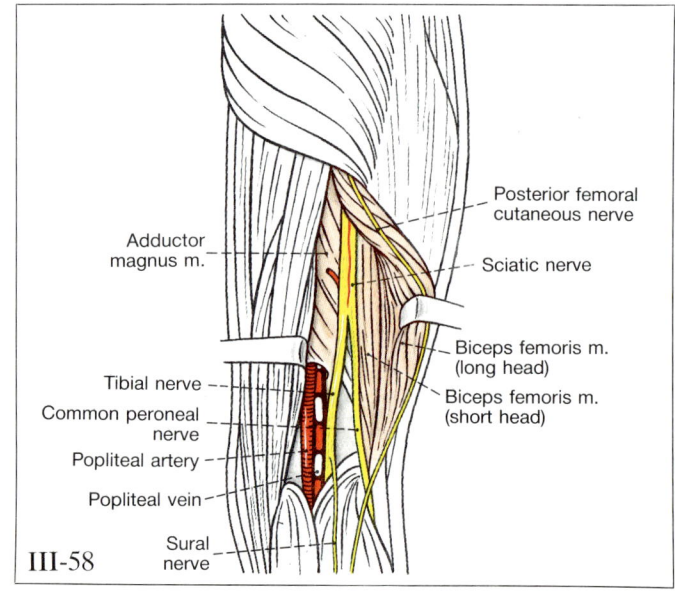

III-58

Shaft of the Femur — Posterior Exposure

4. Retract the sciatic nerve and the popliteal vessels to the lateral and medial sides, respectively. Ligate the transversely running blood vessels, and elevate the adductor magnus muscle and the short head of the biceps muscle subperiosteally.
5. Displace the adductor magnus muscle with the blood vessels medially and the short head of the biceps with the dividing sciatic nerve laterally. Pass a Hohmann retractor under the shaft of the femur (Fig. III-59). The distal two thirds of the femur are now exposed.

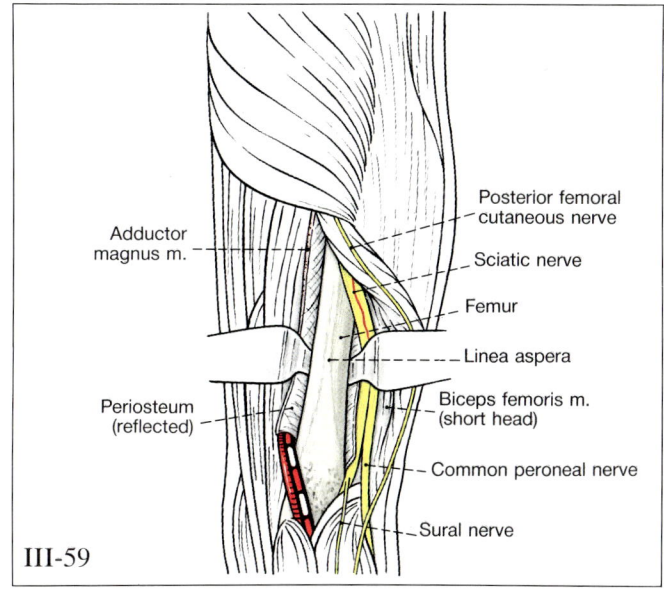

III-59

Distal Shaft of the Femur

Posterior Exposure

Indications

1. Tumors
2. Inflammatory processes
3. Fractures of the distal third of the femur

Operative Steps

1. Begin the skin incision about 8 cm proximal to the medial femoral condyle and extend it distally across the popliteal fossa to the inside of the fibula (Fig. III-60).
2. Incise the superficial and deep fasciae.
3. With blunt dissection, free the vessels and nerves in the region of the popliteal fossa (Fig. III-61).
4. Retract the popliteal vessels and the tibial nerve medially and the common peroneal nerve laterally. This exposes the dorsal distal third of the femur and the dorsal aspect of the joint capsule (Fig. III-62).

Note

This skin incision does not usually lead to keloid formation; neither does it cause a spread of scar tissue. The latter is more apt to occur with a straight skin incision in the popliteal region.

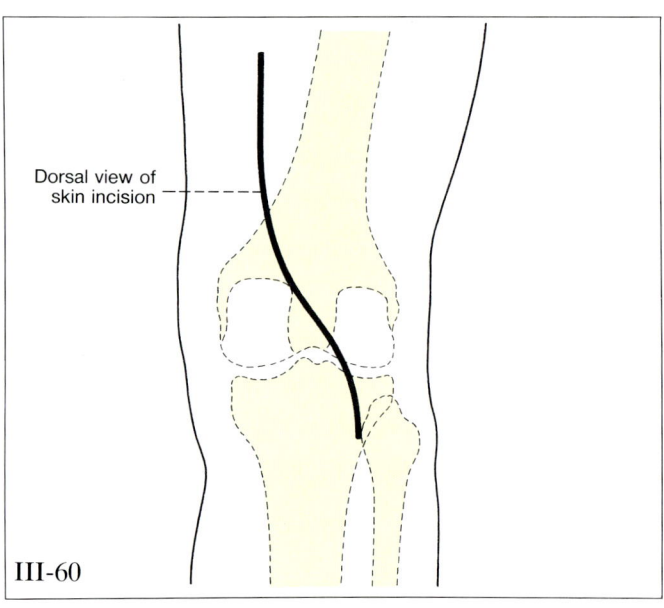

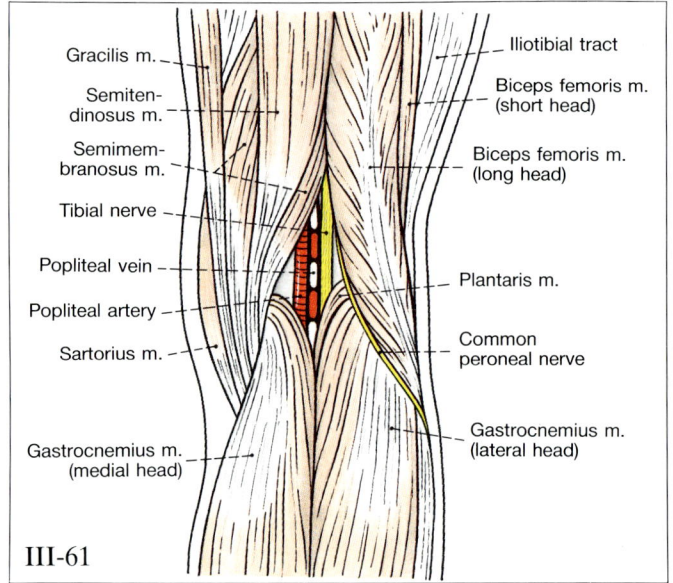

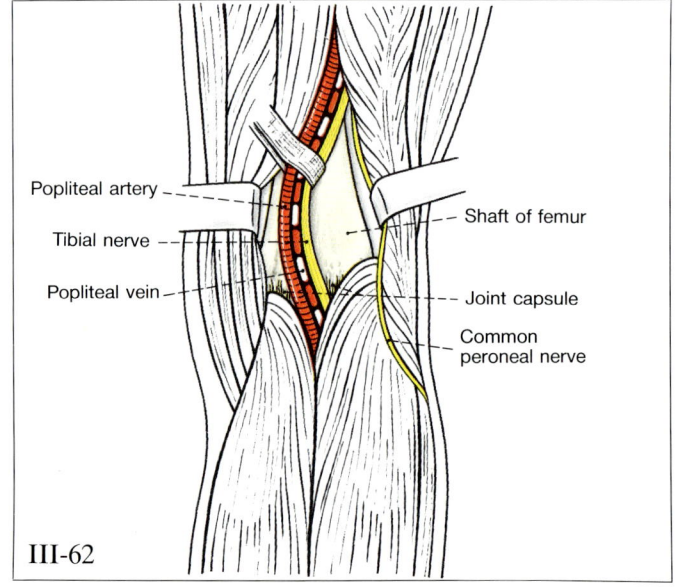

C. Knee Region

Knee Joint

Applied Anatomy

Surface anatomy (Fig. III-63).
Anterior muscle layer (Fig. III-64).
Schematic illustration of the synovial lining of the knee joint in a front view (Fig. III-65).

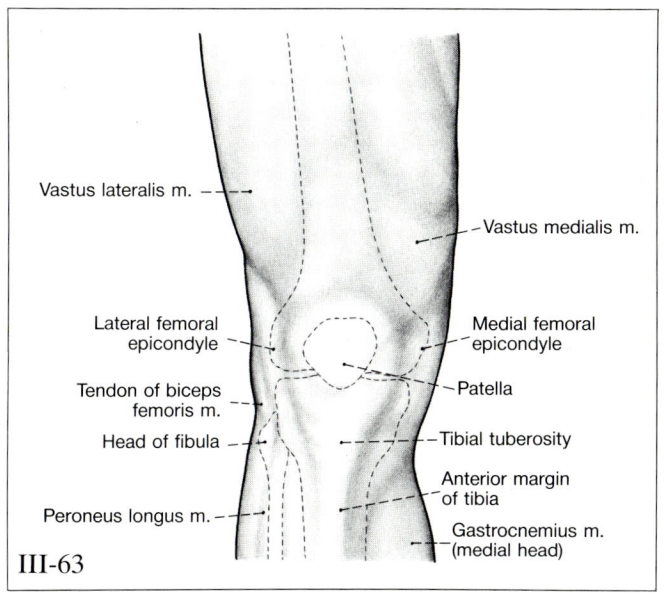

III-63

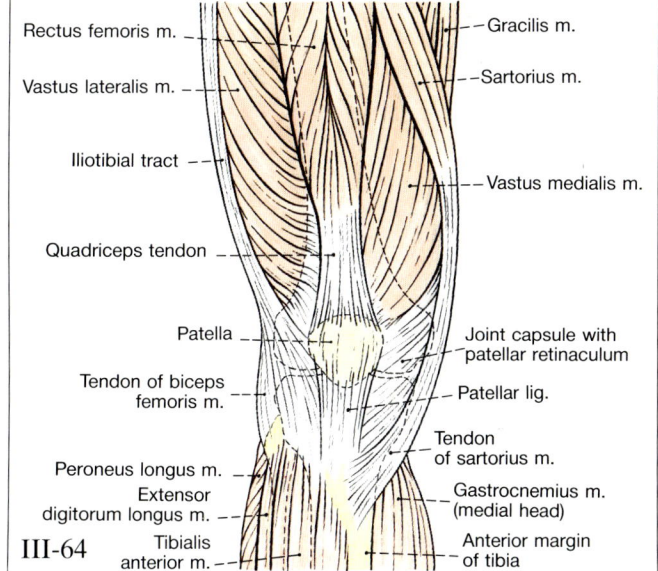

III-64

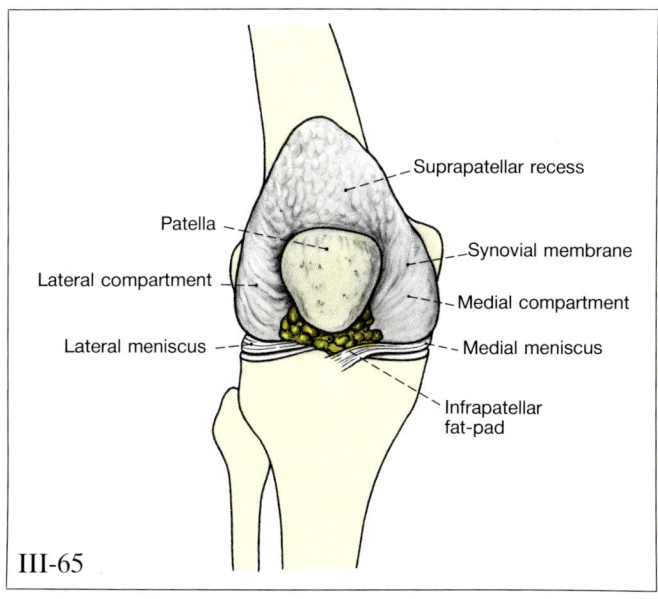

III-65

Arteries of the Knee Joint

The most important arterial anastomoses are illustrated in Figs. III-66 and III-67. If the inferior lateral or inferior medial genicular artery is severed and not ligated during the operation, a large hemarthrosis of the knee joint can develop and interfere with wound healing.

Notes

1. Operations on the knee joint, leg, and foot should, if possible, be performed under bloodless conditions with a pneumatic cuff after unwrapping the limb from the toes to the middle of the thigh.
2. A partly exsanguinated limb is sometimes preferred for better visualization of the different structures. It can be achieved by simply elevating the limb to a vertical position for 3–6 minutes. Then apply a pneumatic cuff.
3. The required cuff pressure depends on the degree of muscular development but should be about 300 mm Hg.

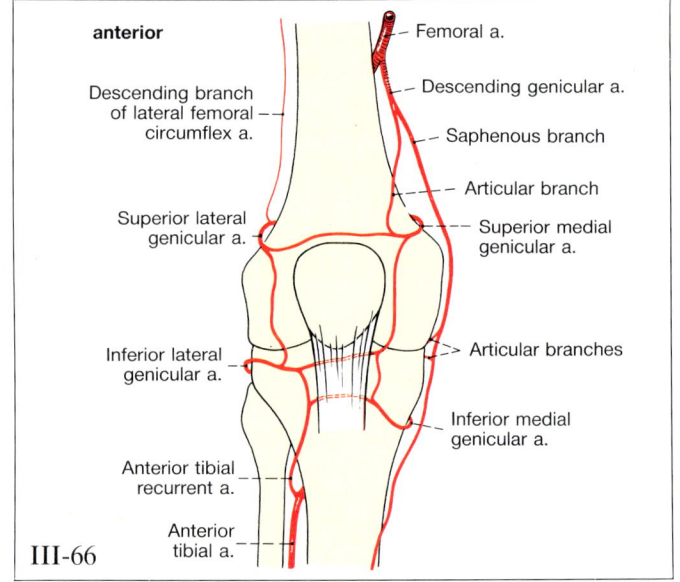

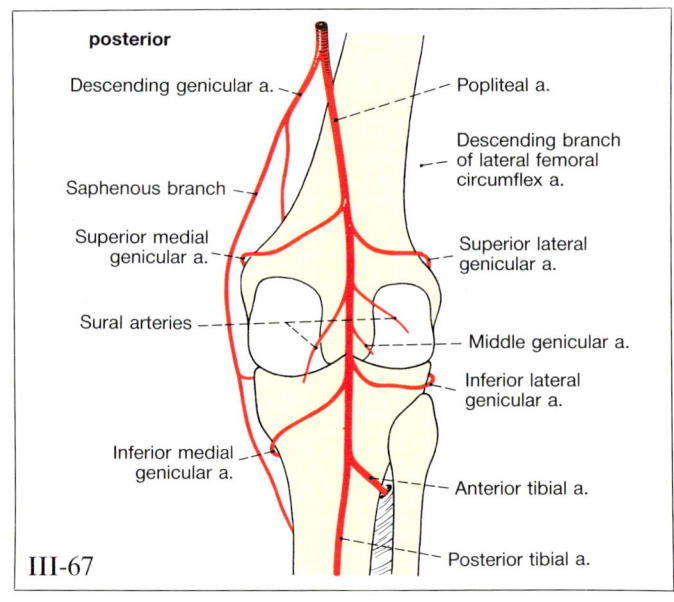

Anteromedial Exposure

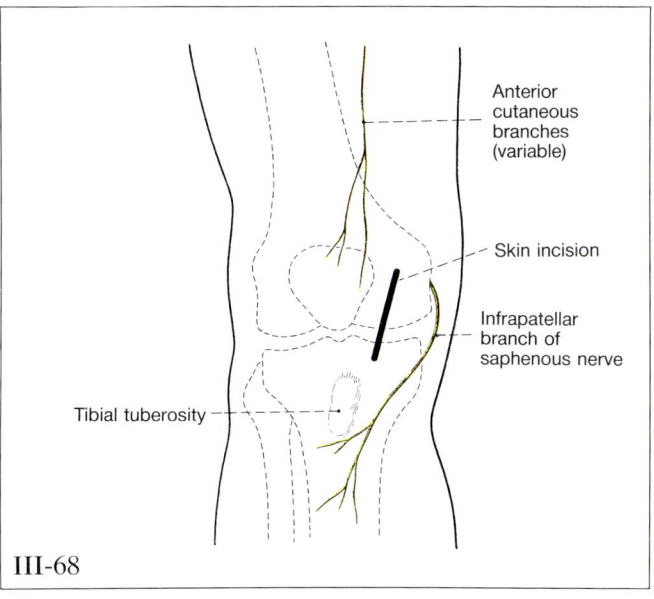

III-68

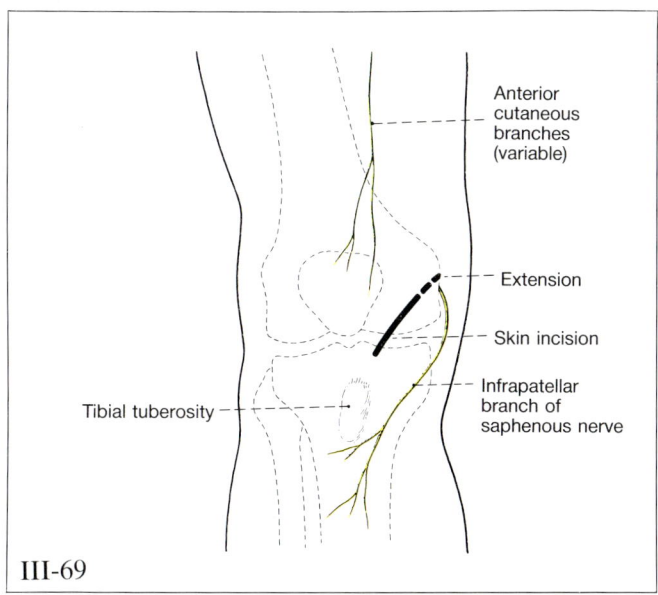

III-69

Indications

1. Removal of the medial meniscus
2. Removal of loose bodies from the joint
3. Exploration of osteochondrosis dissecans

Operative Steps

1. Make a 5-cm, slightly oblique longitudinal incision beginning 2–4 cm medial to the patella and ending distally at the medial border of the patellar ligament (Fig. III-68, alternatively, Fig. III-69). The apex of the patella is usually situated over the joint line and thus provides a good landmark.
2. Reflect the skin.
3. Incise the medial aspect of the joint capsule longitudinally (Fig. III-70). This reduces the danger of injury to the infrapatellar branch (of the saphenous nerve).
4. Reflect the capsule and make an incision in the synovial membrane similar to that used for the capsule.
5. Open the joint with the knee flexed (under certain circumstances at right angle). This can be done by drawing the limb up or by removing the support of the leg so it can hang freely (so-called "hanging knee").

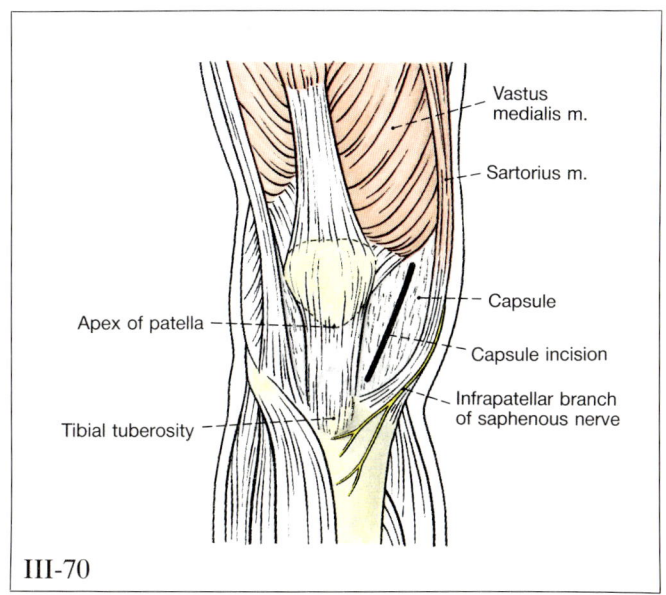

III-70

6. Additional lateral bending of the lower leg in valgus position will augment the exposure.
7. Retract the skin, capsule, and synovial membrane with deep, narrow retractors (Fig. III-71).
8. This exposes the cruciate ligaments, the medial femoral condyle, and the anterior two thirds of the medial meniscus (Fig. III-71).
9. Close the wound in layers with the knee joint extended or slightly flexed.

Notes

1. If possible, the opening of the knee joint should be planned so as to provide a good overview for the evaluation of the synovial membrane, the menisci, the cartilaginous lining, and the condition of the articular surfaces of the patella.
2. Injury of the infrapatellar branch leads readily to the formation of a painful neuroma.
3. By extending the incision (Fig. III-69) in the direction of the medial epicondyle and adding a longitudinal capsular incision (Fig. III-72) behind the medial border of the tibial collateral ligament, it is possible to inspect the posterior compartment of the joint and the posterior horn of the medial meniscus. The skin incision can be stretched toward the back.
4. If the meniscus is to be removed and there is limited help from assistants, the hanging knee position with the leg freely suspended is preferred because, for example, a valgus position is more readily obtained. The thigh rests at the end of the table or on a support padded with foam rubber.
5. In the hanging knee position, it is important that the popliteal region remains unobstructed. The thigh should not be immediately above the edge of the table but should extend somewhat beyond. Otherwise, the popliteal artery may be compressed against the posterior aspect of the capsule and injured during the procedure.

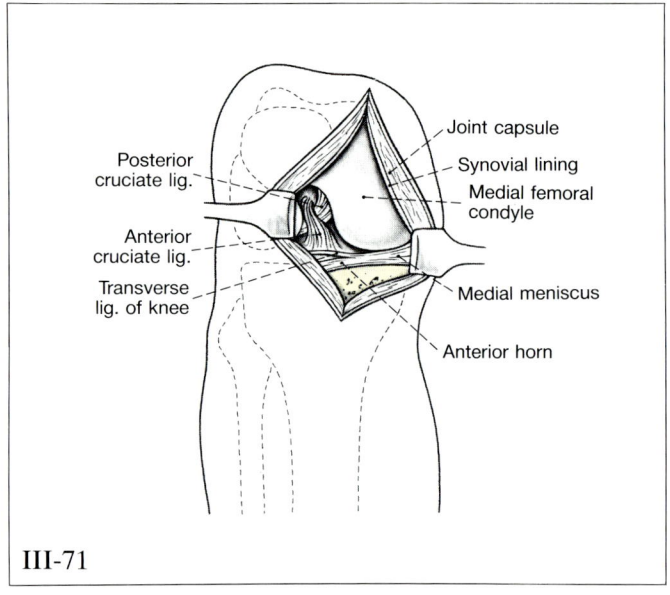

III-71

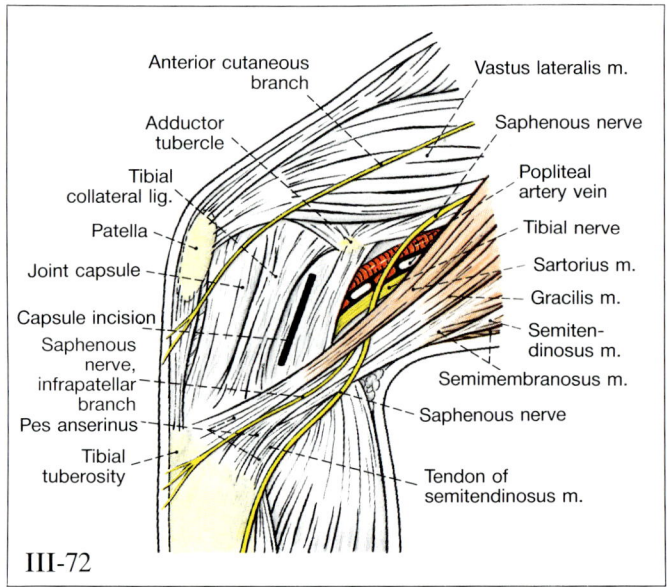

III-72

Knee Joint — Medial Curved Incision

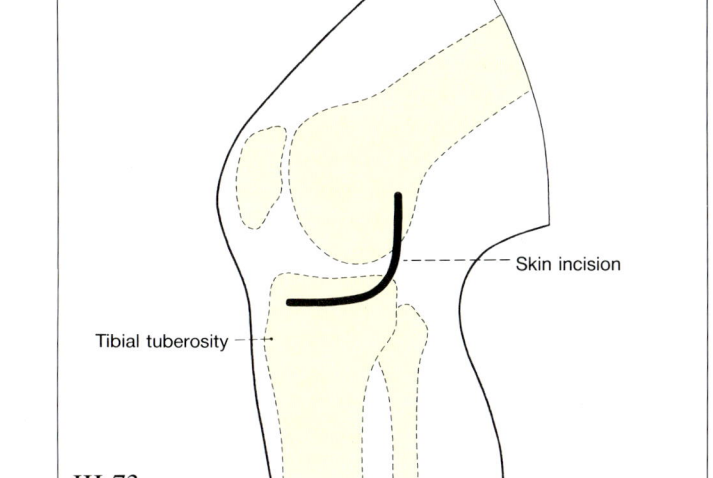

III-73

Medial Curved Incision

Indications

1. Total removal of the medial meniscus
2. Removal of loose joint bodies
3. Exploration or repair of tibial collateral ligament

Operative Steps

1. Make a curved incision from a point 4 cm medial and dorsal to the middle of the patella, continuing distally and anteriorly to the medial border of the patellar ligament (Fig. III-73).
2. Make two longitudinal incisions in the fiber direction of the joint capsule, about 2–3 cm apart (Fig. III-74).
3. Retract the capsule forward and backward to expose the anterior and posterior portions of the medial meniscus (Fig. III-75).

Note

Watch out for the infrapatellar branch of the saphenous nerve when making the posterior incision of the capsule.

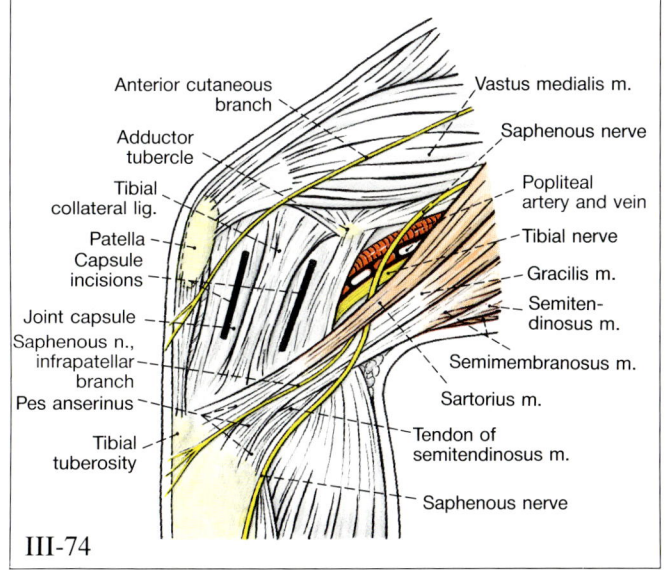

III-74

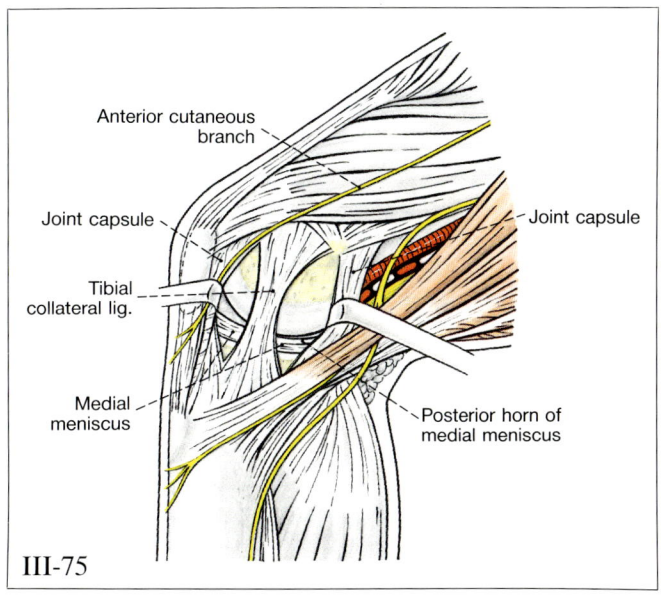

III-75

183

Alternative

Medial S-Incision or Anteroposterior Exposure from the Medial Side

Indication

Rupture of the tibial collateral ligament combined with tears of the anterior cruciate ligament and the medial meniscus (unhappy triad).

Operative Steps

1. The S-shaped incision (Fig. III-76) or the continuous anteroposterior incision (Fig. III-77) is suited for an extensive exploration of the joint.
2. The joint is then opened in front of the collateral ligament and proximally, from the border of the vastus medialis muscle.

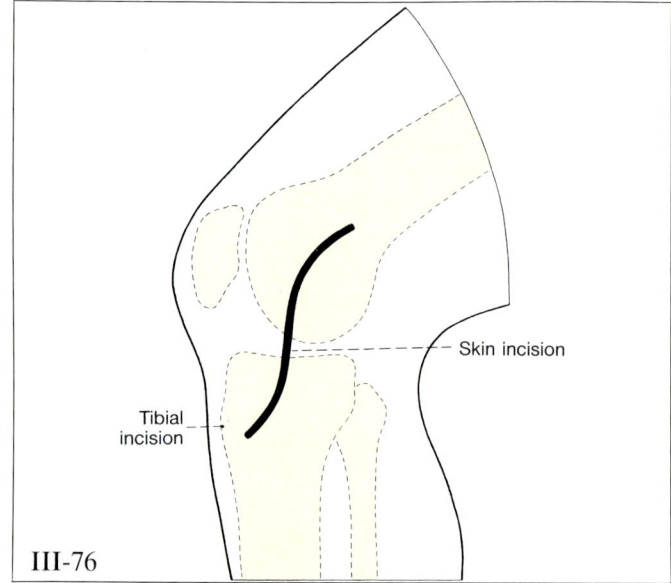

III-76

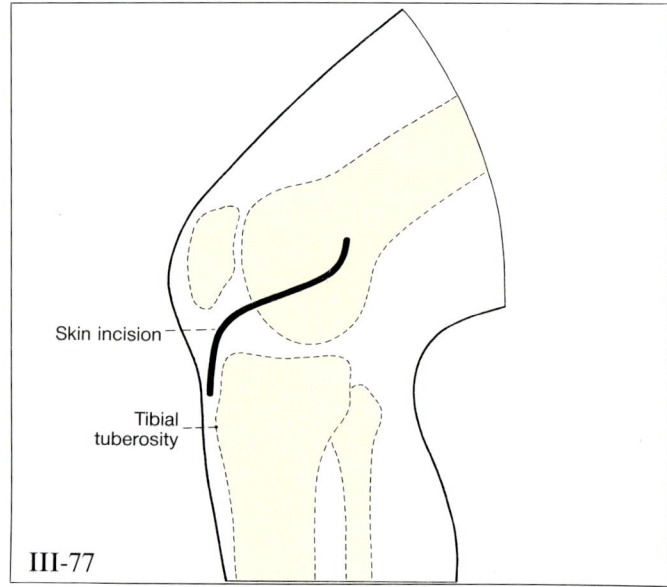

III-77

Posteromedial Exposure (1)

Indications

1. Removal of loose bodies from the posterior compartment of the knee joint
2. Resection of the posterior horn of the medial meniscus

Operative Steps

1. Make a 3- to 4-cm longitudinal incision on the inside the knee joint, forward and distally, from a point dorsal to the femoral epicondyle to the medial tibial condyle (Fig. III-78).
2. Reflect the skin to expose the joint capsule.
3. Incise and reflect the joint capsule to bring into view the dorsomedial compartment of the knee joint (Fig. III-79).

Note

The infrapatellar branch of the saphenous nerve should be closely watched.

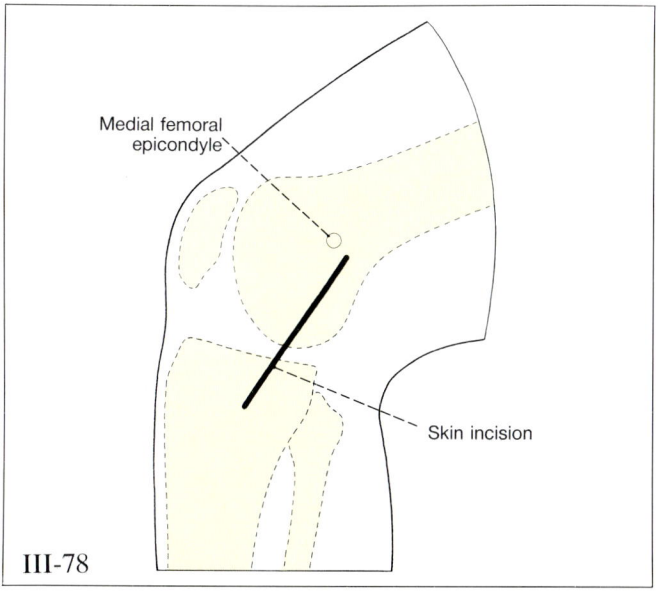

III-78

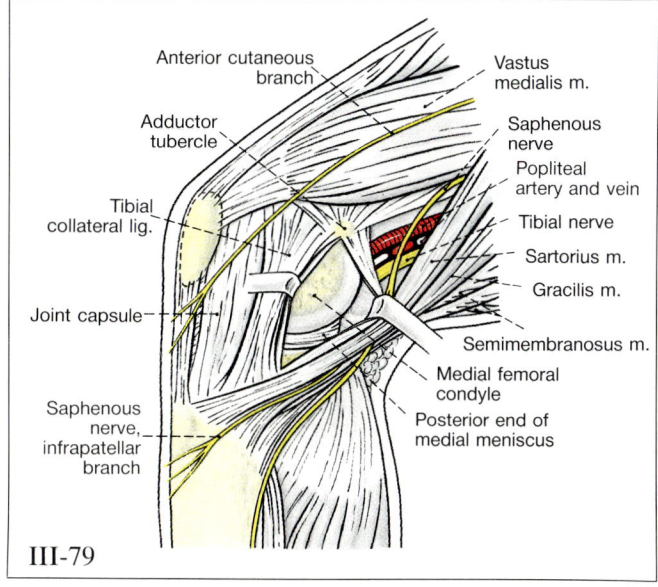

III-79

Anteromedial Exposure
Short Medial *Payr* Incision or
Long Medial *Payr* Incision

Indications

1. Synovectomy of the knee joint
2. Removal of the medial meniscus
3. Exploration of arthrosis deformans
4. Arthrodesis of the knee joint
5. Arthroplasty
6. Endoprosthetics

Operative Steps

1. Make an approximately 12-cm-long curved incision along the medial edge of the quadriceps tendon, beginning about 7 cm above the patella and continuing distally to the medial border of the tibial tuberosity (Fig. III-80, short *Payr* incision).
2. Alternatively, for an augmented exposure use the long incision (Fig. III-81, long *Payr* incision).
3. Reflect the skin.

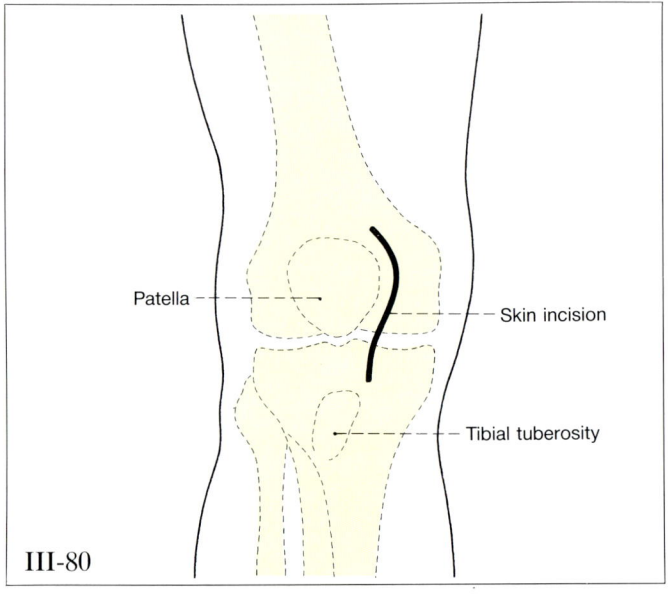

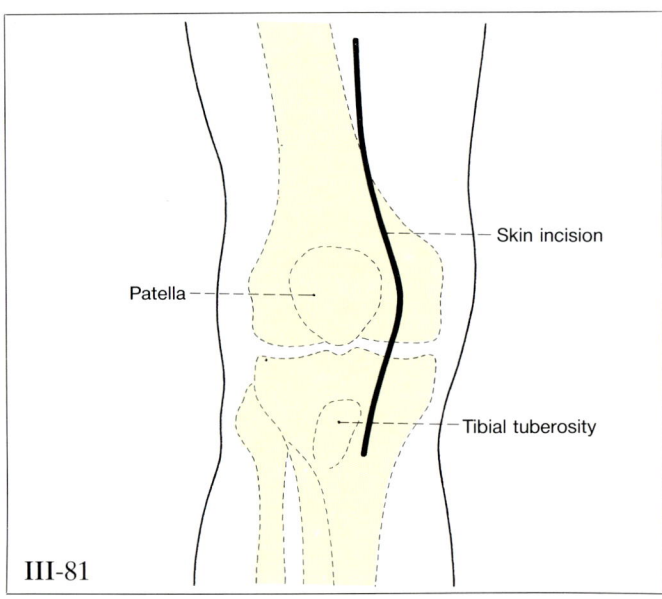

4. Separate the vastus medialis muscle from the quadriceps tendon (Fig. III-82).
5. Cut through the capsule and the synovial membrane 1.5 cm away from the medial border of the patella and the patellar ligament.
6. Flex the knee at a right angle and displace the patella to the outside (Fig. III-83).
7. This affords a good overview of the distal end of the femur, the cruciate ligaments, the menisci, and the articular surfaces of the patella (Fig. III-83).
8. Close the wound with the knee joint extended.

Notes

1. This is a commonly used exposure.
2. Portions of the incision can be used for a limited exposure or an inspection of the knee joint and may be augmented as needed.
3. An laternative longitudinal incision directly over the patella is also feasible. This prevents injury to the infrapatellar branch of the saphenous nerve.
4. Two parapatellar incisions are frequently preferred for synovectomy (Fig. III-84).

Medial Parapatellar Exposure and Lateral Parapatellar Exposure

Indication

Synovectomy

Operative Steps

1. Make approximately 8-cm-long curved medial and lateral parapatellar longitudinal incisions 1.5 cm away from the respective patellar borders, converging slightly at their proximal ends (Fig. III-84).
2. Make corresponding incisions in the outer joint capsule. The broad tendon of the vastus medialis is only partly cut, i.e., the proximal portion is only undermined.

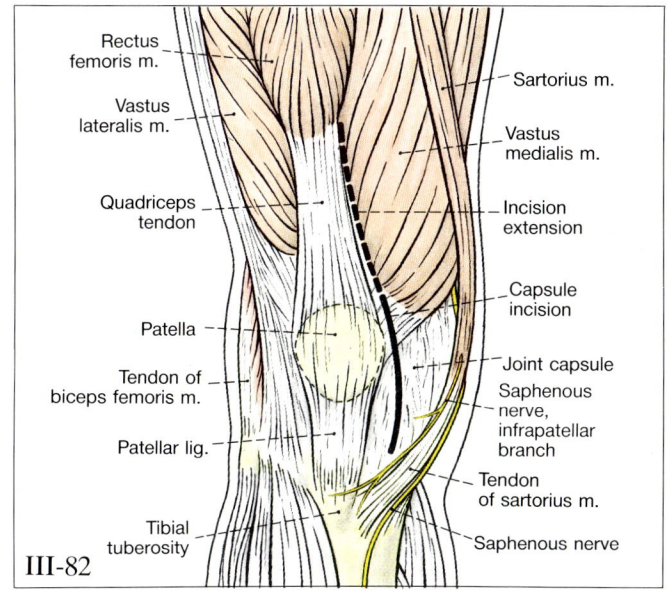

III-82

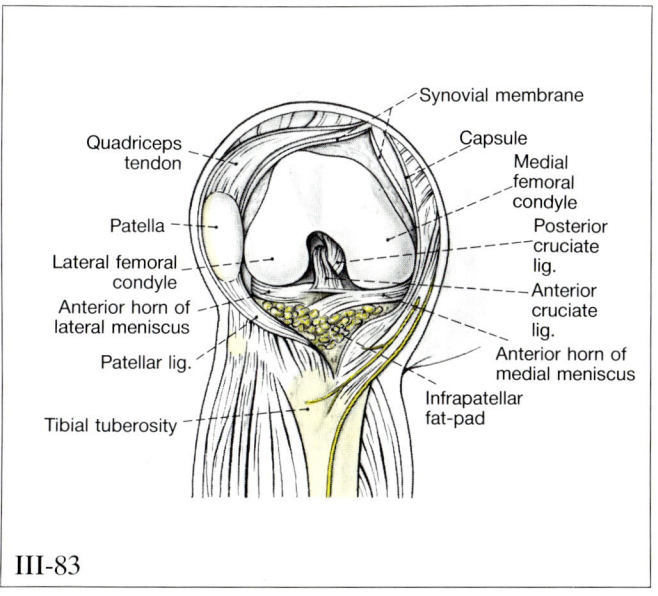

III-83

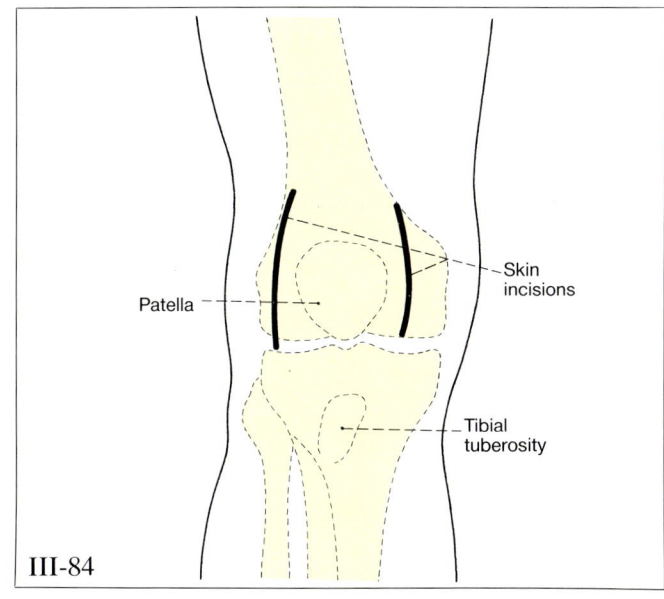

III-84

Knee Joint

Anteromedial Exposure of Coonse-Adams

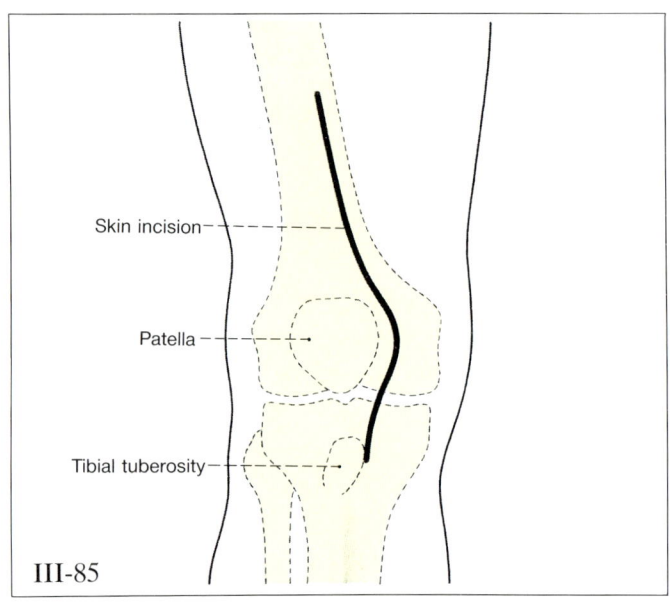

III-85

Indications

1. Synovectomy and exploration of joint
2. Arthroplasty

Operative Steps

1. Make a 15- to 18-cm curved skin incision, beginning at the medial border of the quadriceps tendon about 8 cm above the patella. Continue the incision around the medial border of the patella to the inner margin of the tibial tuberosity (Fig. III-85).
2. Remove the skin from the patella.
3. Split the quadriceps tendon down the middle, beginning at the muscle-tendon junction.
4. At a point about 1.5 cm above the upper pole of the patella, continue the incision on the medial and lateral sides of the patella and distally along the sides of the patellar ligament (Fig. III-86).
5. Reflect the patella and the patellar ligament downward (Fig. III-87).
6. Reflect the capsule medially and laterally to expose the distal end of the femur.
7. Flexion of the knee affords a good overview of the distal end of the femur, the knee joint, the menisci, and the ligaments.

Note

The exposure is not practical and has been generally abandoned.

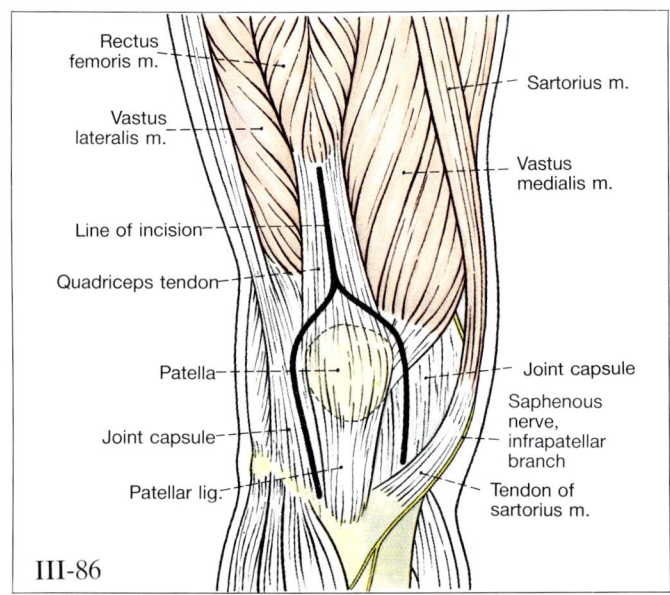

III-86

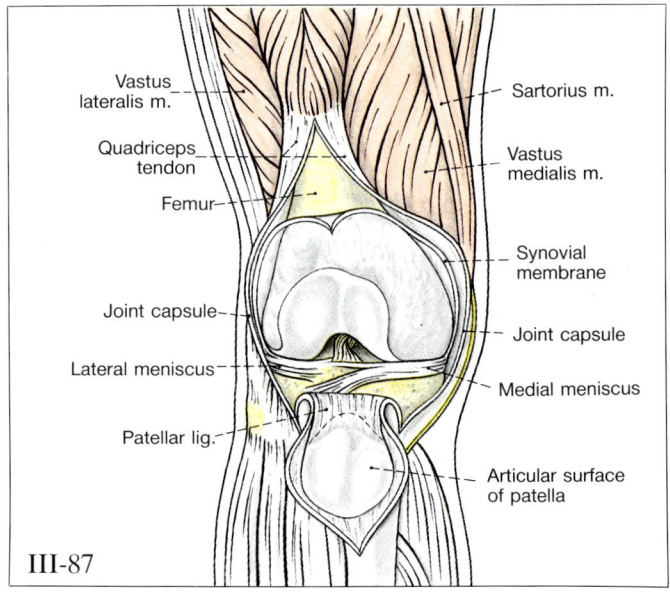

III-87

Anterior Curved Incision

Textor Incision

Indications

1. Patellar fractures
2. Arthroplasty
3. Insertion of knee prosthesis

Operative Steps

1. Make a U-shaped, distally convex skin incision, beginning at the medial femoral condyle. Cross the midline at the level of the tibial tuberosity and continue the incision to the lateral femoral condyle (Fig. III-88).
2. Retract the skin proximally to expose the patella, the patellar ligament, and the anterior aspect of the joint capsule.

Notes

1. For arthroplasty of the knee joint, the incision of the capsule and the patellar ligament corresponds to the skin incision.
2. This line of incision (*Textor* incision) may be rejected in favor of the anteromedial (*Payr* incision) or the anterolateral approach.

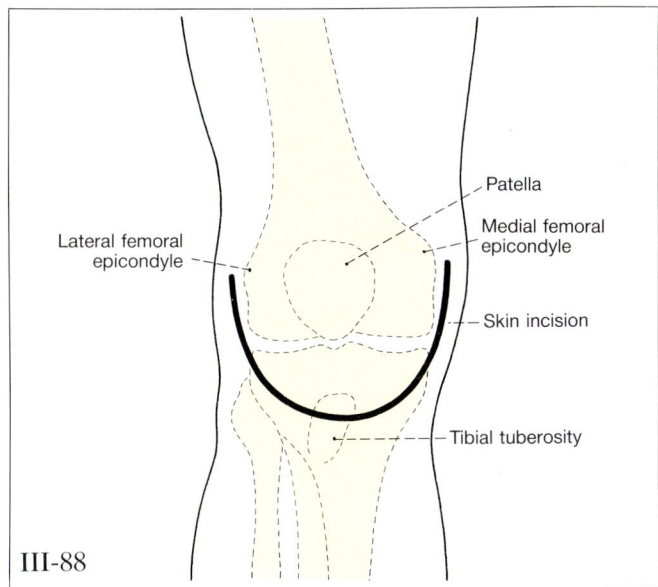

III-88

Anterolateral Exposure
Short Anterolateral Incision or Long Anterolateral Incision

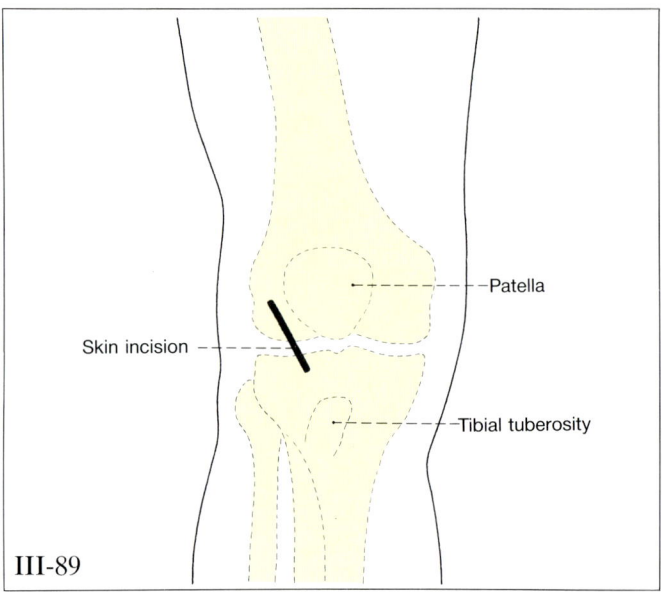

III-89

Indications
1. Removal of loose joint bodies
2. Excision of the lateral meniscus
3. Genu varum endoprosthetics

Operative Steps
1. Begin an approximately 5-cm-long, slightly oblique longitudinal incision 2–4 cm away from the lateral margin of the patella. Continue the incision distally and medially to the lateral margin of the patellar ligament (Fig. III-89, short anterolateral incision).
2. As an alternative for an augmented exposure, begin the incision over the vastus lateralis muscle, about 5 cm above and lateral to the upper edge of the patella, and carry it distally and medially to the inferior limit of the tibial tuberosity (Fig. III-90, long anterolateral incision).
3. Or: Make a longitudinal incision over the vastus lateralis muscle from a point about 1.5 cm above and lateral to the upper edge of the patella. Continue distally in a straight line, ending approximately 1.5 cm below the tibial tuberosity (Fig. III-91).

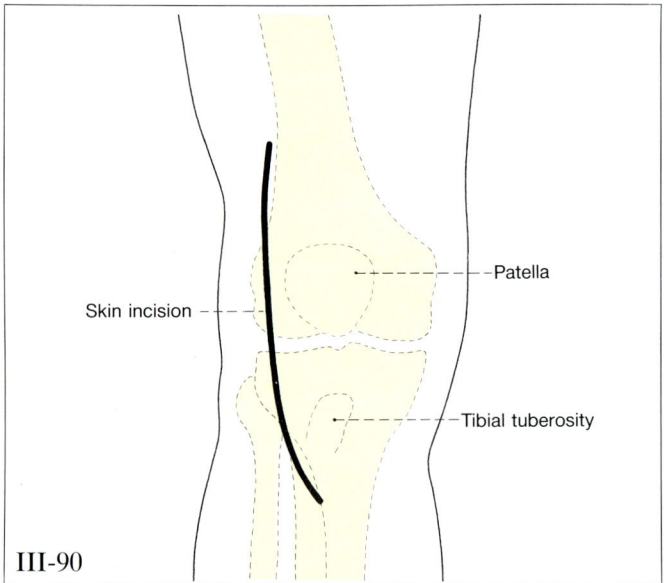

III-90

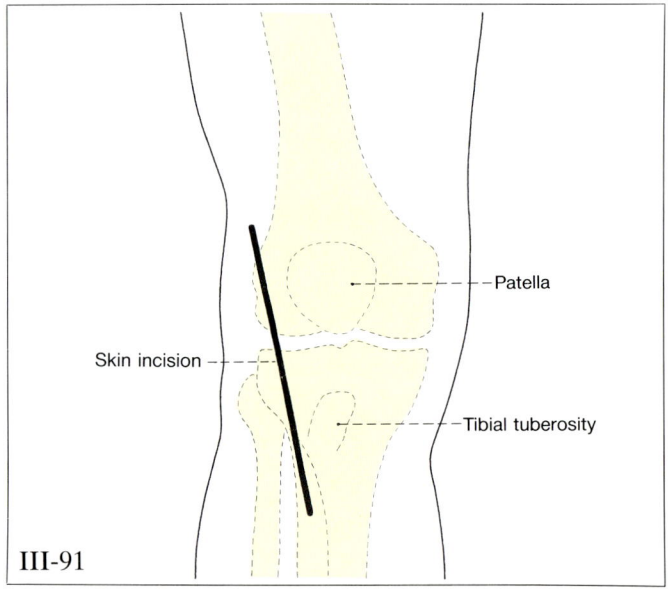

III-91

Knee Joint — Anterolateral Exposure

4. Incise the joint capsule and the synovial membrane in the same direction as the skin, about 1.5 cm lateral to the edge of the patella (Fig. III-92).
5. Flex the knee at a right angle.
6. Retract the capsule and the tibialis anterior muscle laterally, and the patella and the patellar ligament medially. This brings into view the lateral femoral condyle and the lateral meniscus, as well as the proximal and lateral aspect of the tibia (Fig. III-93).

Notes

1. The short anterolateral line of incision can be considered the standard approach, e.g., for removal of the lateral meniscus.
2. Frequently, only the upper portion of the long anterolateral incision will be sufficient for adequate exposure.
3. The curved long incision is also designated as a lateral *Payr* incision (Fig. III-90).
4. The lateral inferior genicular artery, which runs parallel to the lower border of the lateral meniscus, can be severed when using these incisions. One must make certain that it is ligated or cauterized during wound closure.
5a. Exploration of the menisicus is best achieved in the "hanging knee" position, because the joint can be opened so readily.
5b. The leg support on the operating table is then removed.
5c. It is important that the popliteal fossa remains unobstructed. This implies that the end of the thigh does not merely overlie the edge of the table but extends beyond it. The posterior aspect of the capsule is therefore free and the popliteal artery will not be compressed or injured during the operation.

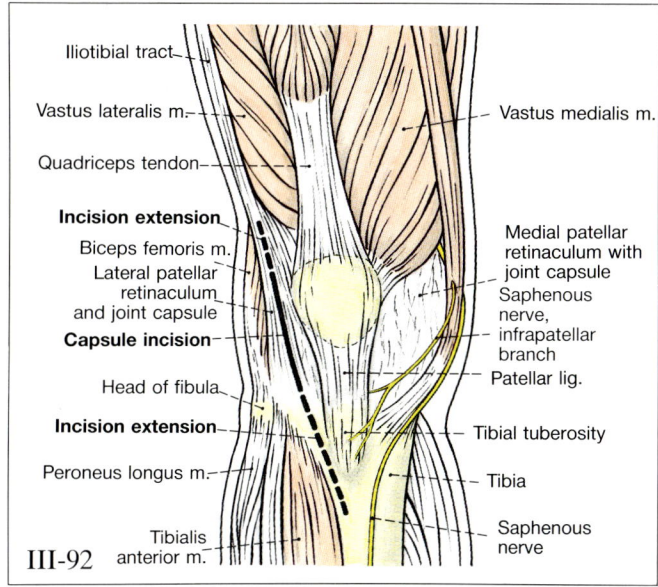

III-92

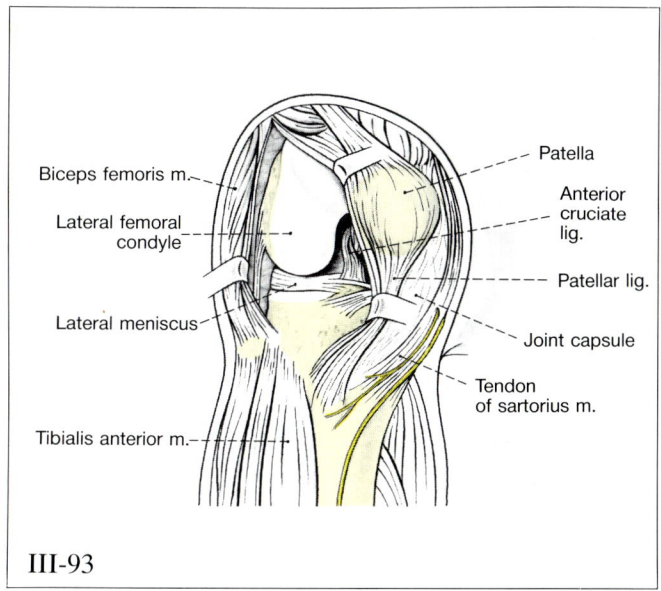

III-93

Knee Joint — Lateral Exposure

Lateral Exposure
Transverse Incision

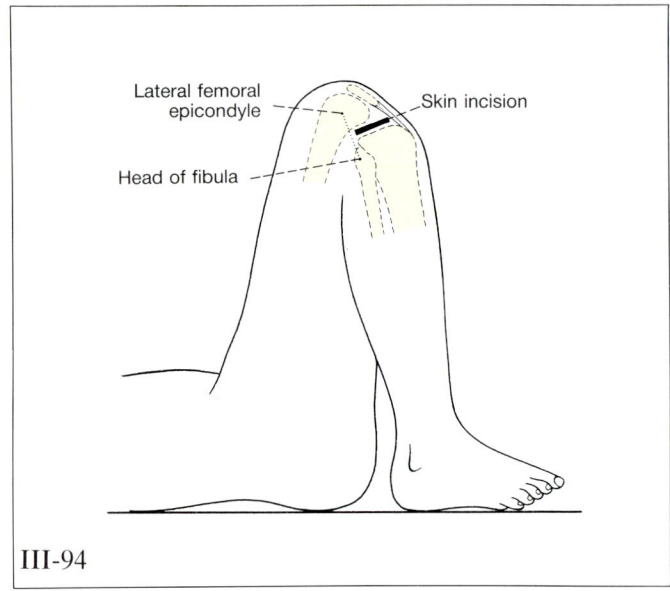

III-94

Indications

1. Removal of the lateral meniscus
2. Removal of loose bodies from the lateral compartment of the knee joint

Operative Steps

1. Position the knee fully flexed with the foot on the table and the heel against the buttock.
2. Make a skin incision on the lateral side of the knee joint 0.5 cm above the surface of the tibial condyle from the lateral margin of the patellar ligament to the anterior border of the fibular collateral ligament (Fig. III-94).
3. Reflect the skin to expose the fibers of the iliotibial tract. These fibers run almost parallel to the skin incision and the joint line.
4. The incision in the dorsal half of the fascia must be done with special care because it is made directly over the stretched collateral ligament (Fig. III-95).
5. Reflect the incised fascia to bring into view the lateral meniscus as well as the lateral inferior genicular artery, which runs just distal and parallel to the lateral meniscus (Fig. III-96).
6. Extend the knee joint after removal of the lateral meniscus. This facilitates suturing of the split fascia.

Notes

1. The line of incision is particularly well adapted for exposure of the lateral components of the knee joint.
2. It is reemphasized that this exposure is facilitated by maintaining the knee joint in full flexion with the foot on the table and the heel placed up against the buttock.
3. If the lateral inferior genicular artery should be accidentally cut, the ends must be ligated or cauterized to prevent a hemarthrosis.

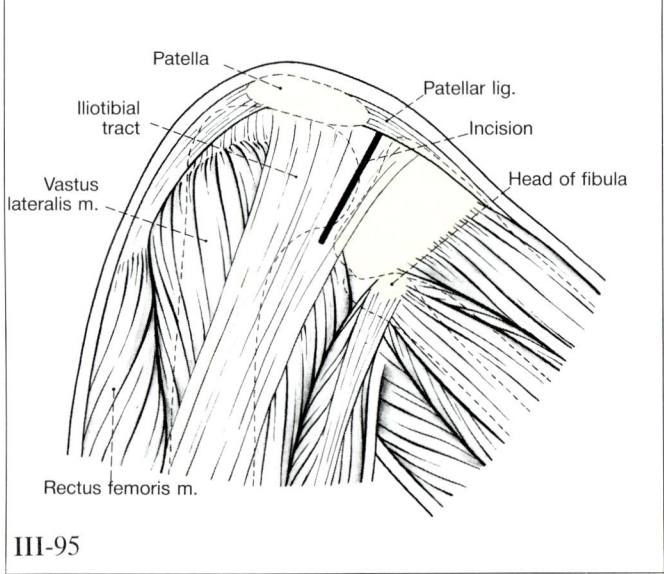

III-95

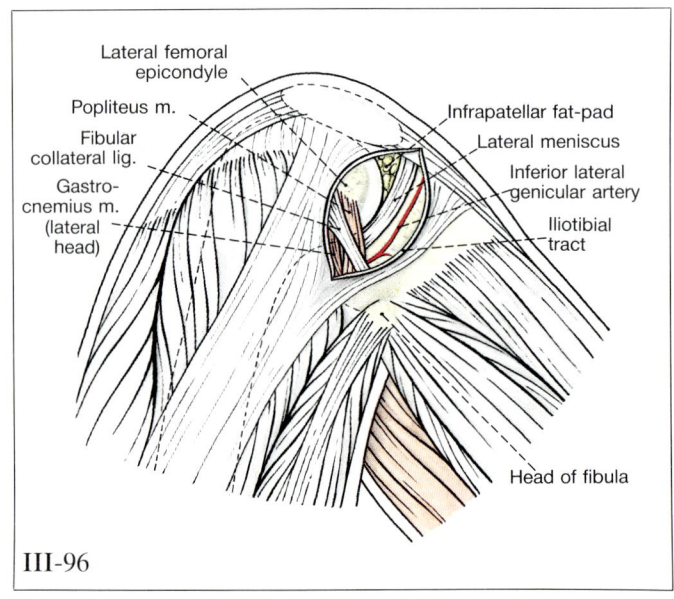

III-96

Knee Joint — Posterolateral Exposure

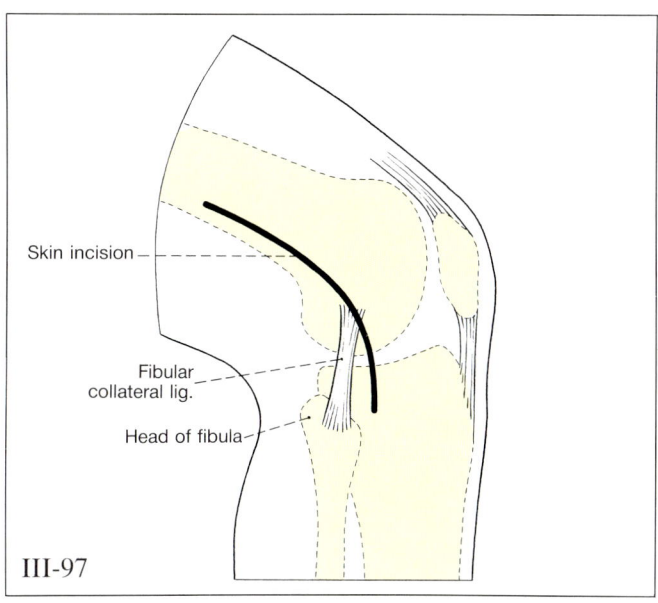

III-97

Posterolateral Exposure

Indications

1. Loose bodies in the posterior compartment of the knee joint.
2. Removal of the posterior horn of the lateral meniscus.

Operative Steps

1. Make an approximately 8-cm-long longitudinal incision on the lateral side of the knee joint in front of the head of the fibula and the biceps tendon (Fig. III-97).
2. Continue the incision through the iliotibial tract (Fig. III-98).
3. Incise the capsule in a longitudinal direction behind the lateral collateral ligament, which can be readily palpated by flexing and adducting the leg.
4. Reflect one part of the capsule forward and the other part, with the biceps femoris muscle, dorsally. This exposes the posterolateral aspect of the knee joint (Fig. III-99).

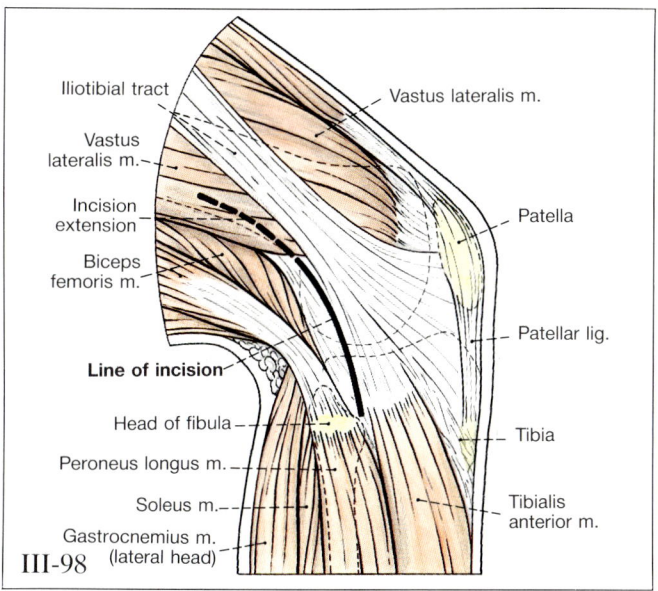

III-98

Notes

1. When opening the capsule, the tendon of the popliteus muscle is in jeopardy because of its intimate topographical relationship. It should be displaced forward.
2. The common peroneal nerve runs behind the biceps tendon, so it is only exposed during an extensive exploration.
3. Injury to the lateral inferior genicular artery should be considered a possibility since it runs immediately below the margin of the lateral meniscus.
4. By extending the skin incision and making a separate oblique anterior incision in the capsule, it is possible to expose simultaneously the anterior horn of the lateral meniscus.

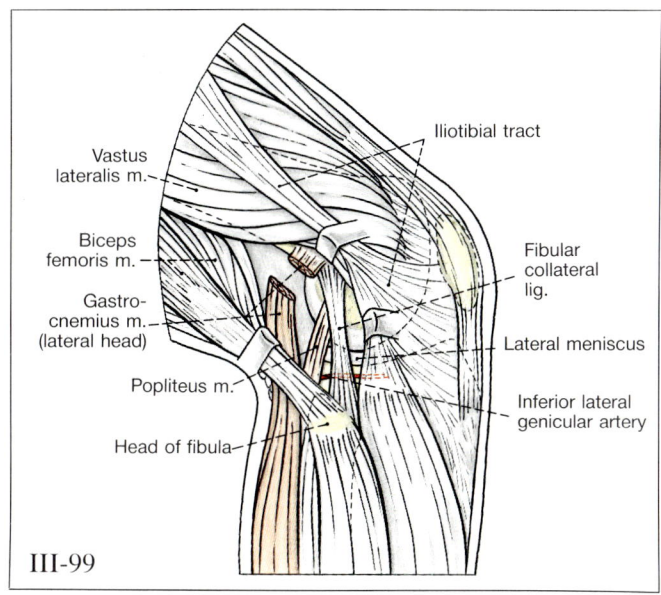

III-99

Alternative Anteroposterior Exposure from Lateral Side

The anteroposterior line of incision is useful in an extensive lateral exploration of the joint (Fig. III-100).

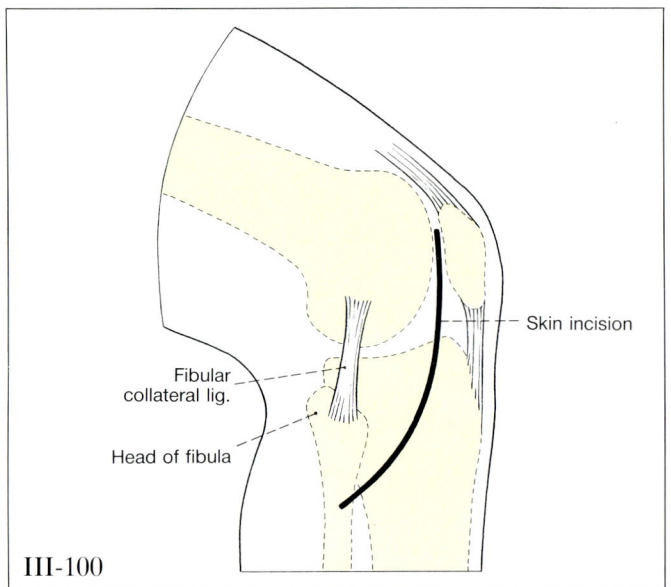

Posteromedial Exposure (2)

Indications

1. Removal of loose bodies from the dorsomedial compartment of the knee joint.
2. Removal of tumors from the distal portion of the medial femoral condyle.

Operative Steps

1. Make a 10-cm longitudinal incision over the medial side of the popliteal fossa (Fig. III-101). The midpoint of the incision is approximately at the level of the joint line.

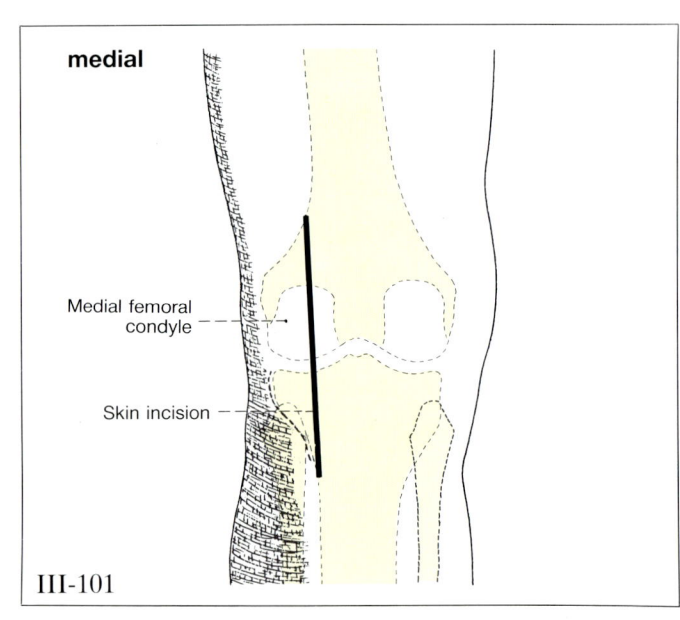

Knee Joint — Posteromedial Exposure

2. As an alternative, make a bayonet-shaped incision (Fig. III-102).
3. Cut through the subcutaneous fascia.
4. With blunt dissection, develop the space between the semitendinosus and the medial head of the gastrocnemius muscles (Fig. III-103).
5. Displace the semitendinosus muscle to the medial (tibial) side and the gastrocnemius muscle to the lateral (fibular) side. This exposes the capsule over the medial femoral condyle.
6. Incise the capsule in a longitudinal direction down to the popliteus muscle (Fig. III-104).
7. Incise the synovial membrane to expose the medial femoral condyle, the posterior horn of the medial meniscus, and the dorsal part of the head of the tibia.

Note

Although this approach to the dorsomedial structures of the knee joint is not frequently chosen, it is nevertheless a good one because no important nerves or arteries enter the operative field.

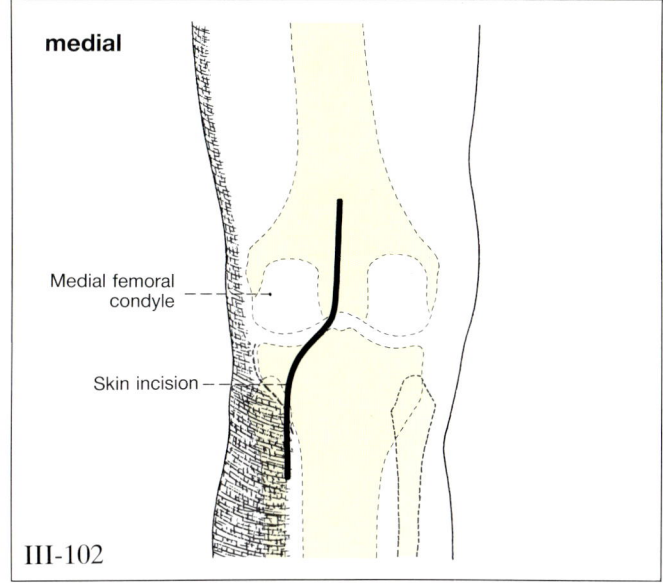
III-102

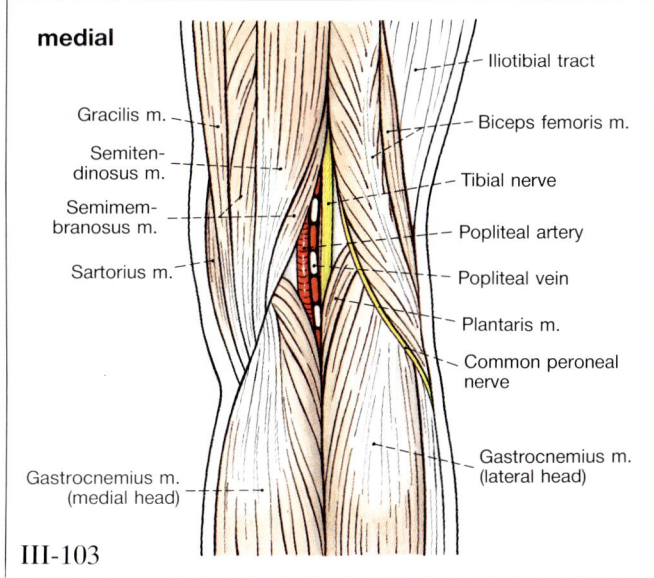
III-103

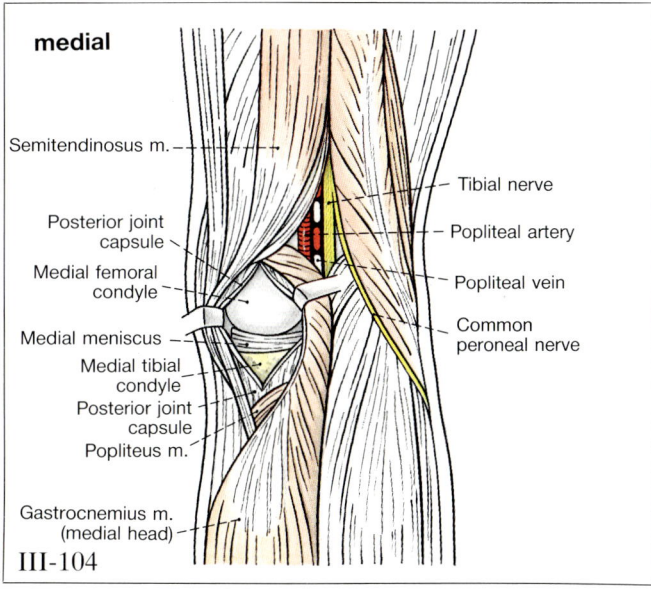
III-104

Knee Joint — Posterocentral Exposure/Safe Zone of Distal Femur

Posterocentral Exposure

Indications

1. Exploration of the neurovascular bundle
2. Excision of Baker's cyst
3. Exploration of the attachment of the posterior cruciate ligament

Operative Steps

1. Make a transverse incision along the flexor fold of the popliteal region (with the ends turning in a longitudinal direction) (Fig. III-105).
2. The incision is suitable for exploration of various structures in the popliteal fossa (Fig. III-103). A longitudinal incision has the disadvantage of eventually causing scar contracture.

Note

The medial sural cutaneous nerve (farther distally, the sural nerve) must be protected during exploration of the popliteal fossa. It is a branch of the tibial nerve and runs lateral to the lesser saphenous vein.

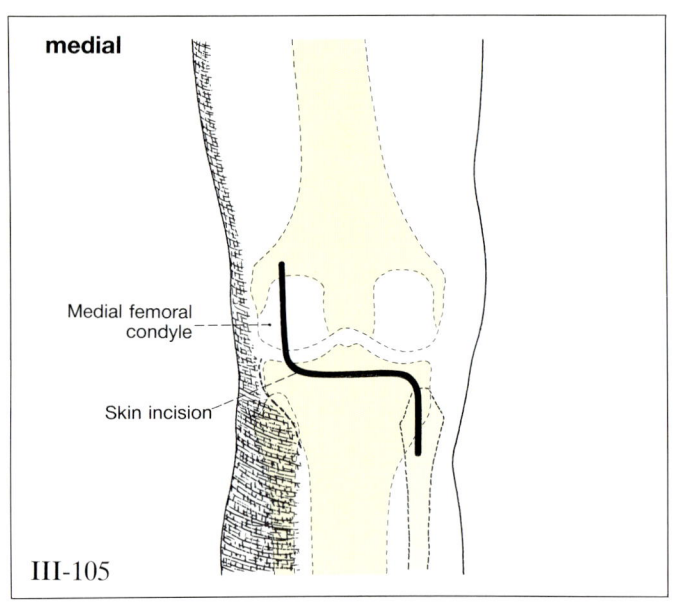

III-105

Safe Zone of the Distal Femur

To determine the safe zone at the distal end of the femur, draw a line dorsally from the upper pole of the patella to a point of intersection with a vertical line passing in front of the fibular head. The intersection indicates the safe zone in which Kirschner wires and Steimann nails can be attached (Fig. III-106).

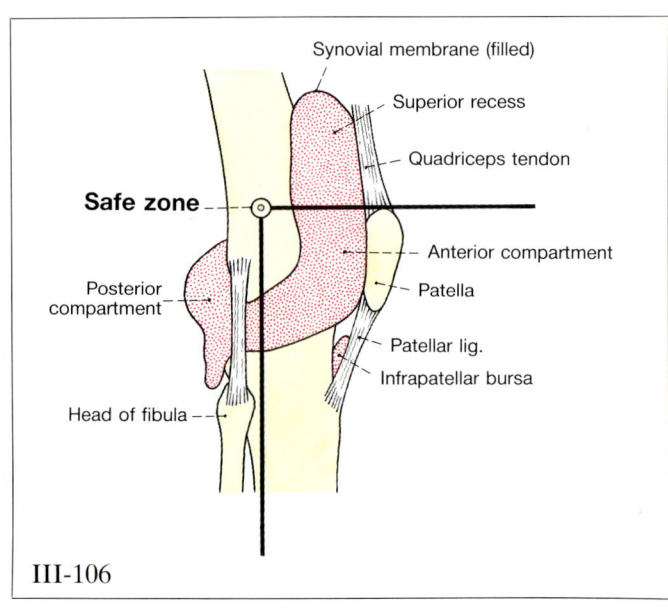

III-106

Head of Tibia with Knee Joint

Anterior Exposure

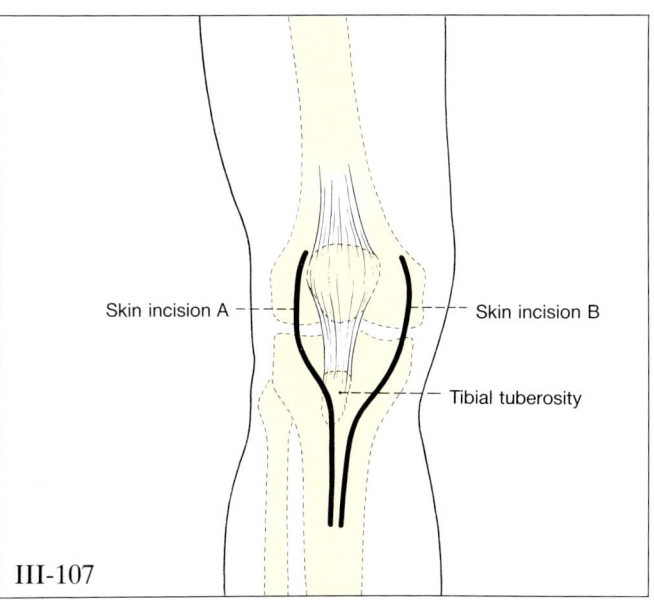

III-107

Indication

Fractures of head of tibia

Operative Steps

1. To expose the head of the tibia and explore the joint, choose the lateral skin incision A or the medial skin incision B in Fig. III-107.
2. The line of incision in Fig. III-108 makes possible an extensive exposure of the tibial head and the knee joint.
3. If necessary, the patellar ligament can be cut transversely or in a Z-shaped fashion and reflected proximally with the patella.
4. The star-shaped incision in Fig. III-109 for bilateral exposure of the tibial head and the joint is also available.

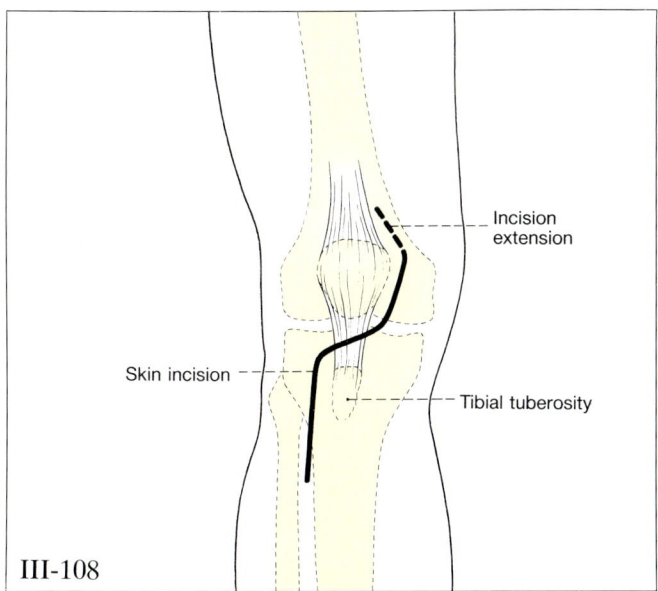

III-108

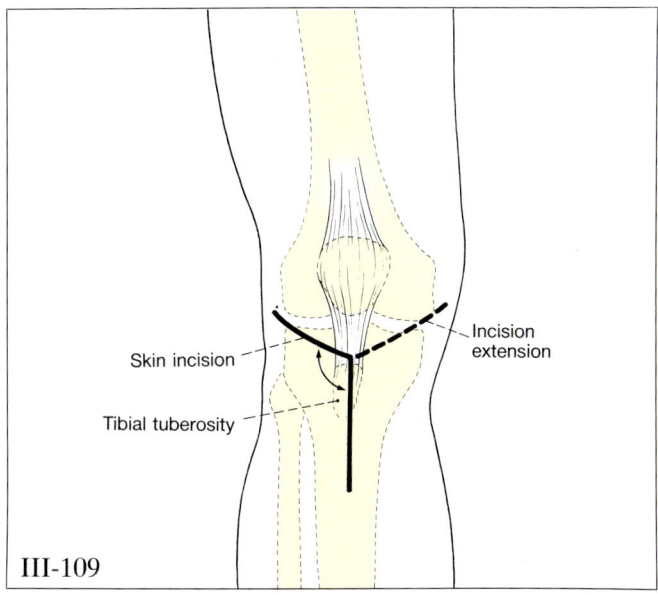

III-109

Head of Tibia

Anterior Exposure

Indications

1. High osteotomy of the tibia
2. Tumors and inflammatory processes

Operative Steps

1. Make a medial and/or a lateral oblique incision on the sides of the anterior aspect of the head of the tibia (Fig. III-110).
2. Expose and free the deep surface of the patellar ligament so it can be elevated.
3. Displace the soft tissues and the periosteum from the head of the tibia, on the back side with a curved rasp.
4. Detach the tibiofibular ligaments, too, if necessary.
5. Elevate and support the lower leg with a thickly folded cloth to permit posterior displacement of the soft popliteal tissues away from the operative field.

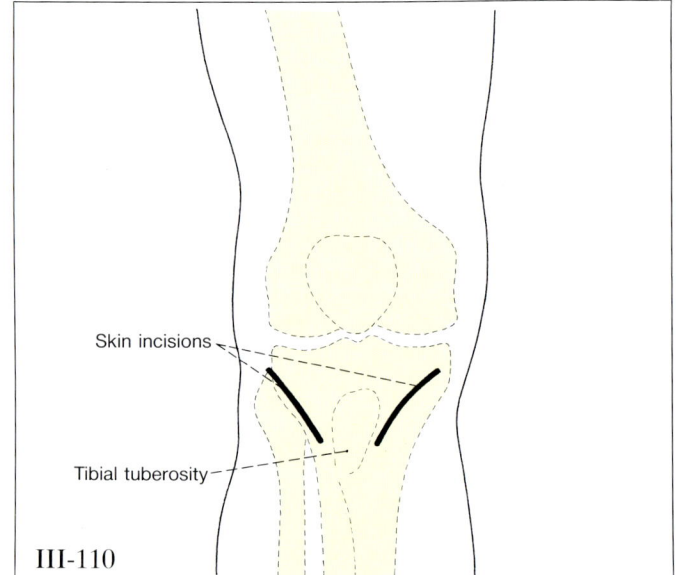

D. Leg

Tibia

Anterolateral Exposure

Anterior Exposure

Indications

1. Reduction and osteosynthesis of tibial fractures
2. Bone tumors
3. Osteotomy of tibia with osteosynthesis

Operative Steps

1. Begin a slightly curved, laterally convex skin incision below the tibial tuberosity and continue it distally to a point above the lower end of the tibia (Fig. III-111).
2. Reflect the skin flap medially.

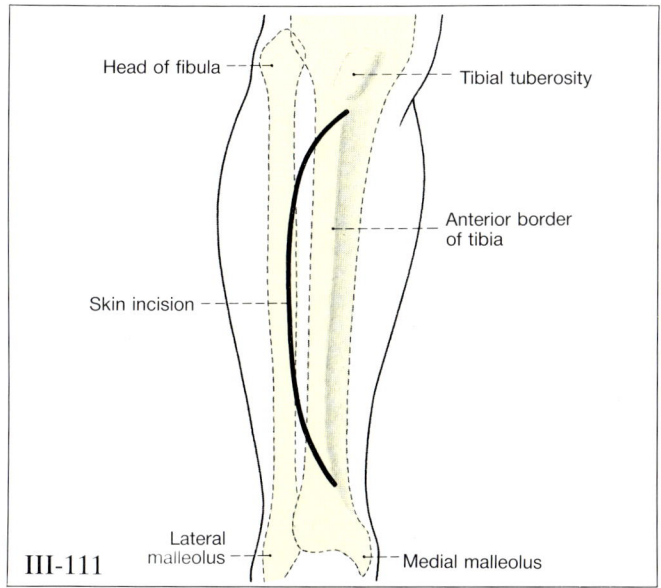

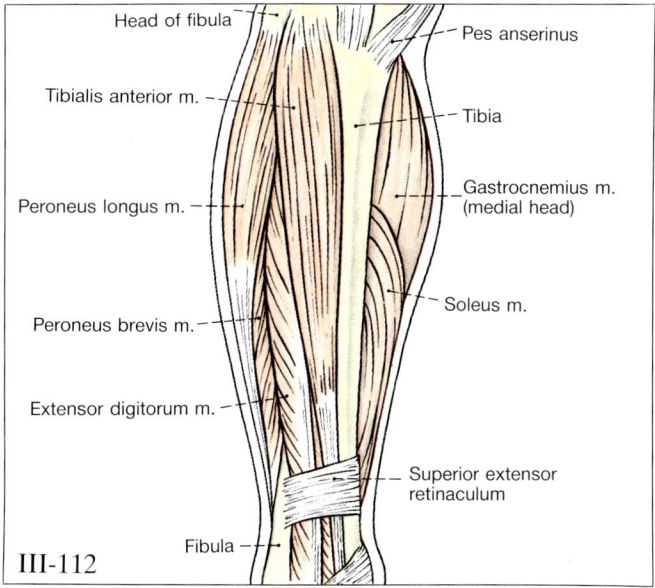

Tibia — Anterolateral Exposure

3. Retract the tibialis anterior muscle laterally to expose the lateral and medial aspects of the tibial shaft (Fig. III-113).
4. As an alternative, a straight incision parallel to and immediately lateral to the anterior tibial border may be chosen (Fig. III-114). An extension of the incision toward the medial malleolus is possible.
5. A schematic illustration of the anterolateral exposure is shown in a cross section of the leg (Fig. III-115).

Notes

1. This is a standard approach.
2. The position of the superficial peroneal nerve is variable. Not infrequently it is found lying against the fibula or it is embedded in muscle.

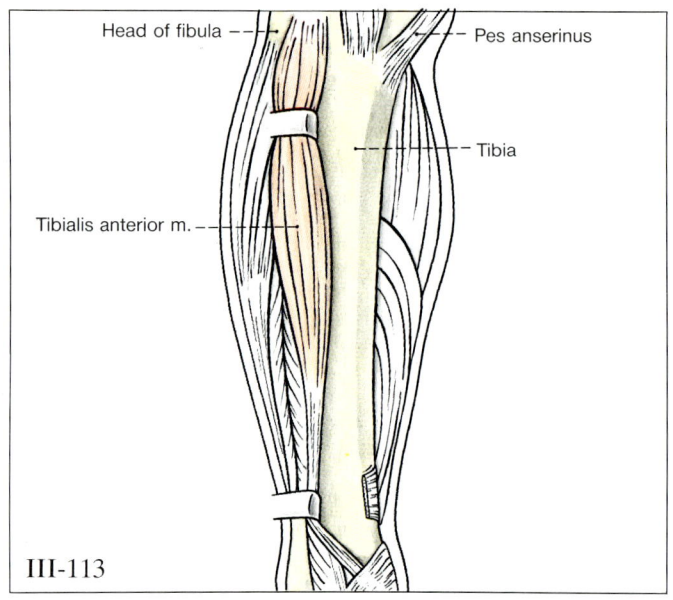

III-113

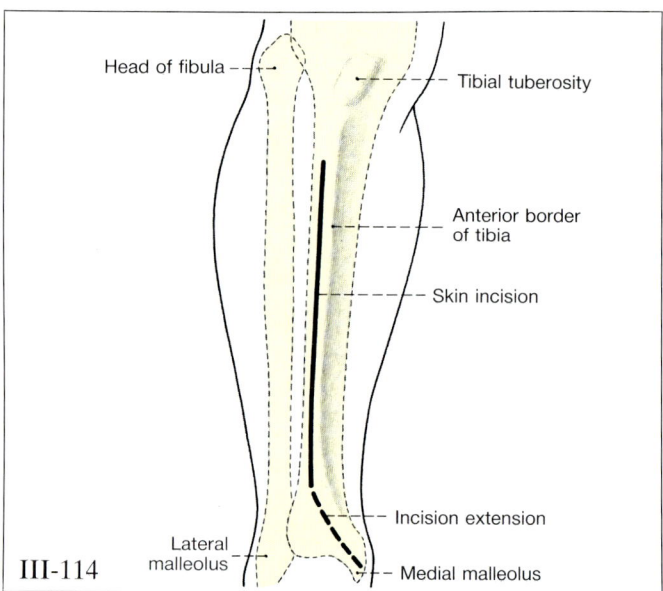

III-114

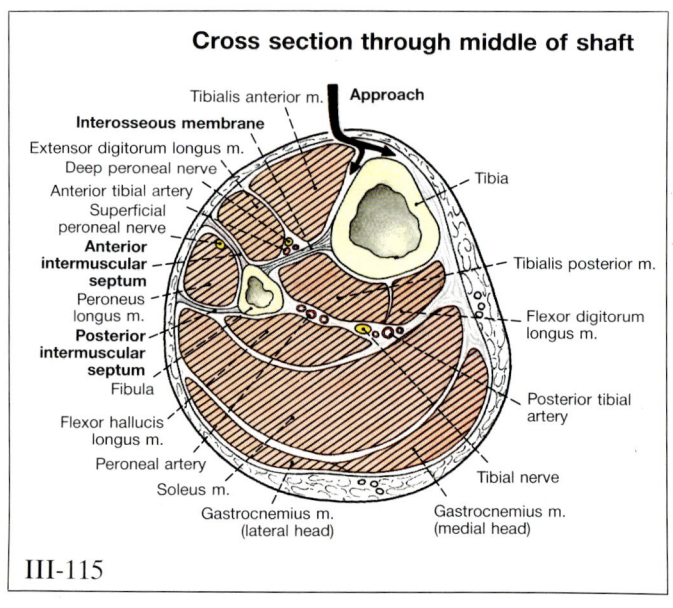

III-115

Medial Exposure

Indications

1. Reduction and osteosynthesis of tibial shaft fractures
2. Bone tumors
3. Corrective osteotomy of tibia with osteosynthesis

Operative Steps

1. Make a longitudinal incision over the middle of the medial surface of the tibia, if necessary, from the head of the tibia to the medial malleolus (Fig. III-116). The course of the infrapatellar branch of the saphenous nerve should be watched in the proximal part of the incision.

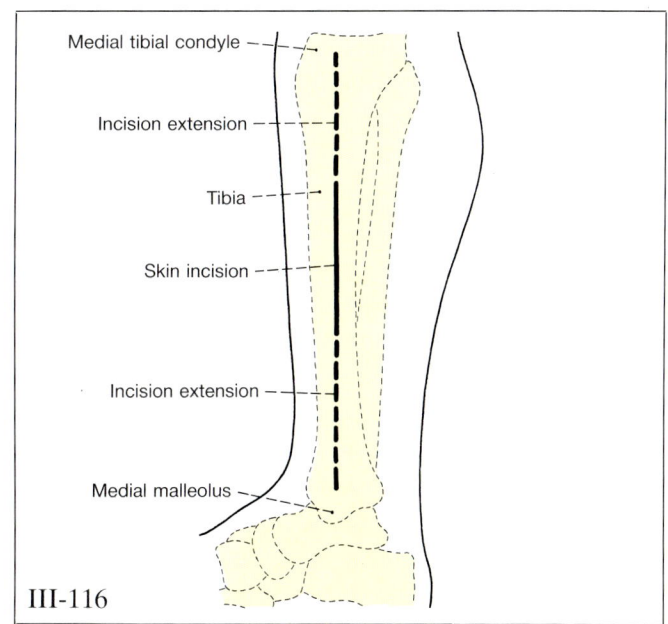

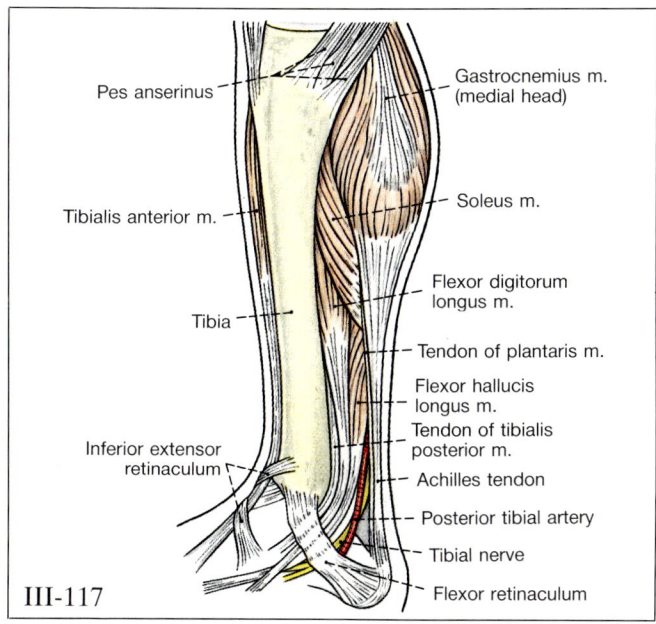

Tibia — Medial Exposure

2. Reflect the tibialis anterior muscle forward and the dorsal musculature toward the back to expose the medial and dorsal surfaces of the tibial shaft (Fig. III-118).
3. A schematic illustration of the exposure is seen in a cross section of the leg (Fig. III-119).

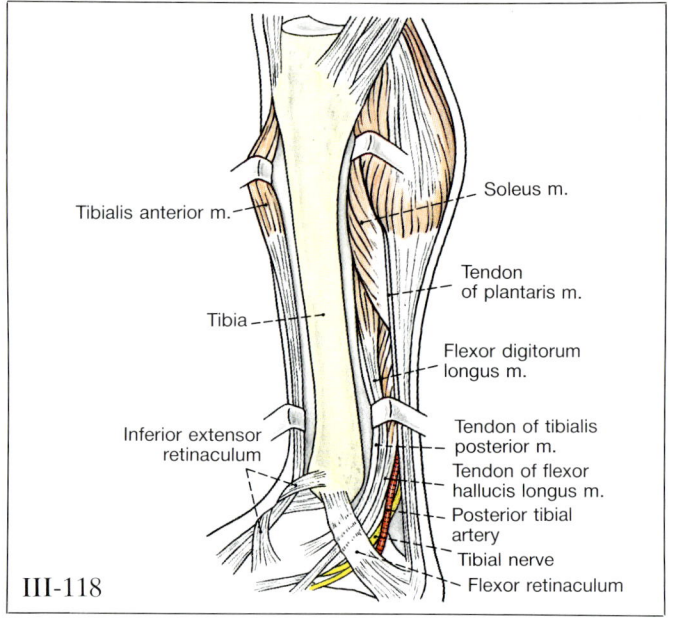

III-118

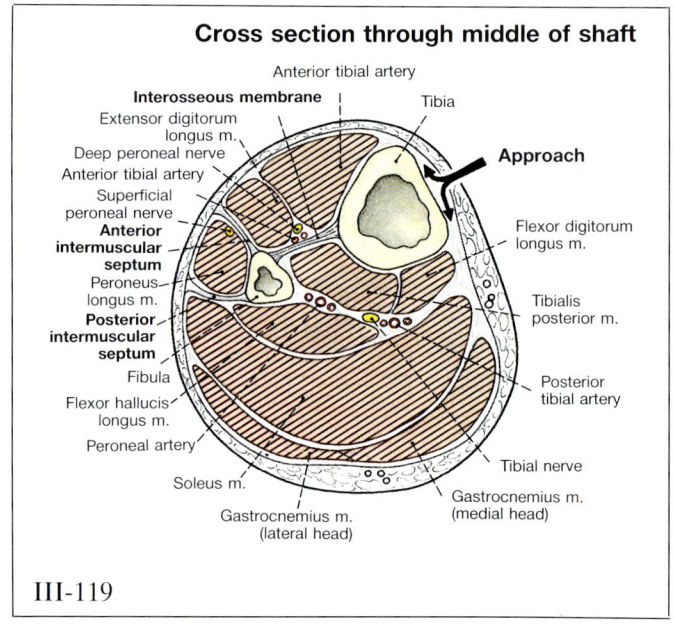

III-119

Posteromedial Exposure

Indication

Dorsal plate osteosynthesis in tibial shaft fractures

Operative Steps

1. Make a curved incision, slightly convex dorsally, on the inside of the leg. In the middle third, the incision reaches the midpoint of the leg's circumference (not that of the tibia) (Fig. III-120).
2. The posteromedial approach is indicated in the cross section of the leg in Fig. III-121.
3. The alternative approach in Fig. III-121 is primarily applicable to the proximal and distal ends of the incision.

Note

The posteromedial exposure is also called a mailbox approach because the soft tissues are elevated like a lid.

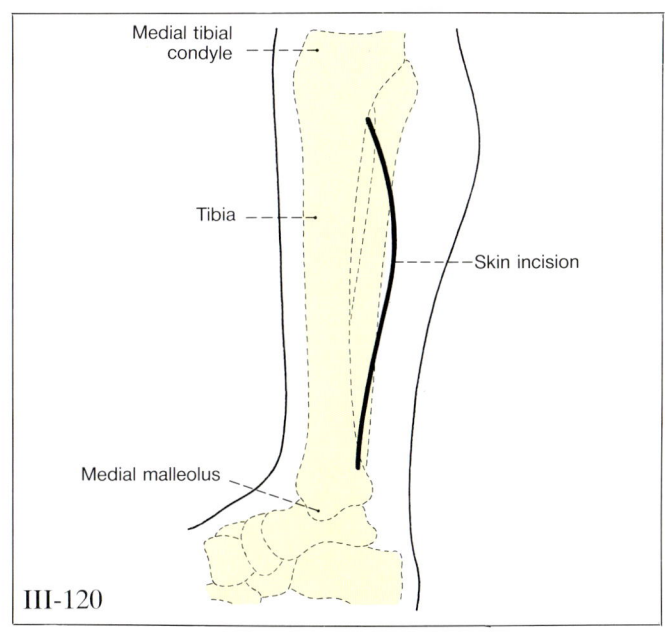

III-120

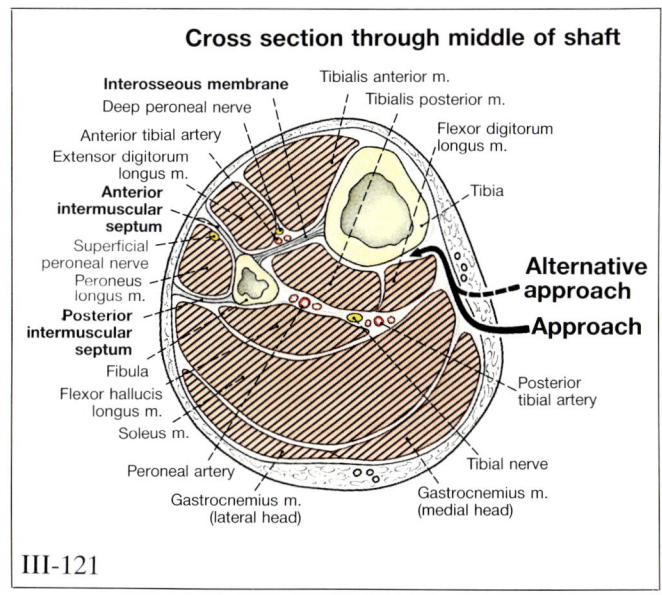

III-121

Fibula

Lateral Exposure

Indications

1. Fibular fractures
2. Inflammatory processes
3. Bone tumors
4. Resection of fibula
5. Exploration of the peroneal nerve

Operative Steps

1. Make a longitudinal incision along the dorsal margin of the fibula from just below the head of the fibula down to the lateral malleolus (Fig. III-122). Extensions of the incision are possible both proximally and distally (Fig. III-122).
2. Cut through the superficial and deep fasciae.
3. Expose the common peroneal nerve, which lies behind the tendon of the biceps femoris muscle in the upper portion of the incision, and retract it forward (Fig. III-124).
4. Separate that part of the peroneus longus muscle which attaches to the lateral surface of the head of the fibula and prevents displacement of the peroneal nerve anteriorly over the head (Fig. III-124).
5. Detach the soleus muscle from the fibula and reflect it backward.
6. Detach the peroneus brevis muscle from the fibula and reflect it forward with the peroneus longus muscle so that the shaft of the fibula is exposed.

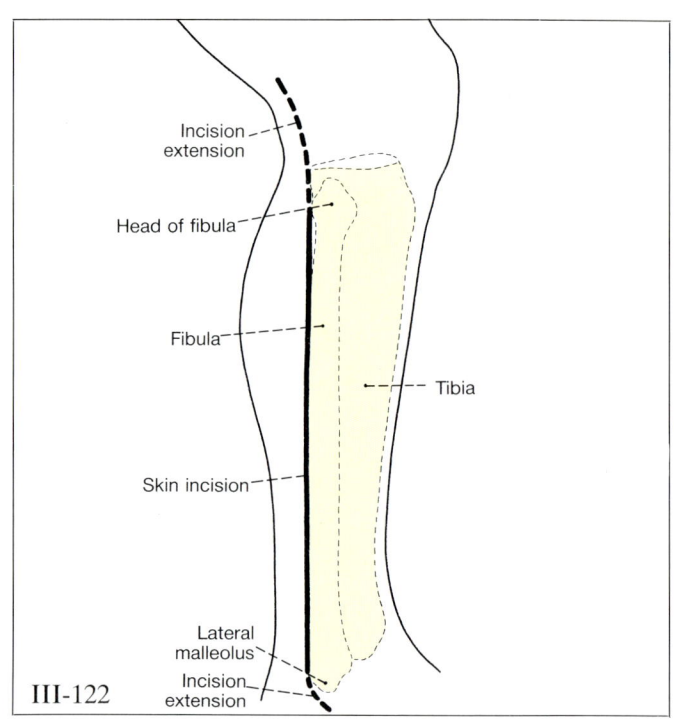

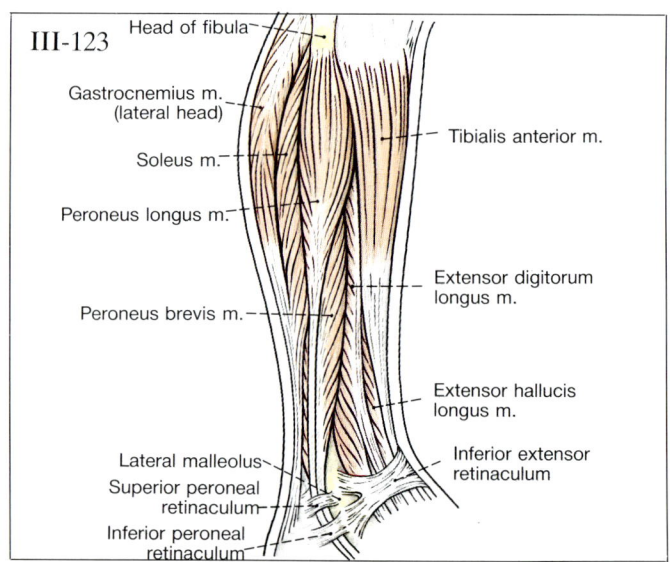

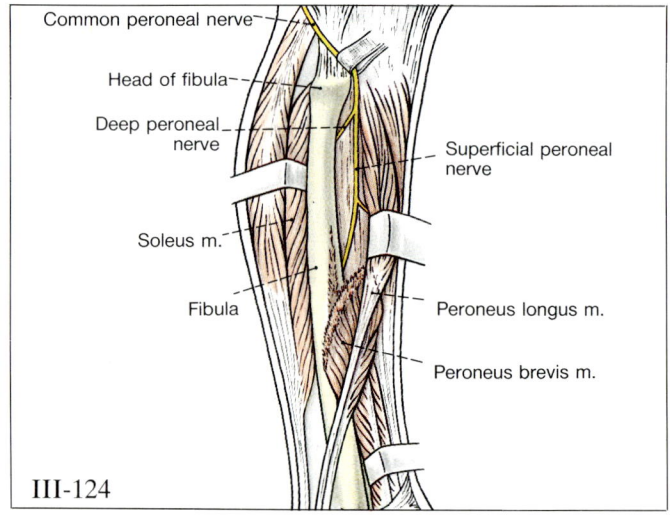

Fibula | Alternative Exposures

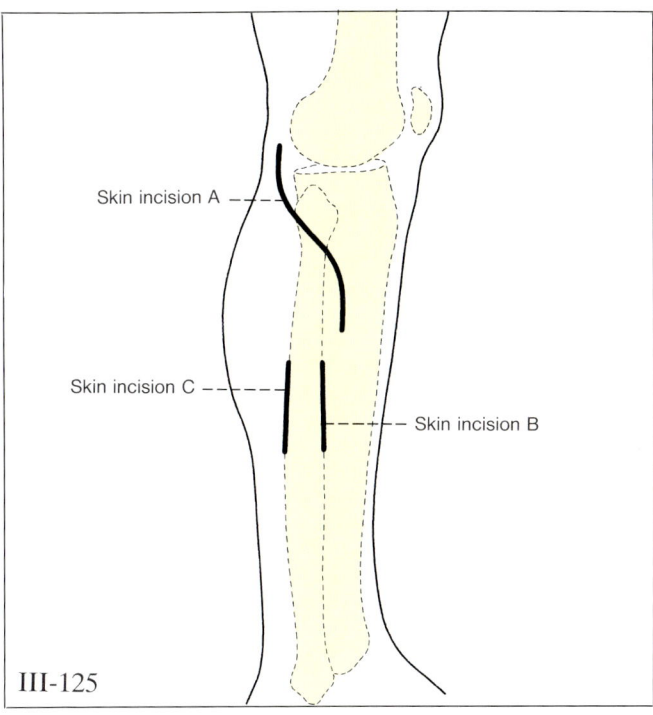

Alternative Exposures

1. Frequently, only portions of the incisions described under the lateral approach to the fibula are required, and these can be modified to fit the demands.
2. To expose the head of the fibula and the proximal third of its shaft, an S-shaped incision from dorsal to ventral is suitable (Fig. III-125, skin incision A). An augmented operative field requires the identification and exposure of the peroneal nerve. This begins in the area adjacent to the popliteal fossa.
3. A schematic illustration of the approach and of the critical structures is seen in a cross section of the leg at the level of the tibial tuberosity (Fig. III-126).
4. In the middle third of the fibula, the choice is between skin incision B and C (Fig. III-125). Skin incision C is preferred for fibular osteotomy.
5. The approach to the fibula is then blunt dissection between the ventral extensors and the peroneal musculature on one side and the dorsal calf musculature on the other side.
6. A schematic illustration of approach B and C is seen in cross section through the middle of the fibular shaft (Fig. III-127).

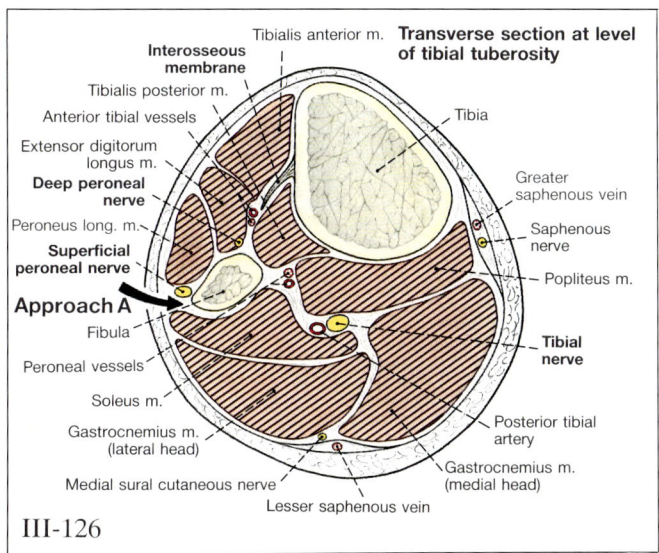

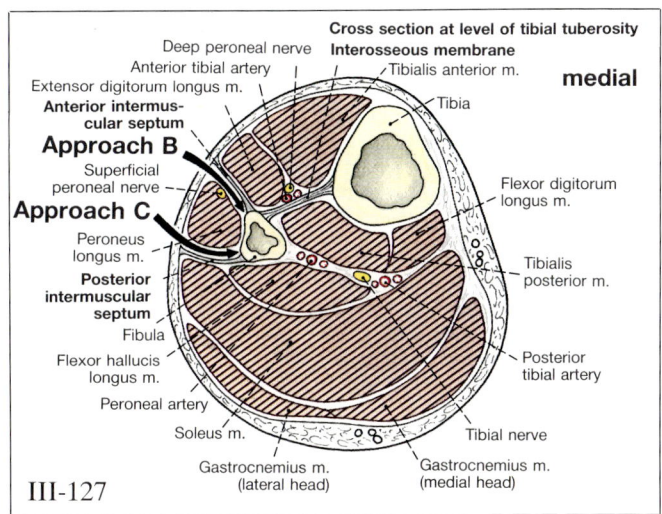

Fibula and Tibia

Lateral Exposure

Operative Steps

1. The exposure of both fibula and tibia is also possible with just one incision.
2. Make a lateral incision over the fibula as indicated in Fig. III-128.
3. Further development of the exposure along the anterior intermuscular septum is illustrated in the schematic cross section of the leg (Fig. III-129).

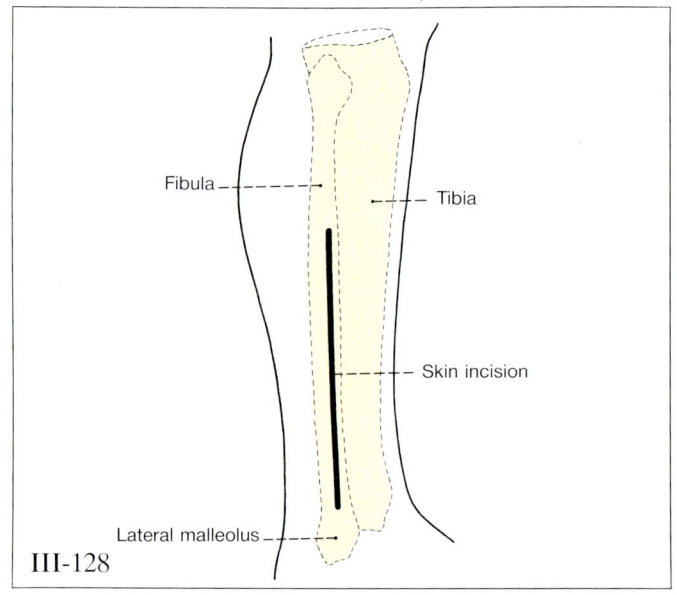

III-128

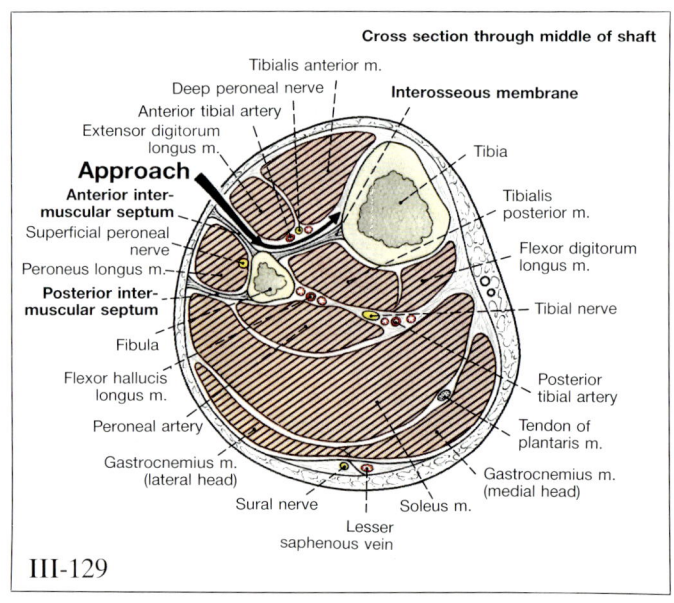

III-129

Leg Compartments

Anterolateral Exposure and Posteromedial Exposure

Indication

Compartment syndrome

Operative Steps

1. See Fig. III-130 (after *Lanz-Wachsmuth*) for an illustration of the four compartments of the leg formed by the connective tissue septa, the interosseous membrane, and the crural fasciae. Distinguish between: a) anterior compartment, b) lateral compartment, c) superficial posterior compartment, and d) deep posterior compartment.
2. Access to all compartments is possible through two lines of incision, as indicated in Fig. III-131. The anterior and lateral compartments are approached by splitting the fascia on the anterolateral aspect (approach A of Fig. III-131). Both posterior compartments are opened by a posteromedial incision (approach B of Fig. III-131).
3. As an alternative, the dorsal compartments can also be accessed through a posterolateral approach (see page 5; Fig. III-127), but dorsally to the posterior intermuscular septum.

Note

Frequently only the anterior compartment is opened. This is often inadequate.

---

* After J. Lanz, W. Wachsmuth: Bein und Statik. 2nd edition, Springer-Verlag, Berlin–Heidelberg–New York, 1972

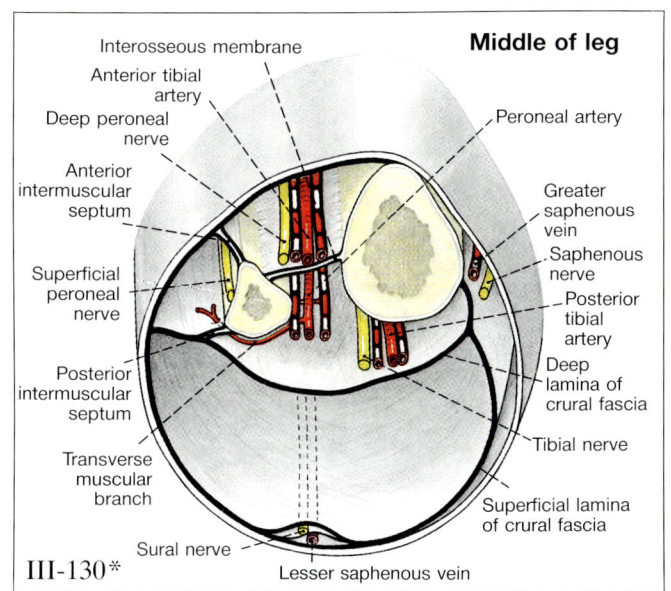

III-130*

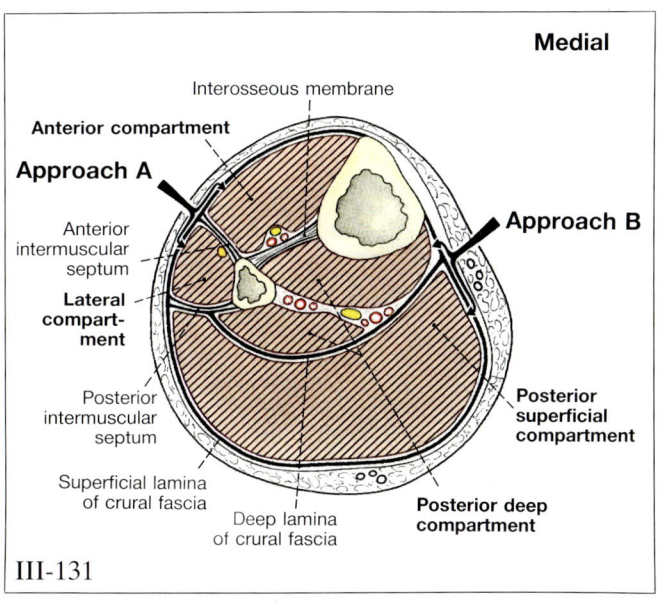

III-131

Plantaris Tendon

Posteromedial Exposure

Indication

Removal of the tendon of the plantaris muscle for use as a free tendon transplant.

Operative Steps

1. Make a short, straight incision along the medial border of the Achilles tendon behind the medial malleolus (Fig. III-132).
2. Split the superficial layer of the crural fascia and find the plantaris tendon immediately medial to or somewhat in front of the Achilles tendon (Fig. III-133).
3. By exerting peripheral traction on the plantaris tendon, its course can be palpated through the skin. Make short transverse incisions as indicated in Fig. III-132.
4. Alternatively, detach the plantaris tendon distally and follow it upward with a vein stripper. Proximally, it enters the calf musculature between the gastrocnemius and soleus muscles.

Note

The plantaris tendon is missing in about 7% of individuals.

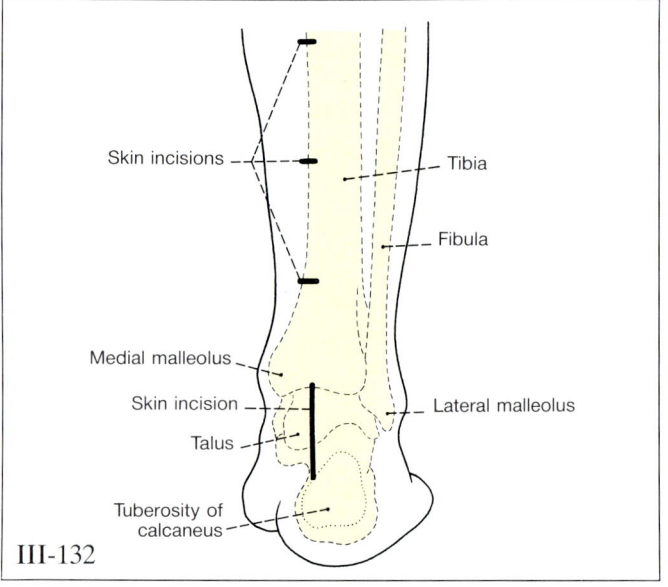

III-132

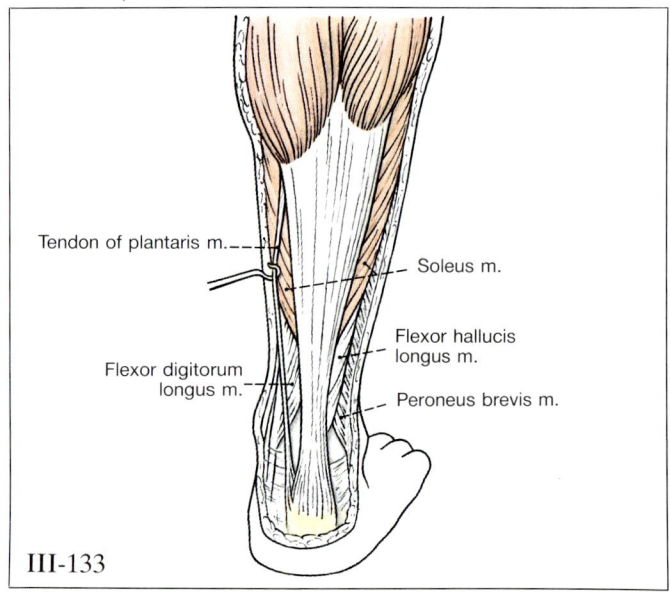

III-133

Sural Nerve/Achilles Tendon

Sural Nerve

Posterolateral Exposure

Indication

Removal of sural nerve for transplant purposes

Operative Steps

1. Expose and dissect free the sural nerve before it divides by making a short transverse incision behind the lateral malleolus (Fig. III-134).
2. By exerting firm traction on the nerve, its course proximally can be traced through the skin. Make short transverse incisions as illustrated in Fig. III-134.

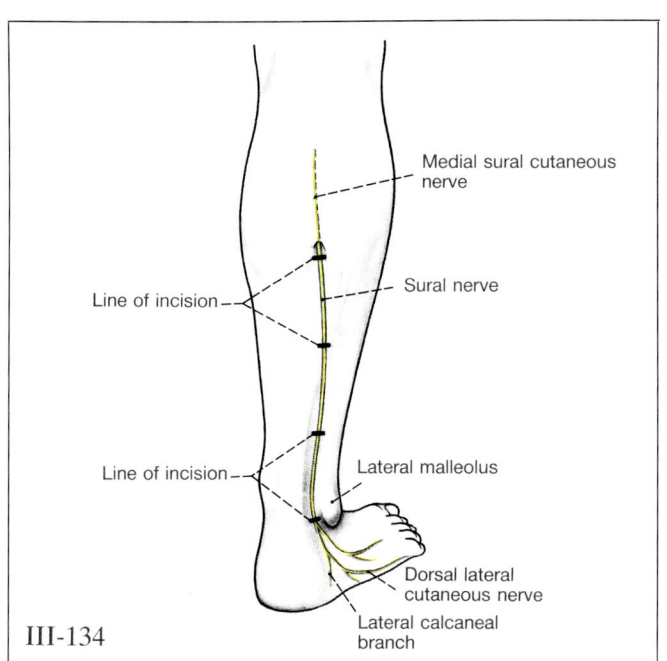

III-134

Achilles Tendon

Posteromedial Exposure or
Posterior Exposure

Indications

1. Extensive lengthening of the Achilles tendon
2. Repair of Achilles tendon rupture

Operative Steps

1. Make a medial incision parallel to the Achilles tendon and, if needed, angle the incision laterally across the insertion of the tendon (Fig. III-135, skin incision A).
2. An augmented view is possible by making a W-shaped incision beginning distally lateral to the insertion of the Achilles tendon (Fig. III-135, skin incision B).

Note

In the posterior approach, the sural nerve must be carefully guarded (see Fig. III-134).

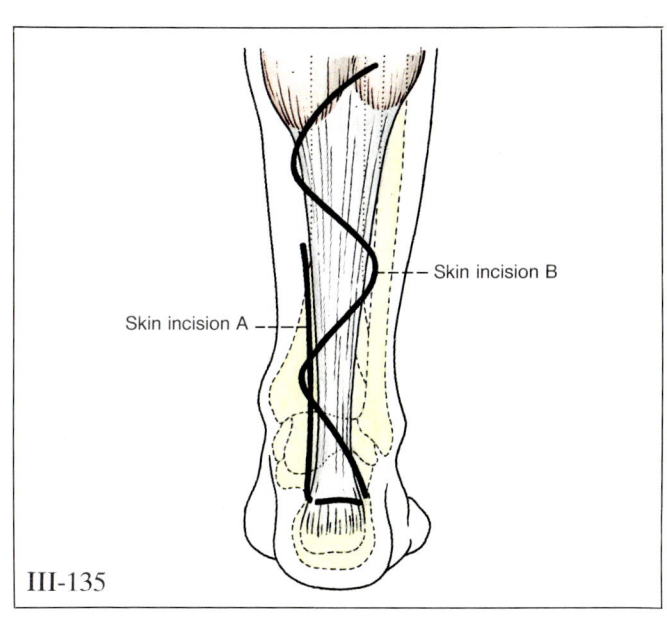

III-135

E. Malleolar Region

Talocrural Joint (1)

Anterior Exposure

Indications

1. Arthrodesis
2. Removal of loose bodies
3. Reduction of fractures of the anterior distal end of the tibia
4. Synovectomy
5. Tenosynovectomy
6. Talus excision

Operative Steps

1. Make an approximately 10-cm-long midline incision longitudinally over the talocrural joint, with the midpoint of the incision at the level of the joint line (Fig. III-136).
2. Avoid cutting the superficial branches of the peroneal nerve which pass diagonally across the operative field (Fig. III-137).
3. Incise the superficial and deep fasciae.
4. Cut through the superior and inferior extensor retinacula.

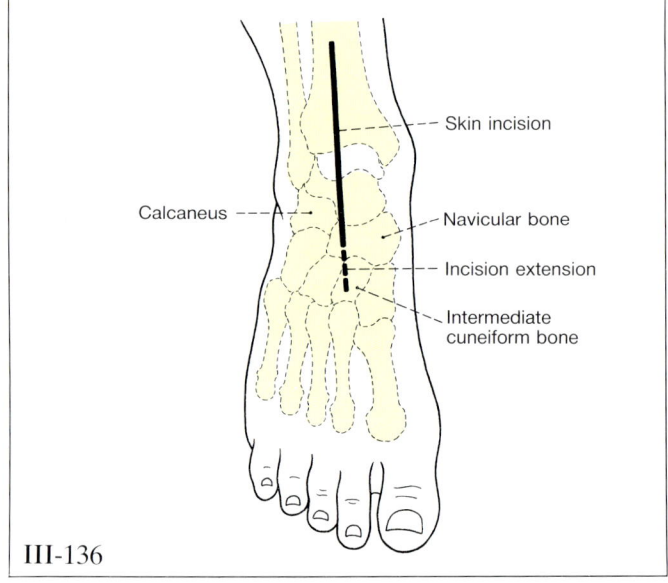

III-136

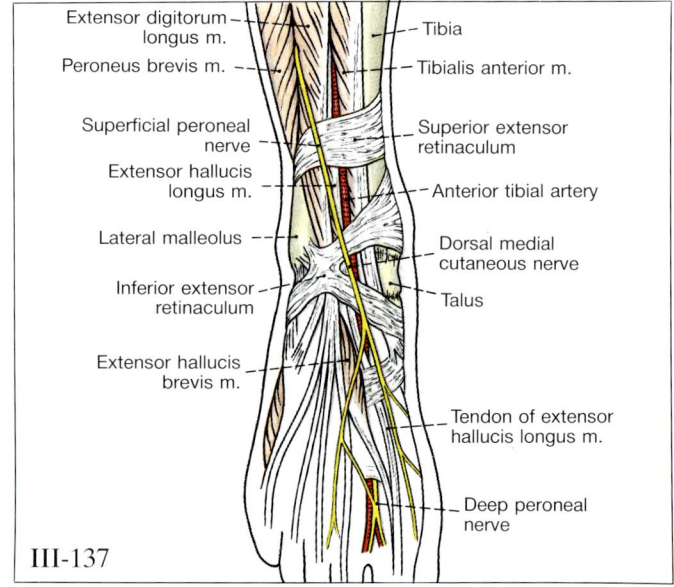

III-137

Talocrural Joint — Anterior Exposure

5. Retract the tibialis anterior muscle to the medial side and the superficial and deep peroneal nerves, the anterior tibial artery, and the tendons of the extensor digitorum longus and extensor hallucis longus muscles to the lateral side (Fig. III-138).
6. Split the joint capsule longitudinally to expose the anterior aspect of the talocrural joint and some of the tarsal bones.
7. The talocrural joint also can be reached through a space created by retracting the neurovascular bundle and the tendons of the tibialis anterior and extensor hallucis longus muscles to the medial side and the extensor digitorum longus tendons to the lateral side.

Notes

1. The anterior approach permits a wide exposure of the talocrural joint from the medial to the lateral malleolus.
2. It is important to avoid injury to the neurovascular bundle and the superficial peroneal nerve.

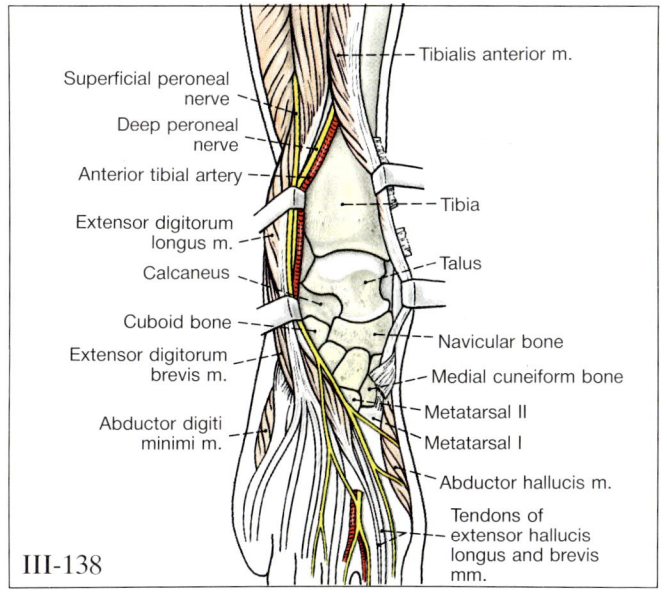

III-138

Alternative

A curved incision from lateral to medial (Fig. III-139) can be used instead of the longitudinal incision (Fig. III-136). This is particularly useful for synovectomy associated with tenosynovectomy of the extensor tendons.

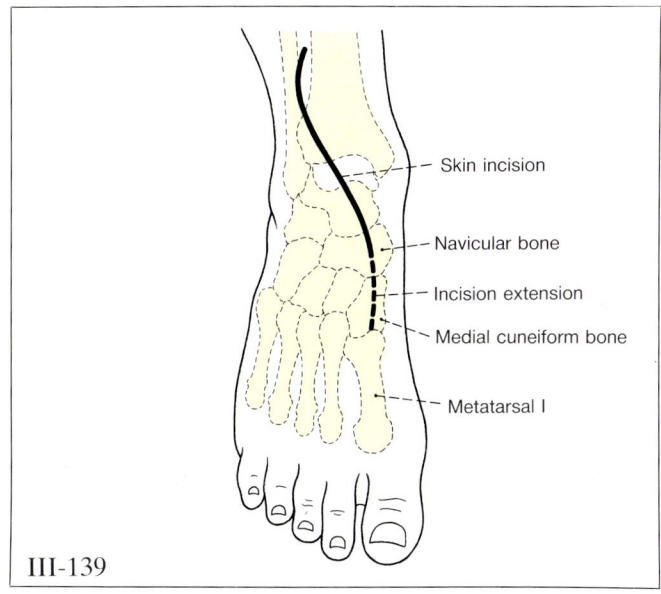

III-139

Anterolateral Exposure

Indication

Joint exploration

Operative Steps

1. Begin the skin incision about 6 cm above the talocrural joint and continue it parallel to the fibula in front of the anterior border of the latter. At the level of the talocrural joint, angle the incision onto the dorsum of the foot in the direction of the lateral cuneiform bone (Fig. III-140).
2. Identify and protect the dorsal intermediate nerve, a branch of the superficial peroneal nerve (see Fig. III-151).
3. Cut the extensor retinacula.
4. Retract the soft structures medially.
5. Open the capsule of the talocrural joint through the corresponding skin incision. The capsule may also be freed from its attachments.
6. Extend the incision distally and detach the extensor digitorum brevis muscle or split it in the direction of its fibers.

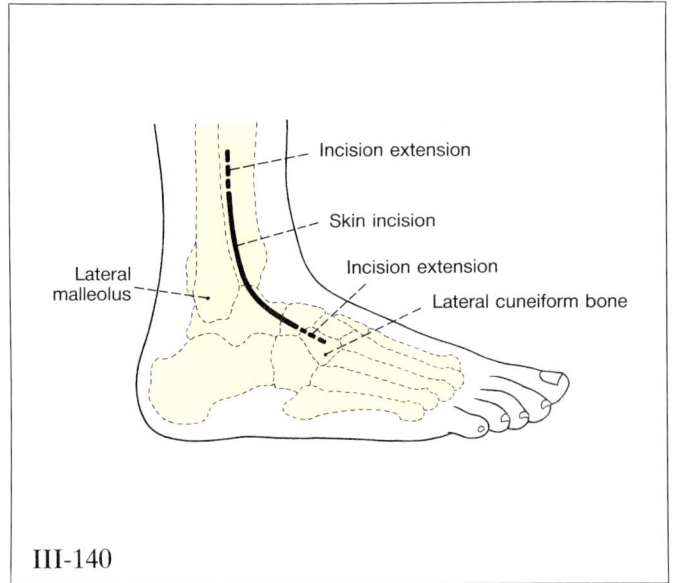

III-140

Notes

1. This line of incision offers the advantage of leaving the soft structures (nerves, anterior tibial artery, and tendons) intact by being retracted to the medial side.
2. Frequently it is not possible to prevent cutting the lateral tarsal artery, which is a branch of the dorsalis pedis artery that contributes to the arterial arch on the dorsum of the foot. This is particularly true if the incision is extended distally.

Talocrural and Subtalar Joint (1)

Posteromedial Para-achillar Exposure
Posterolateral Para-achillar Exposure

Indications

1. Reattachment of a dorsal tibial fragment (Volkmann's triangle)
2. Arthrodesis
3. Capsulotomy

Operative Steps

1. Make an approximately 10-cm-long incision along the medial or lateral border of the Achilles tendon (skin incision A or B). The midpoint of the incision should be at the level of the talocrural joint (Fig. III-141).
2. Incise the superficial and deep fasciae.
3. If the para-achillar exposure is not adequate, divide the Achilles tendon proximally and distally with a Z-cut in the sagittal or the frontal plane (Fig. III-143 and Fig. III-144).

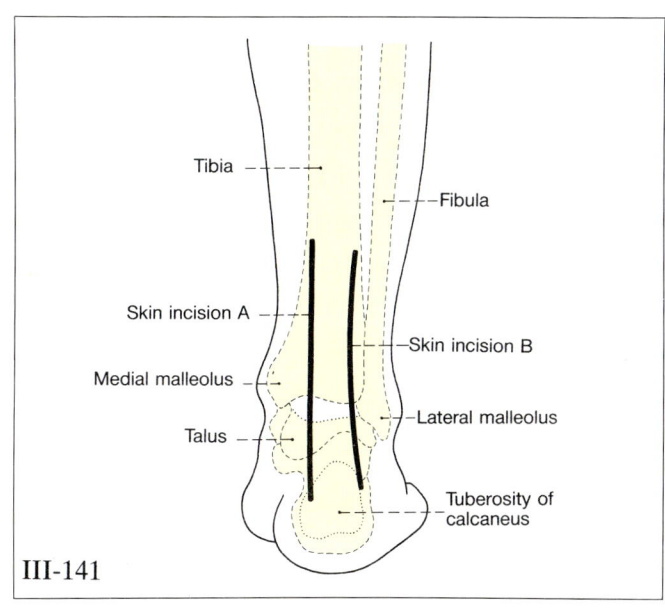

III-141

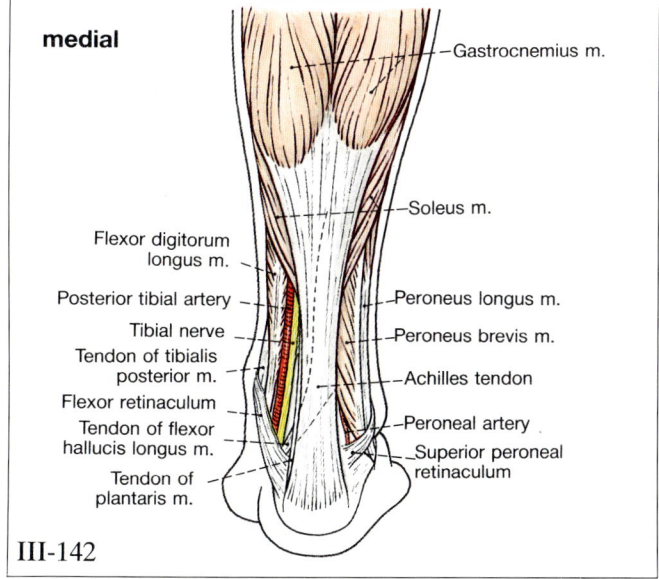

III-142

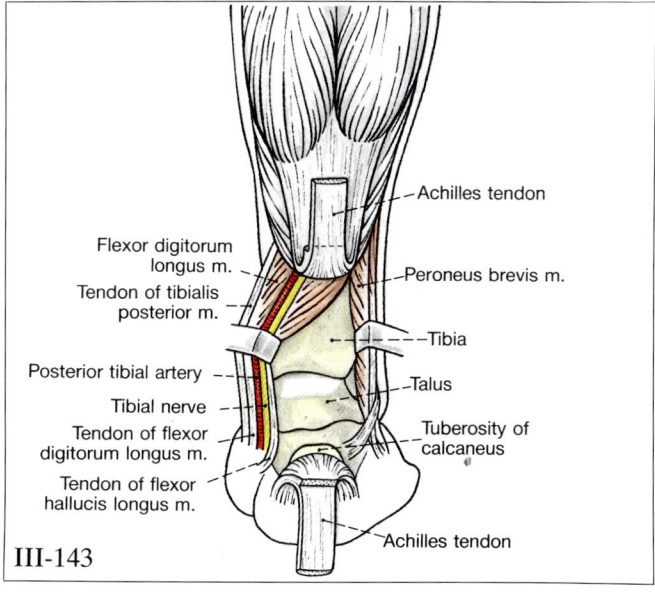

III-143

Talocrural and Subtalar Joint — Posterolateral Exposure

4. Retract the tendons of the peroneus longus and brevis muscles to the lateral side. Displace the posterior tibial artery, the flexor digitorum longus and flexor hallucis longus muscles medially (Fig. III-143). This exposes the distal dorsal aspect of the tibia and the dorsal parts of the capsule of both the talocrural and subtalar joints.

Notes

1. The sural nerve should be watched when making the posterolateral incision (Fig. III-146).
2. The neurovascular bundle with the posterior tibial artery and the tibial nerve must be protected when placing the posteromedial incision (Fig. III-142).

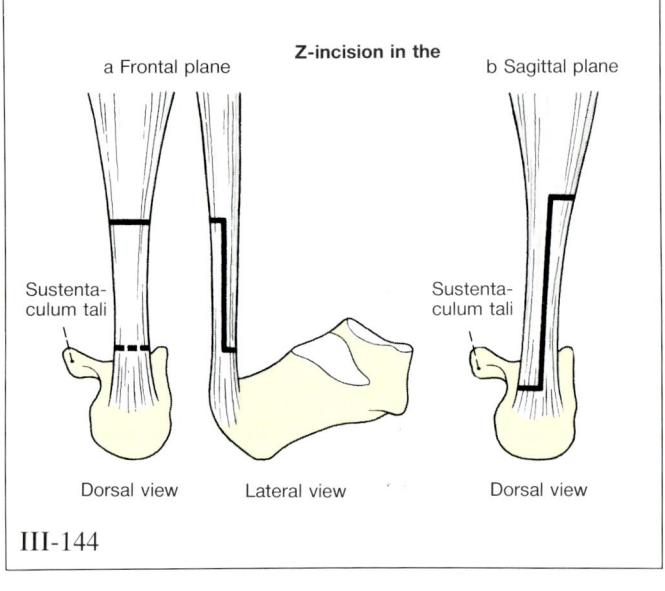

III-144

Posterolateral Exposure

Indications

1. Fractures of the lateral malleolus
2. Exploration of the dorsal components of the talocrural joint

Operative Steps

1. Make an approximately 10-cm-long incision over the back side of the fibula, beginning 7–8 cm above the tip of the lateral malleolus and ending distally at the lateral margin of the tuber calcanei (Fig. III-145).
2. Cut the deep fascia and find the space between the muscle bellies of the flexor hallucis longus and the peroneus brevis muscle (Fig. III-146).

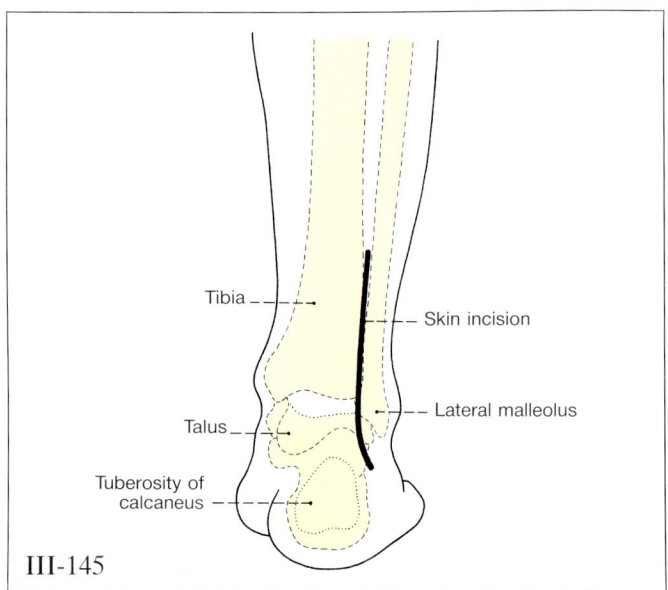

III-145

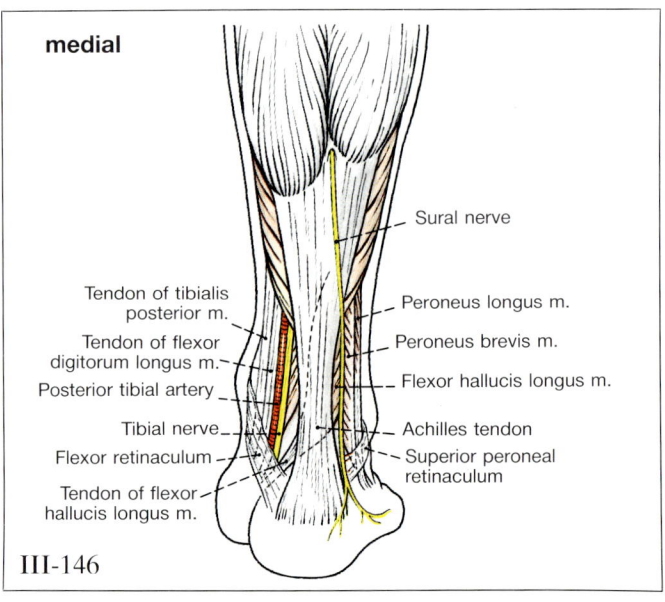

III-146

Talocrural and Subtalar Joint — Posterolateral Exposure/Applied Anatomy

3. Reflect the flexor hallucis longus muscle and the Achilles tendon medially and the peroneus brevis muscle laterally to expose the dorsal components of the joints and the fibula (Fig. III-147).
4. If necessary, the peroneal retinacula can be detached.

Notes

1. The incision is well suited for exposure of the posterior aspect of the syndesmosis in case of fracture of the fibula and a distorted Volkmann's triangle.
2. The superficially situated sural nerve and the lesser saphenous vein behind the medial malleolus must be protected in this incision.

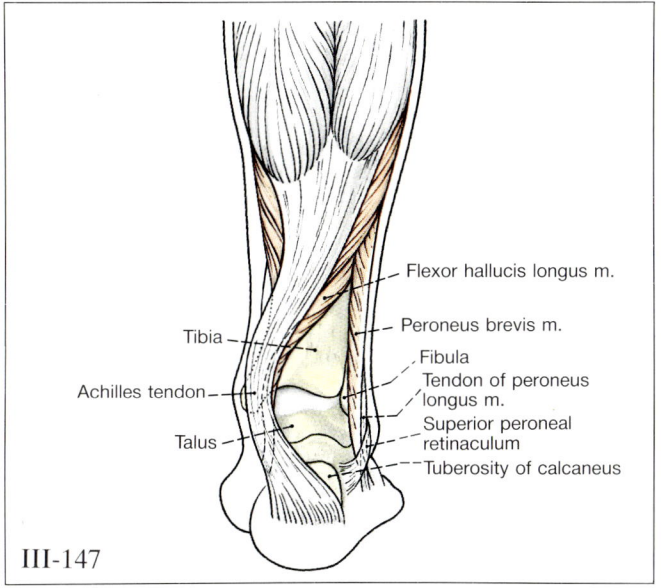

III-147

Applied Anatomy

1. The lateral ligaments of the talocrural and subtalar joints are illustrated in Fig. III-148. The anterior fibulotalar ligament and the fibulocalcaneal ligament are particularly important from a practical viewpoint.
2. The posterior ligaments are shown in Fig. III-149. Here the posterior part of the deltoid ligament is of special importance.

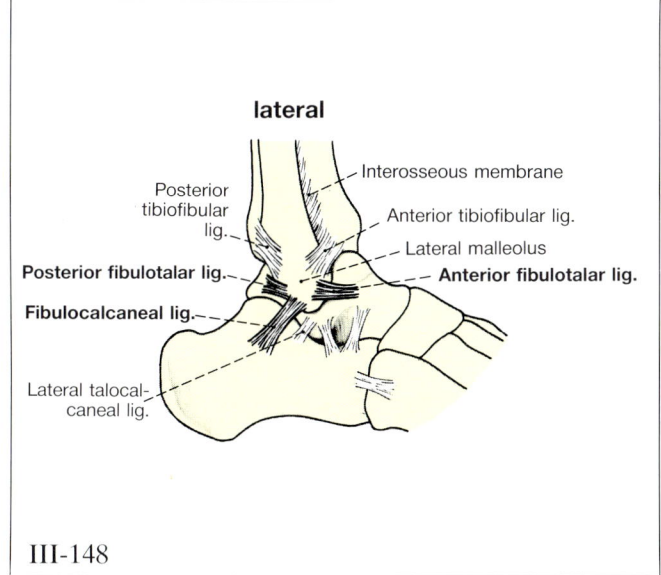

III-148

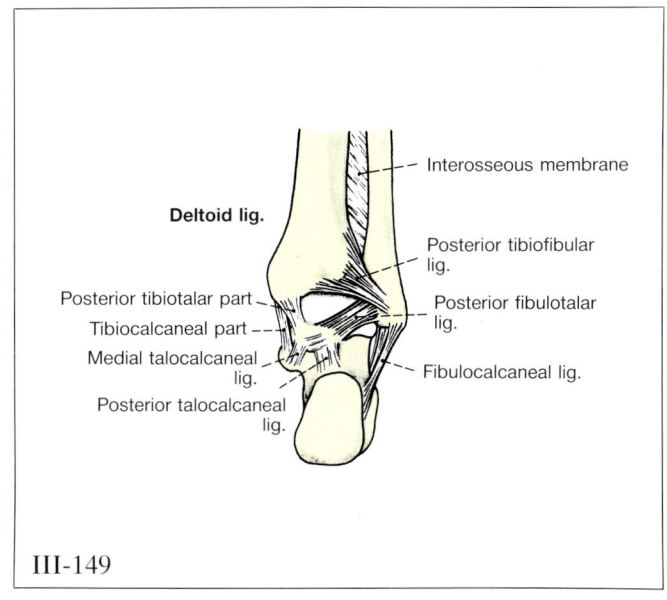

III-149

Ankle Joints – Lateral Malleolus

Lateral Exposure

(*Kocher* Incision)

Indications

1. Arthrodesis
2. Talus fractures
3. Dislocations of ankle joint
4. Ruptures of lateral ligaments
5. Exploration of peroneal tendons

Operative Steps

1. Begin the curved lateral incision 5–8 cm above the tip of the malleolus between the Achilles tendon and the dorsal margin of the fibula (Fig. III-150). Continue the incision distally to a point about 2 cm below the tip of the malleolus, and angle it forward to the cuboid bone.
2. Reflect the tendons of the peroneus longus and brevis muscles toward the back.
3. Displace the superficial peroneal nerve, the peroneus tertius, and extensor digitorum longus muscles forward.
4. Make a curved incision in the capsule to expose the lateral components of the talocrural and subtalar joints (Fig. III-152).

Notes

1. A wider exposure is obtained by temporarily severing the tendons of the peroneus longus and brevis muscles, using Z-shaped cuts.
2. The branches of the superficial peroneal nerve and the dorsal lateral cutaneous nerve (Fig. III-151), as well as the tributaries to the lesser saphenous vein, must be protected when placing this incision.
3. The long curved incision of *Kocher* frequently can be shortened in its upper portion.

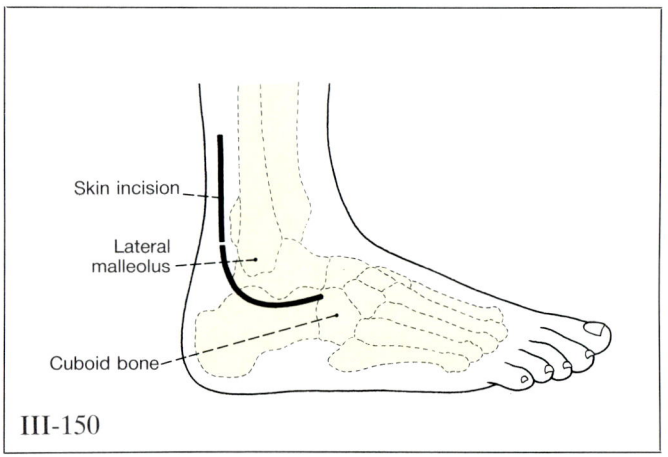

III-150

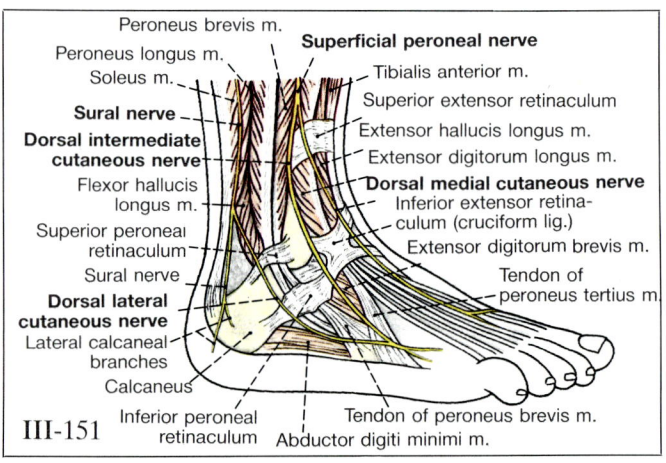

III-151

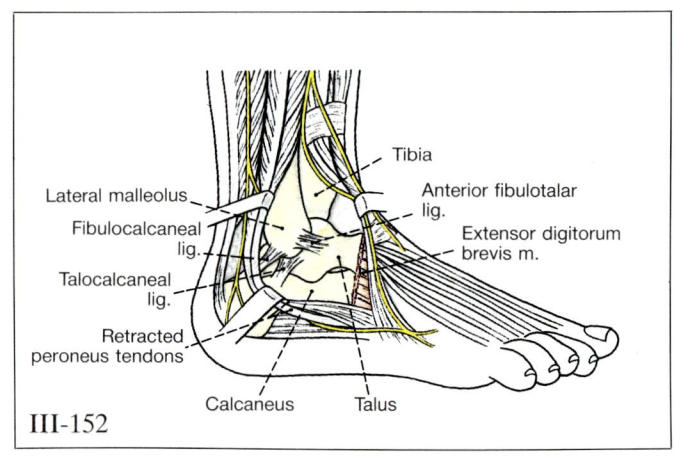

III-152

Talocrural and Subtalar Joint/Lateral Malleolus

Alternative Lateral Exposures

Indications

1. Ruptures of lateral ligaments
2. Fracture of lateral malleolus
3. Sprained syndesmosis
4. Dislocation of peroneal tendons

Operative Steps

1. Alternatively, somewhat different (and also more conservative) lines of incision may be chosen, depending on specific needs.
2. As opposed to the *Kocher* incision, a proximal incision can be used.
3. Begin the skin incision laterally over the margin of the fibula and continue it forward to a point just short of the cuboid bone (Fig. III-153, skin incision A). Alternatively, make a parallel incision over the middle of the fibula (Fig. III-153, skin incision B).
4. Incise the inferior extensor retinaculum (cruciform ligament) immediately in front of the fibula, and displace the digital extensor and the variable peroneus tertius muscles forward.
5. The syndesmosis, the capsule, and the lateral ligaments are now exposed.
6. See Fig. III-154 (skin incisions A and B) for further variations of the incision.
7. For inspection of the anterior fibular ligament in case of rupture, a short curved incision in front of the lateral malleolus is adequate (Fig. III-155).

Alternative Lateral Exposures

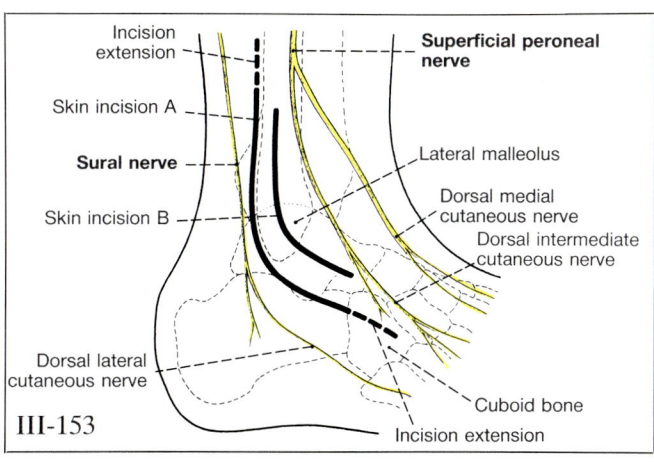

III-153

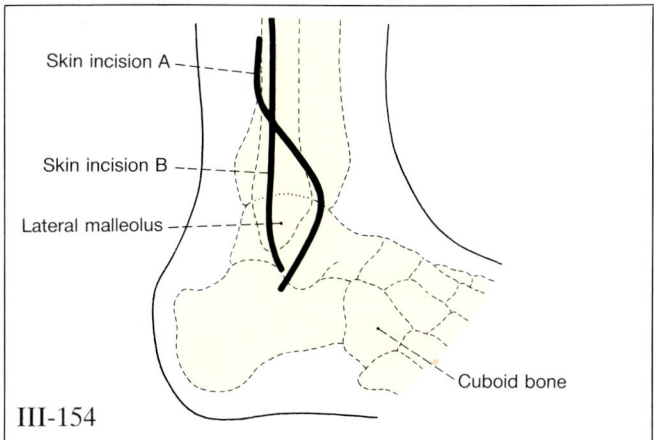

III-154

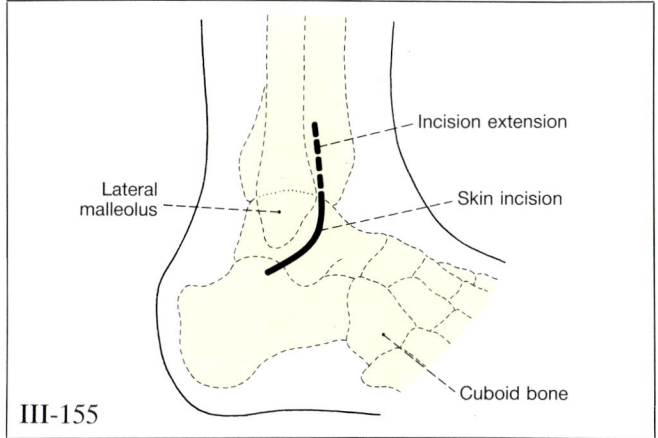

III-155

Notes

1. The intermediate dorsal cutaneous nerve, a branch of the superficial peroneal nerve, should be protected while making these incisions.
2. Occasionally the lateral part of the trochlea of the talus is to be exposed (e.g., in osteochondrosis dissecans) but cannot be exposed from the front. In this case, cut the fibula at the level of the talocrural articulation (beneath the syndesmosis) and turn down the lower end of the fibula.
3. The joint can now be opened from the lateral side.
4. Later fixation of the lateral malleolus is accomplished with the use of two Kirschner wires in a figure-of-eight configuration or an obliquely placed AO-malleolar screw. The drilling of the canal for the screw is best done prior to performing the osteotomy.

Talocrural Joint (2)

Posterolateral Exposure of *Patrick*

Indication

Arthrodesis

Operative Steps

1. Begin the skin incision on the dorsal border of the fibula 8–10 cm proximal to the tip of the fibula. Continue it distally around the malleolus (Fig. III-156).
2. Perform a transverse osteotomy of the fibula at the proximal end of the skin incision (Fig. III-157).
3. Cut the interosseous membrane, the syndesmosis, and the ligamentous connections, and reflect the fibular fragment downward (Fig. III-158) or remove it temporarily.
4. Direct access is now obtained to the talocrural as well as the subtalar joint.

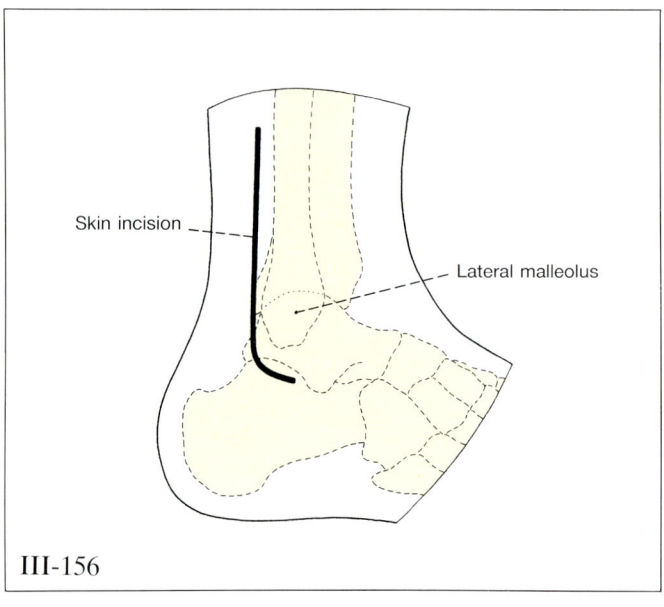

III-156

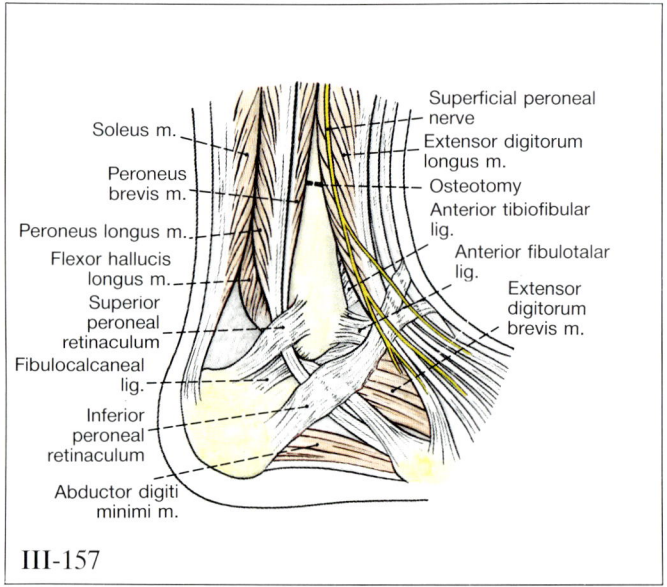

III-157

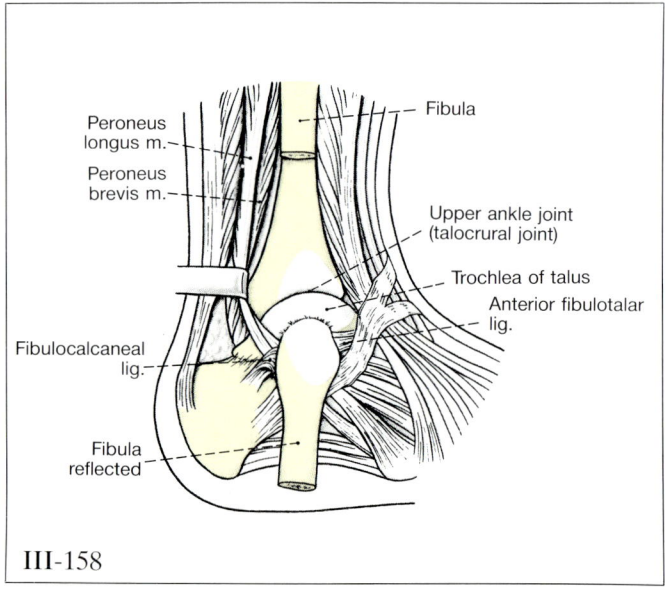

III-158

Subtalar Joint

Lateral Exposure

Short *Kocher* Incisions

Indications

1. Subtalar arthrodesis
2. Fracture of the calcaneus
3. Exploration of the fibulocalcaneal ligament

Operative Steps

1. Make a short, curved incision beginning about 1.5 cm behind the lateral malleolus and continuing approximately 2 cm below the tip of the fibula to the upper border of the cuboid bone (Fig. III-159).
2. If needed, the peroneal retinacula can be cut to displace the peroneal tendons.
3. The pattern of the lateral ligaments is illustrated in Fig. III-148.

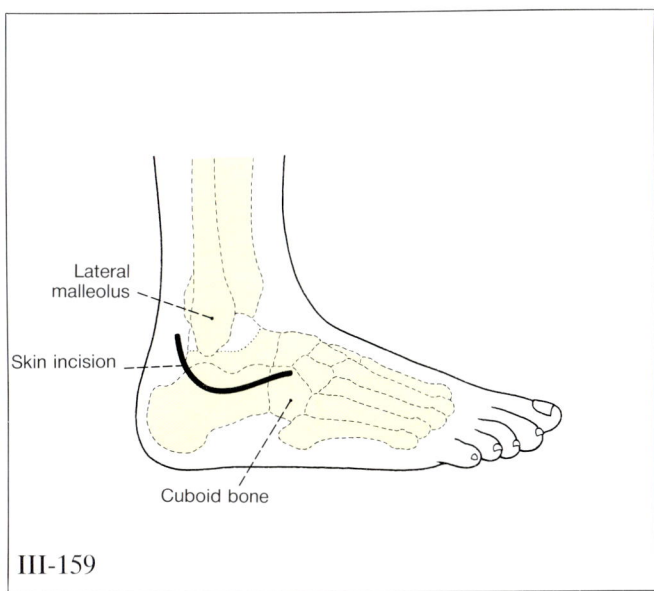

Talocrural and Subtalar Joint (2)

Applied Anatomy

The medial ligaments are illustrated in Fig. III-160.

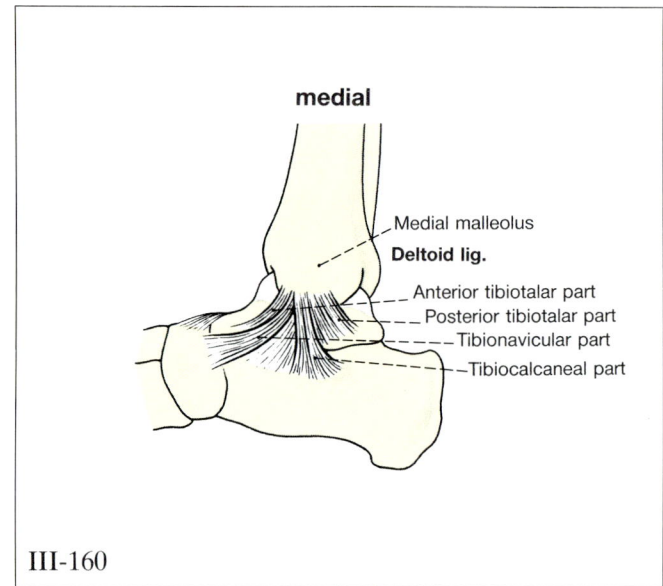

III-160

Subtalar Joint

Medial Exposure

Short Curved Incision
Long Curved Incision

Indications

1. Subtalar arthrodesis
2. Talus fractures
3. Exploration of tarsal tunnel
4. Tenosynovectomy

Operative Steps

1. Make a short curved medial skin incision beginning behind the medial malleolus. Continue the incision under the malleolus and distally to the tuberosity of the navicular bone (Fig. III-161).

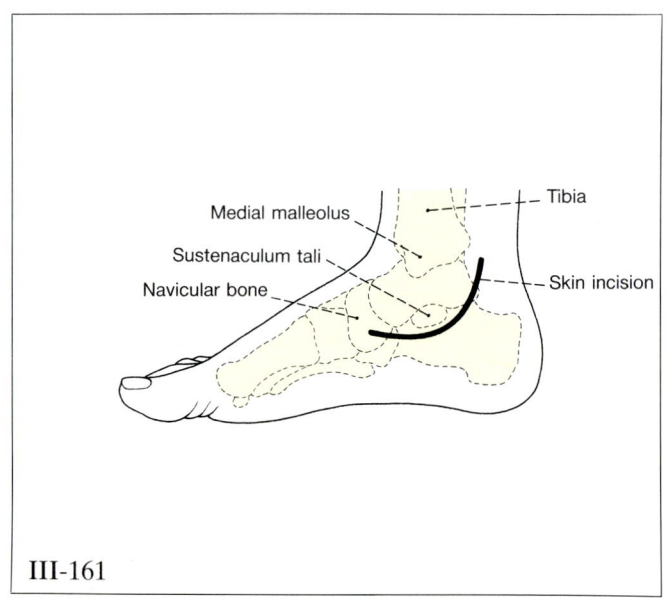

III-161

Talocrural and Subtalar Joint — Medial Exposure

2. Alternative: Make a long curved medial skin incision beginning about 6 cm above the tip of the malleolus, between the dorsal surface of the tibia and the Achilles tendon. Continue the incision around the medial malleolus to the tuberosity of the navicular bone (Fig. III-162).
3. Cut through the flexor retinaculum immediately below its tibial attachment (Fig. III-163, incision A).
4. Retract the tendons of the flexor digitorum longus and the tibialis posterior muscles toward the back, or free them from their compartments and displace them anteriorly (Fig. III-164).
5. Retract the flexor hallucis longus muscle, the tibial nerve, and the posterior tibial artery toward the back (Fig. III-164).
6. Incise the capsule transversely to view the medial components of the joint.

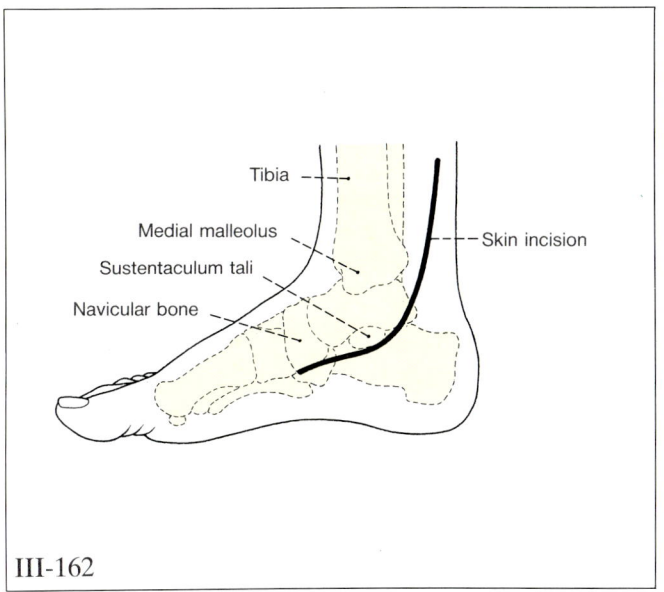

III-162

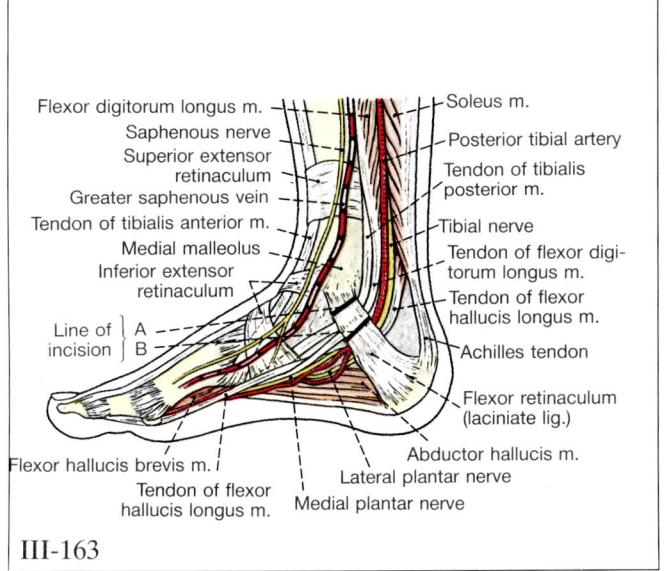

III-163

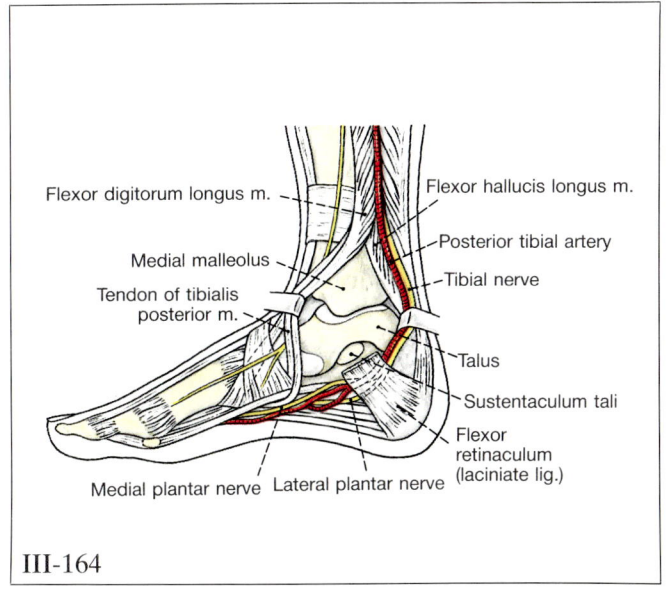

III-164

Talocrural Joint – Medial Malleolus

Medial Exposures

Indications

1. Ruptures of medial ligaments
2. Fracture of the medial malleolus
3. Inspection of the medial part of the trochlea of talus

Operative Steps

1. The line of incision may be made somewhat more proximal in comparison to the exposure of the subtalar joint. Make the curved incision over the medial malleolus from dorsal to ventral (Fig. III-165 or a variation corresponding to skin incision A in Fig. III-166).
2. A curved incision from the front to the back along the margin of the medial malleolus may also be elected (Fig. III-166, skin incision B).
3. This exposes the medial malleolus.
4. For an expanded operative field, cut the flexor retinaculum (laciniate ligament) (Fig. III-163).
5. Free the tendon of the tibialis posterior muscle and the flexor tendons from their compartments, and displace them and the neurovascular bundle from the field.

Notes

1. To expose the trochlea of the talus in case of a fragmented talar margin, cysts, or osteochondrosis dissecans, the medial malleolus can be osteotomized transversely.
2. The joint is then exposed.
3. Reattachment is later accomplished with an AO spongiosa screw or with two AO malleolar screws.
4. The canals for the screws should be drilled prior to performing the osteotomy.
5. The tendon of the tibialis posterior muscle lies immediately behind the medial malleolus and may be endangered during a transverse osteotomy (Fig. III-163).
6. When exposing the medial malleolus (and using skin incision B, especially), the saphenous nerve and the greater saphenous vein must be protected since they lie directly in front of the medial malleolus (Fig. III-163).

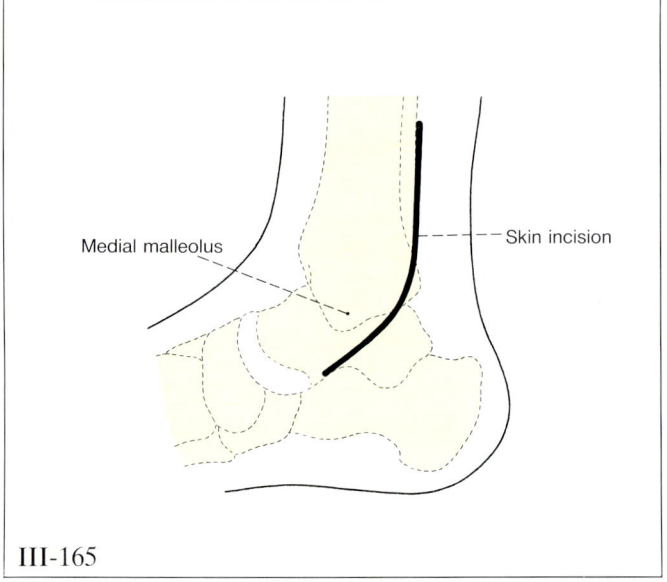

III-165

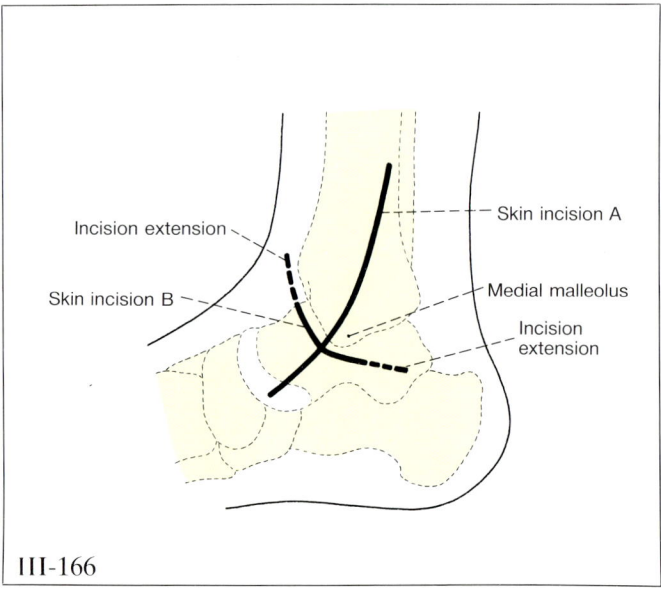

III-166

Tarsal Tunnel

Exposure

Indications

1. Tarsal tunnel syndrome
2. Tenosynovectomy of flexor tendons

Operative Steps

1. For the skin incision see the medial approach to the subtalar joint (Fig. III-161).
2. Split the superficial lamina of the flexor retinaculum as illustrated in Fig. III-163, incision B.
3. Expose the neurovascular bundle to the foot, containing the posterior tibial artery and the tibial nerve with its branches, the medial and lateral planter nerves (Fig. III-167).
4. If only the flexor tendons are to be exposed, incision A in Fig. III-163 can be elected. The tunnel for the neurovascular structures is then left untouched.
5. The flexor tendons (with their synovial sheaths), which tend to run in separate compartments, are exposed by cutting the deep lamina of the flexor retinaculum. For purposes of identification: The tendon of the flexor hallucis longus muscle is frequently associated with some muscle fibers.

Note

The posterior tibial artery is accompanied by an easily injured venous network.

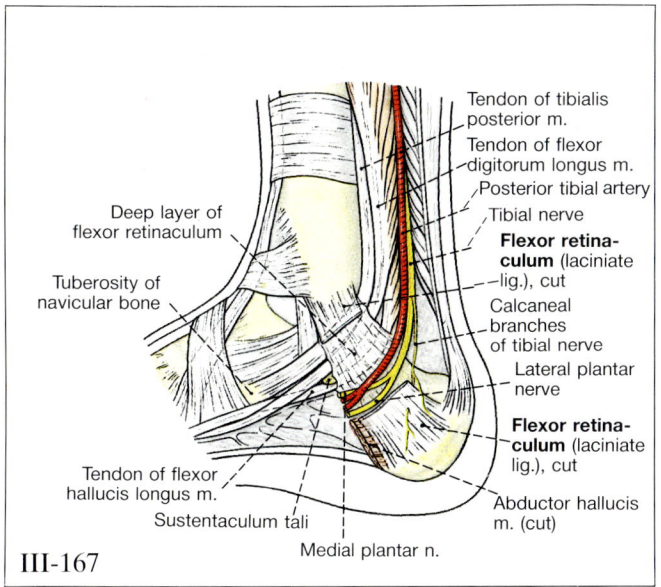

III-167

F. Foot

Calcaneus

Lateral Exposure

Indication

Haglund's disease

Operative Steps

1. Make a lateral, approximately 4- to 5-cm-long and slightly curved incision along the attachment of the Achilles tendon (Fig. III-168).
2. With sharp dissection proceed through the paratendinous tissue down to the bone.
3. For an augmented exposure make a transverse incision over the calcaneus as indicated in Fig. III-172 (skin incision part B) and continue it proximally for about 1–2 cm.

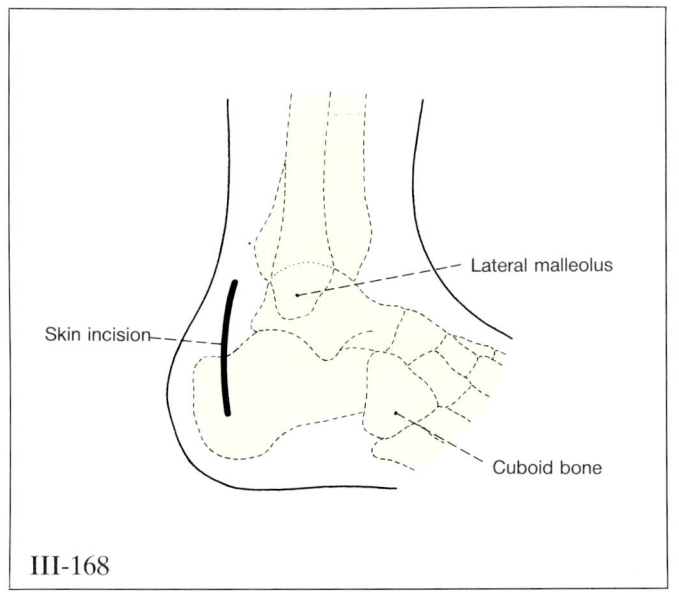

III-168

Alternative Lateral Exposure

Indications

1. Fractures of the calcaneus
2. Calcaneus osteotomy

Operative Steps

1. Make an oblique, slightly curved incision over the outside of the calcaneus (Fig. III-169).
2. With this incision there is no danger of injuring any structures except the sural nerve and the dorsal lateral cutaneous nerve (Fig. III-151).

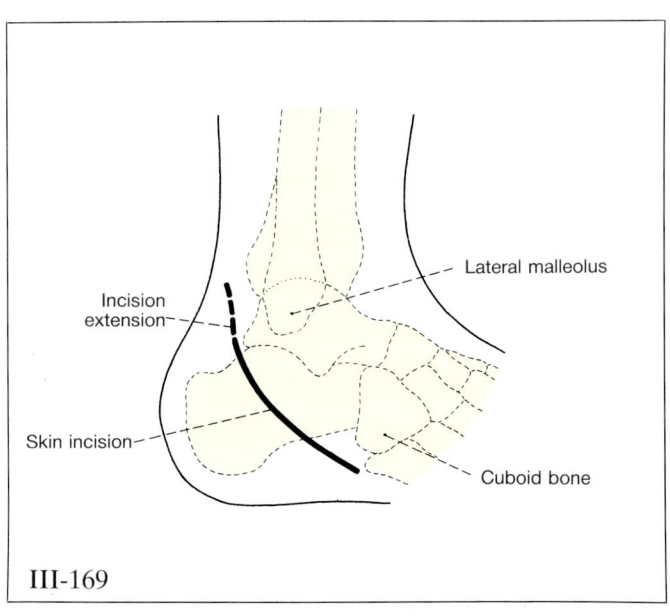

III-169

Lateral Plantar Exposure

Indication

Plantar spur of calcaneus

Operative Steps

1. Make an approximately 4- to 5-cm-long transverse incision on the lateral side over the distal part of the calcaneus parallel to the sole of the foot (Fig. III-170).
2. Dissect through the subcutaneous fat down to the plantar aponeurosis.

Alternative
Medial Plantar Exposure

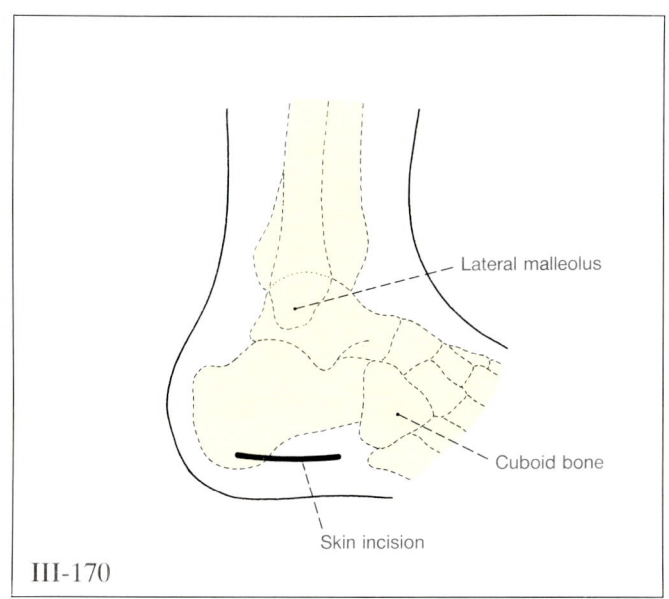
III-170

Operative Steps

1. Make an approximately 4- to 5-cm-long transverse incision on the medial side over the distal part of the calcaneus parallel to the sole of the foot (Fig. III-171).
2. Dissect through the subcutaneous fat down to the plantar aponeurosis.

Notes

1. The course of the medial and lateral plantar nerves should be observed.
2. With the medial exposure it is impossible to avoid cutting a number of small veins running perpendicular to the sole of the foot.

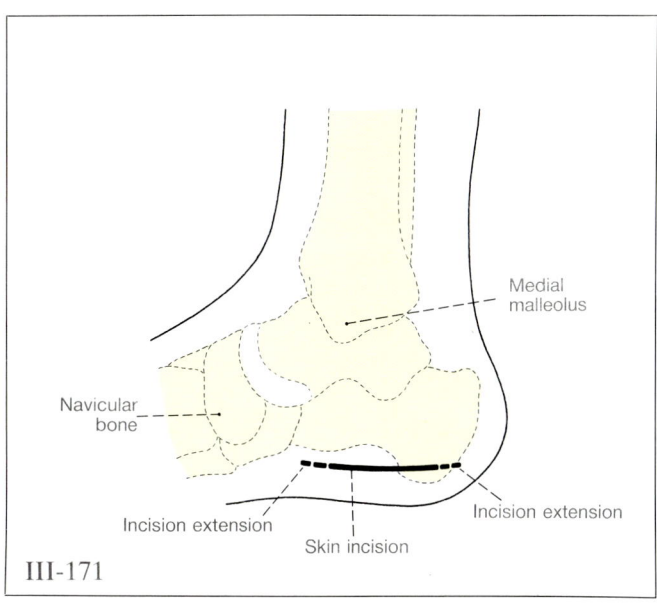
III-171

Calcaneus — Mediolateral Exposure

Mediolateral Exposure

Curved L-Incision of *Kocher*

Indication

Only for an augmented view of the calcaneus

Operative Steps

1. Begin the skin incision 5 cm proximal to the medial malleolus, between the Achilles tendon and the dorsal border of the tibia (Fig. III-172). Continue it distally to the medial edge of the tuberosity of the calcaneus and then anteriorly along the outside of the calcaneus to the tuberosity of metatarsal V (Fig. III-173)
2. Cut through the superficial and deep fasciae.
3. Reflect the taut skin over the calcaneus distally (Fig. III-174).
4. Reflect the proximal skin flap anteriorly with the peroneus longus and brevis muscles.
5. The dorsal and lateral surfaces of the calcaneus are now completely exposed.

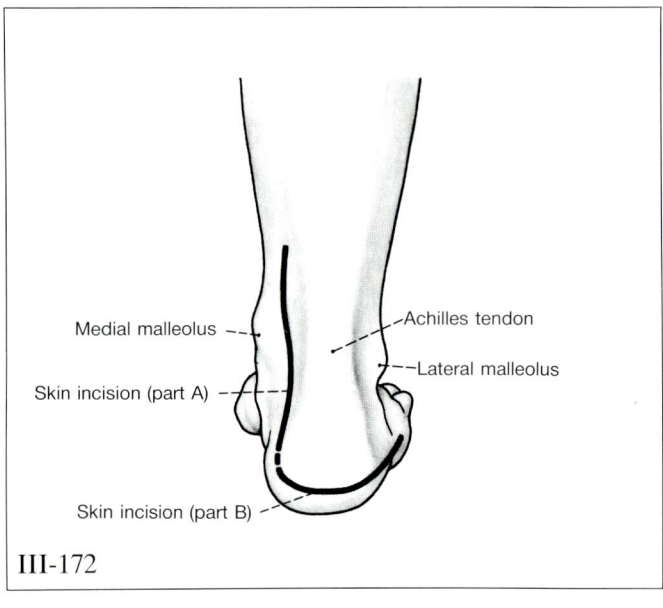

III-172

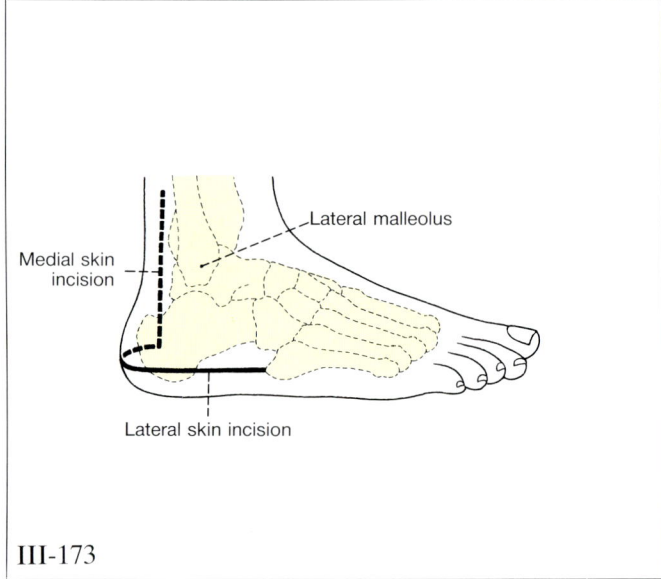

III-173

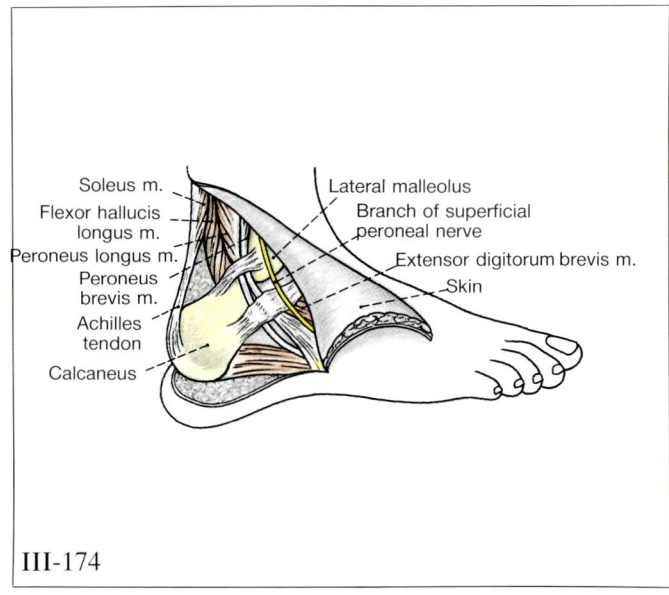

III-174

Plantar Exposure

Indications

1. Tumors
2. Osteomyelitis

Operative Steps

1. Make a 5-cm-long plantar incision longitudinally over the calacaneus in the midline (Fig. III-175).
2. Alternatively, the incision can follow the edge of the sole from the medial side (Fig. III-176) to the posterior aspect.
3. Dissect through the subcutaneous fat down to the plantar aponeurosis.

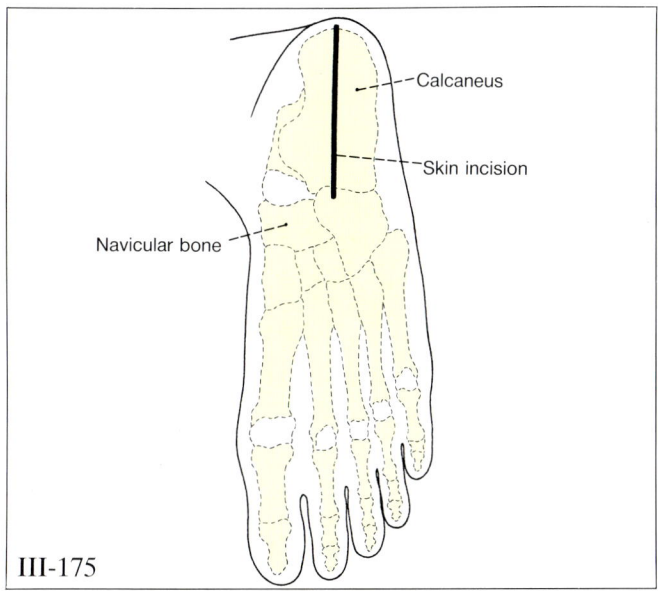

III-175

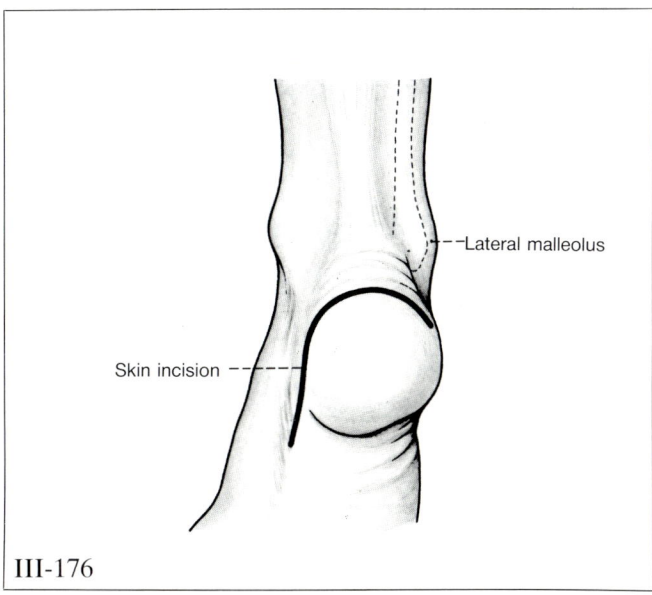

III-176

4. Incise the plantar aponeurosis at its attachment to the calcaneus (Fig. III-177).
5. Injury to the lateral plantar artery and the medial and lateral plantar nerves, which lie medial to the calcaneus, must be avoided.
6. Reflect the plantar aponeurosis and the underlying musculature distally to expose the plantar surface of the calcaneus (Fig. III-178).
7. For an expanded view, the flexor digiti minimi brevis and abductor digiti minimi muscles can be reflected laterally, and the abductor hallucis muscle can be pulled toward the medial side.

Note

Many surgeons hesitate to use this exposure for fear of later scar formation and pain over the calcaneus. In aseptic cases this fear is unwarranted.

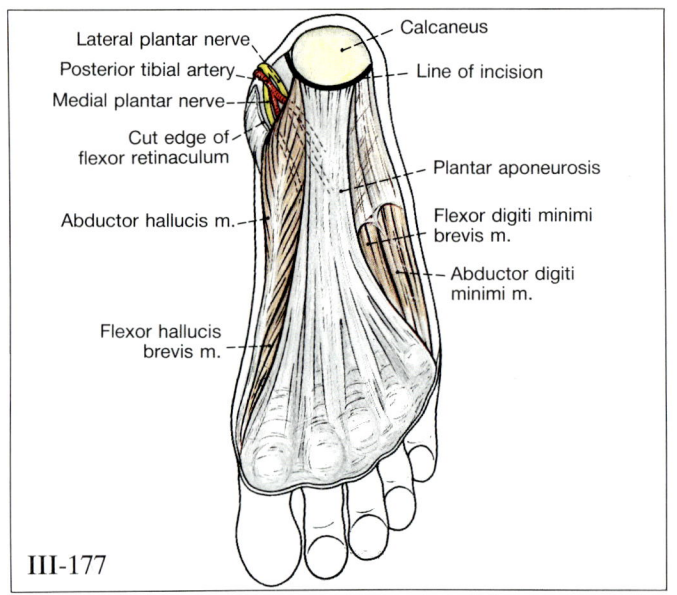

III-177

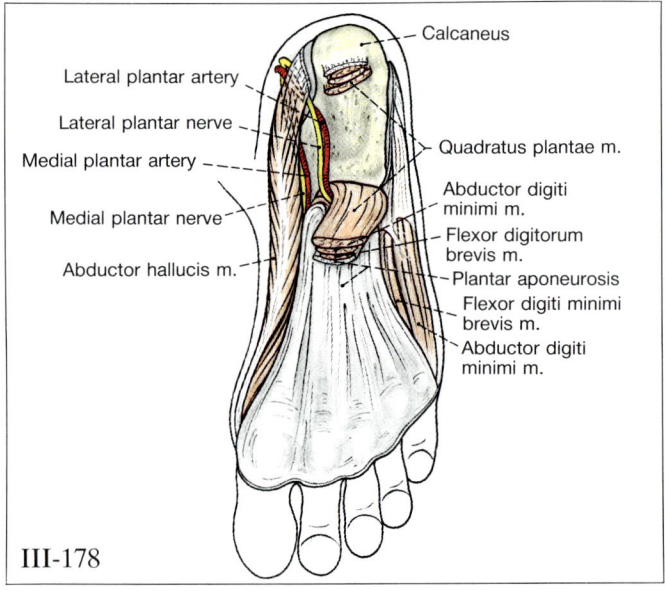

III-178

Tarsus

Medial Exposure

Indications

1. Transverse wedge osteotomy
2. Cornual navicular bone or os tibiale externum
3. Talonavicular arthrodesis
4. Infections of navicular bone

Operative Steps

1. Make an incision along the medial aspect of the foot, beginning at the base of metatarsal I and passing over the talonavicular joint to a point just short of the sustentaculum tali (Fig. III-179).
2. For a more comprehensive exposure, the incision can be extended (Fig. III-179).
3. A corresponding skin incision on the lateral aspect of the foot can be advantageous, particularly in the presence of a very high longitudinal arch.

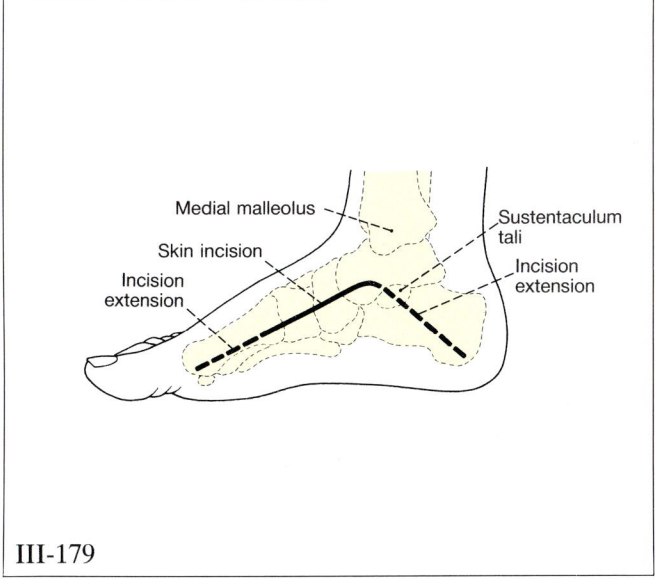

III-179

Anterior Exposure
Ventral Exposure

Indications

1. Wedge osteotomy
2. Arthrodesis

Operative Steps

1. Make a transverse, superficial incision from the medial to the lateral aspect of the foot at the level of the navicular bone (Fig. III-180).
2. Figs. III-137 and III-138 provide additional orientation.
3. Reflect the extensor tendons medially, and detach the origin of the extensor digitorum brevis muscle. The tarsal bones in this region are now exposed.

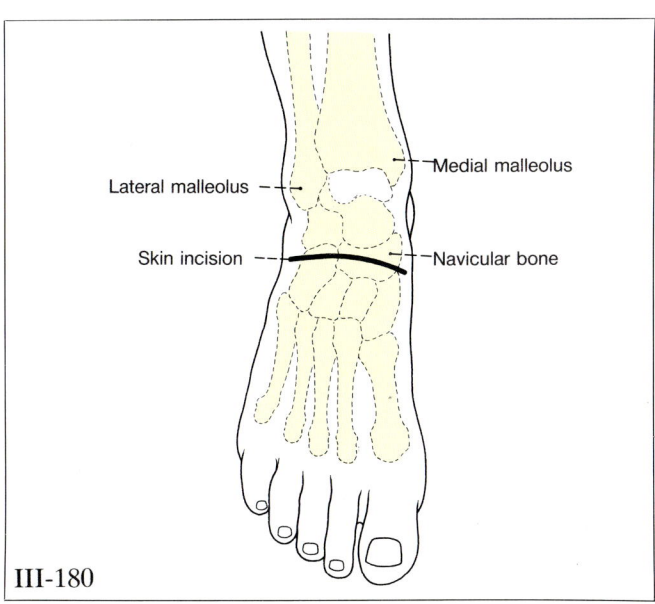

III-180

Tarsus – Metatarsal Bone V

Lateral Exposure

Operative Steps

1. Make an incision along the lateral margin of the foot from the ascending arch of the calcaneus, over the tuberosity of metatarsal V, and along the outer margin of the latter (Fig. III-181, skin incision A).
2. Skin incision B in Fig. III-181 can augment the medial exposure of the tarsus (Fig. III-179).

Metatarsal Bones

Anterior Exposures

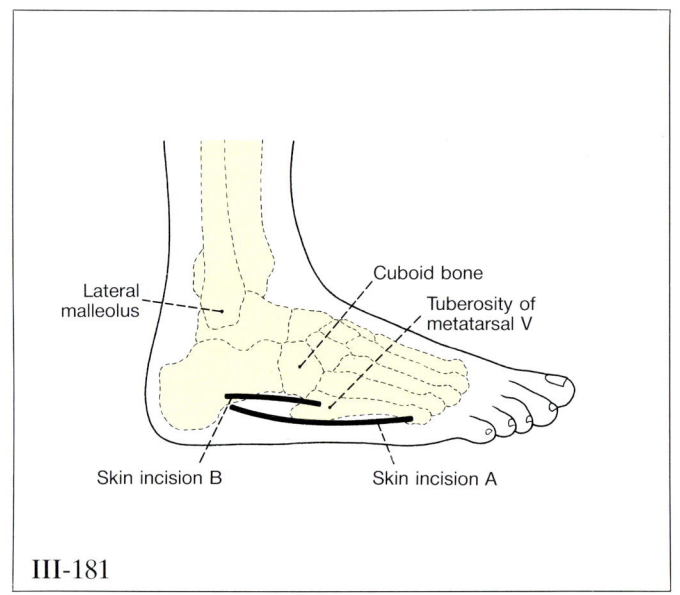

III-181

Indications

1. Fractures of the metatarsals
2. Tumors or inflammatory processes
3. Osteotomies for bone correction

Operative Steps

1. Make the incision along the medial and lateral borders of metatarsal I and V, respectively (Fig. III-182).
2. For the centrally located metatarsals II–IV, make the incision over the middle of the desired bone (Fig. III-182).
3. During further dissection the cutaneous nerve branches, which lie immediately under the skin, and the extensor tendons must be protected (see Fig. III-151).

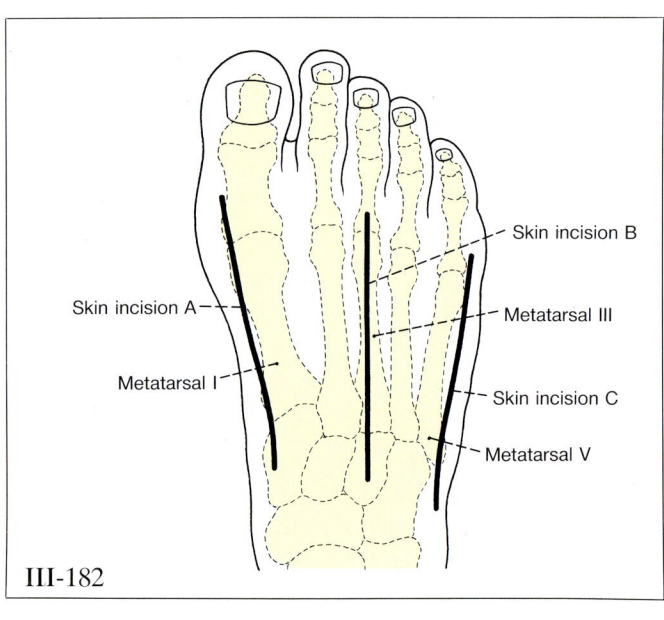

III-182

Sole of the Foot

Median Longitudinal Incision

Indication

Dupuytren's disease

Operative Steps

1. Make a slightly curved median longitudinal incision; the length is commensurate with the requirements (Fig. III-183).
2. A more medially placed incision will endanger the blood supply to the plantar surface of the foot.

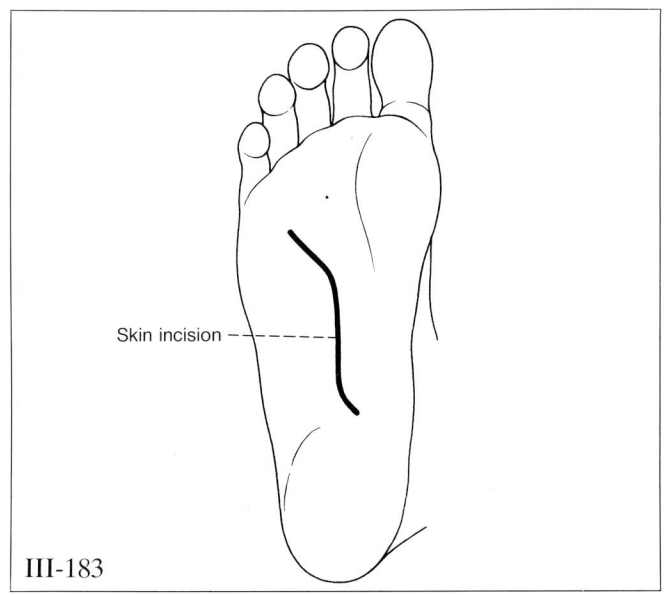

III-183

Applied Anatomy

The sole of the foot with the extent of the plantar aponeurosis is indicated in Fig. III-184.

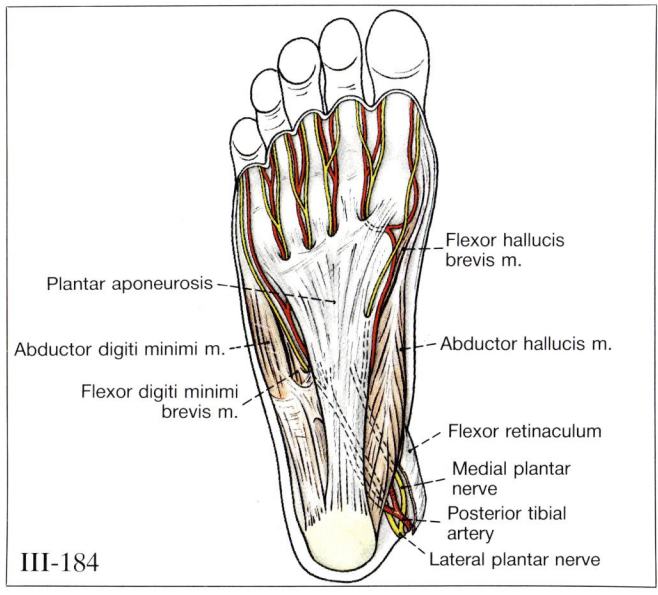

III-184

Plantar Aspect of Forefoot

Plantar Exposure

Indication

Morton's neuralgia

Operative Steps

1. Make a longitudinal incision over the distal sole of the foot toward the web of the toes (Fig. III-185).
2. Split the fascia and carefully dissect the common plantar neurovascular bundle (Fig. III-186).

Notes

1. A thickened inflamed bursa frequently lies over the neurovascular bundle and must be removed.
2. A dorsal approach is also possible by making a corresponding "interdigital" incision. The transverse ligaments of the metatarsal head must then be cut. The operative view is poorer than that gained in a plantar approach.

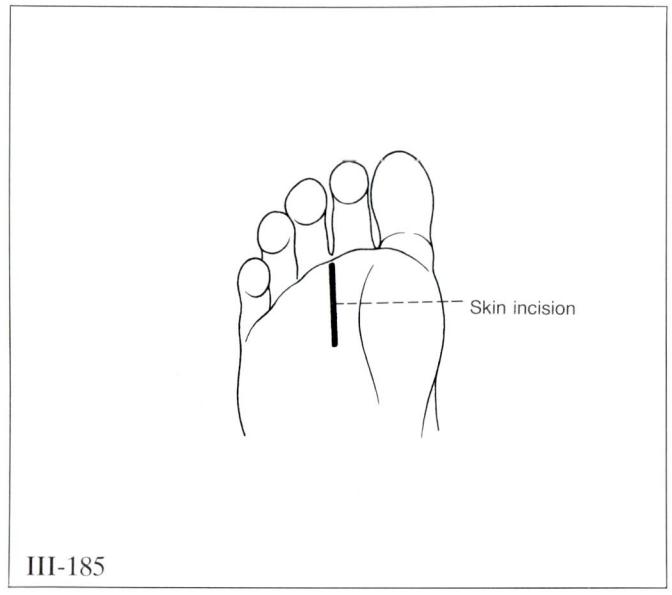

III-185

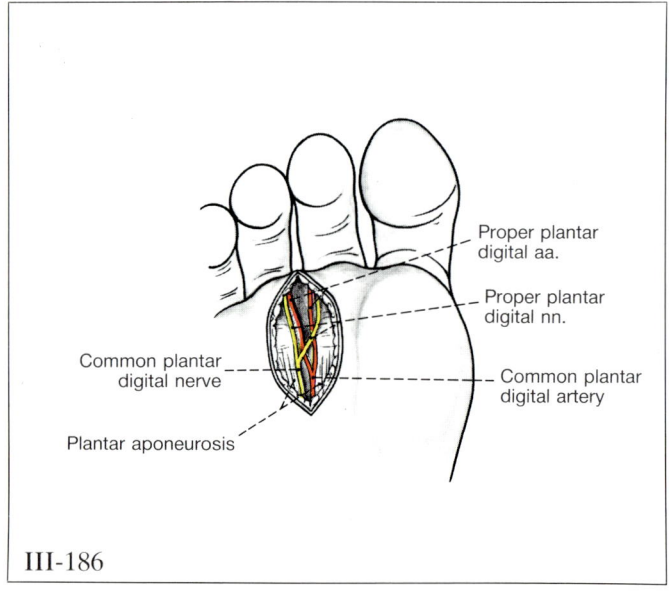

III-186

G. Toes

Metatarsophalangeal Joint of the Big Toe

Medial Exposure

Indications

1. Hallux valgus arthroplasty
2. Arthrodesis

Operative Steps

1. Make an approximately 5- to 8-cm-long skin incision on the medial aspect of the 1st metatarsophalangeal joint, beginning immediately behind the head of the proximal phalanx and continuing proximally across the joint to a point just short of the middle of metatarsal I (Fig. III-187a).
2. Alternatively, curve the incision dorsally (Fig. III-187b).
3. Cut through the superficial and deep fasciae.
4. Incise the capsule (Fig. III-188) longitudinally to expose the metatarsophalangeal joint of the big toe.
5. To augment the exposure of the joint, use a scalpel to detach the capsule from the base of the proximal phalanx and the head of metatarsal I (Figs. III-189 and III-190).

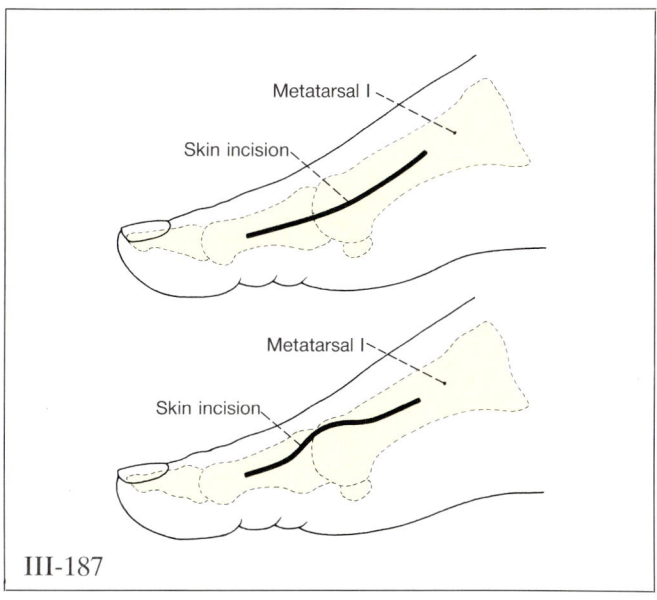

III-187

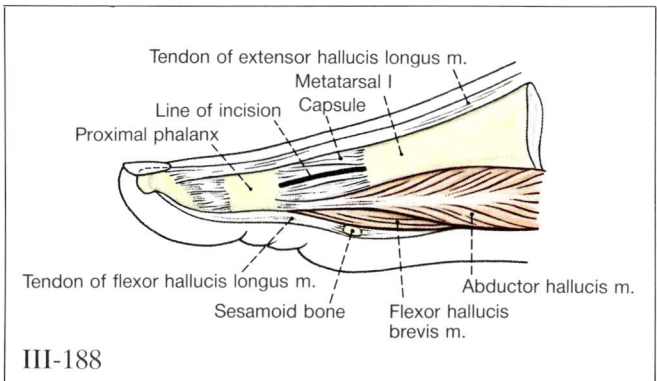

III-188

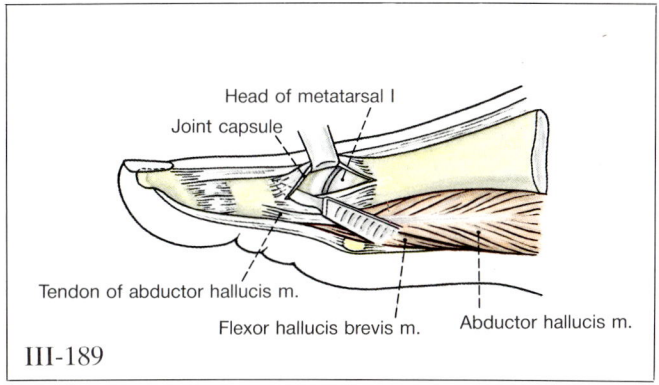

III-189

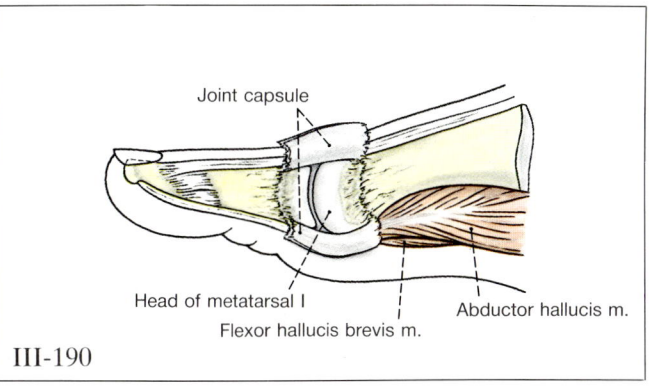

III-190

Anteromedial Exposure

Dorsomedial Exposure

Indications

1. Hallux valgus arthroplasty
2. Arthrodesis
3. Endoprosthetics

Operative Steps

1. Make a somewhat medial, approximately 5- to 6-cm-long curved longitudinal incision on the dorsal aspect of the first metatarsophalangeal joint, beginning immediately behind the head of the proximal phalanx. Continue the incision proximally across the joint to a point short of the middle of metatarsal I, on the medial aspect of the extensor hallucis longus tendon (Fig. III-191a).
2. An oval piece of the superfluous skin to be excised later can be circumscribed as a variation of the incision (Fig. III-191b).
3. Cut through the superficial and deep fasciae.
4. Free the extensor tendons and retract them to either side.
5. Incise the capsule longitudinally to expose the metatarsophalangeal joint of the big toe.

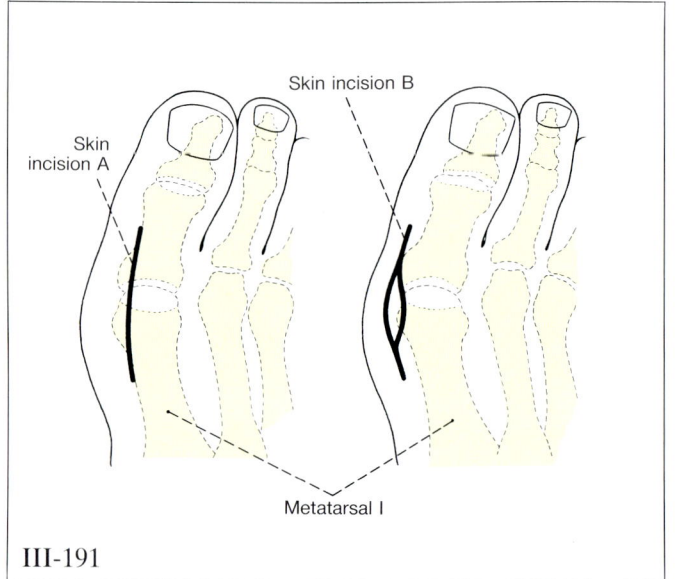

III-191

Note

Dissection of the extensor tendons can be dispensed with to prevent adhesions later.

Toes

Applied Anatomy

1. Dorsal aspect of the toes with the forefoot (Fig. III-192).
2. The big toe is seen in cross section at the level of the proximal phalanx (Fig. III-193). The proper digital nerves are frequently branched.

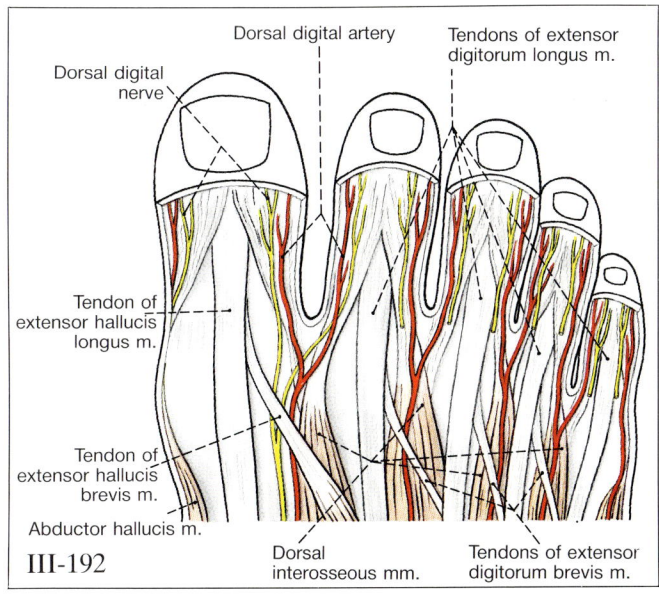

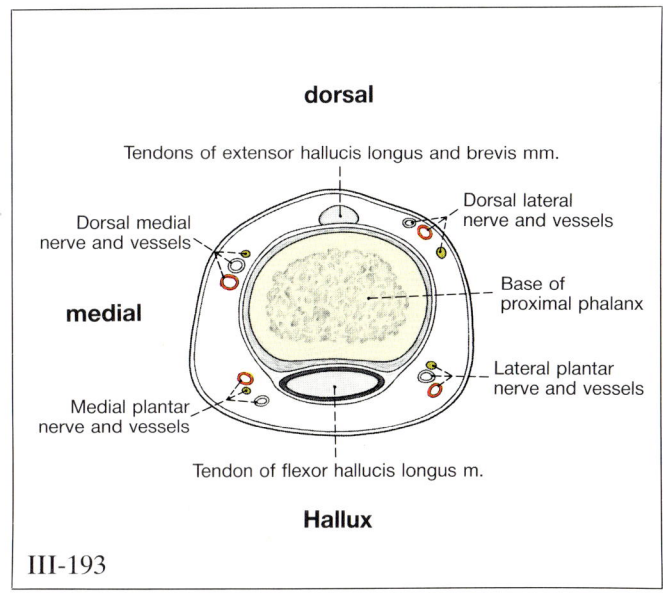

Metatarsophalangeal Joints

Anterior Exposure

Indications

Rheumatic diseases of the forefoot
(Resection of the metatarsal head and the base of the proximal phalanx by the method of *Clayton*)

Operative Steps

1. Make a transverse incision for operations on digits II–V (Fig. III-194).
2. Make a dorsomedial longitudinal incision for the big toe (Fig. III-194).
3. Alternative: Make transverse incisions for operations on digits I–V.

Alternative

1. If exposure of only one metatarsophalangeal joint of digits II–V is required, for example, to do an isolated synovectomy, a Z-incision (Fig. III-195, skin incision A) is indicated.
2. A para-articular longitudinal incision through the web of the toes can also be used by undermining the skin and retracting it (Fig. III-195, skin incision B).
3. The metatarsophalangeal joint of the little toe can be approached through a longitudinal incision on the outside.

Note

The single longitudinal incision over the metatarsophalangeal joint can lead at times to scar contracture and secondary deviation of the toe.

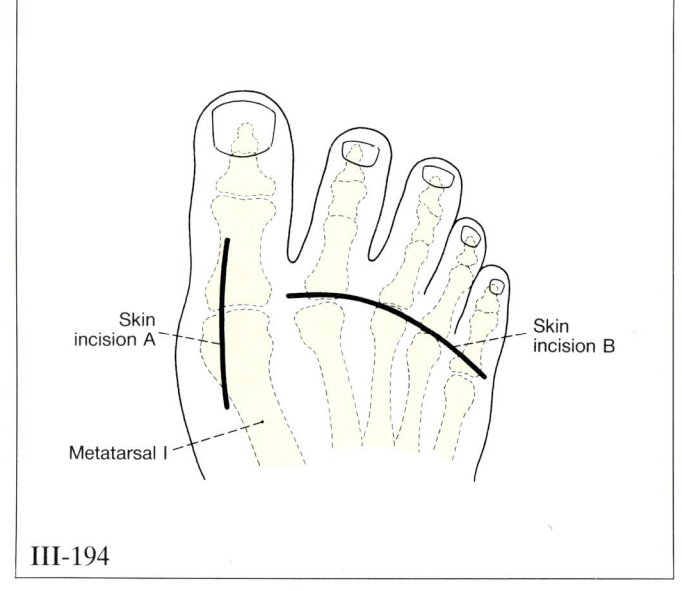

III-194

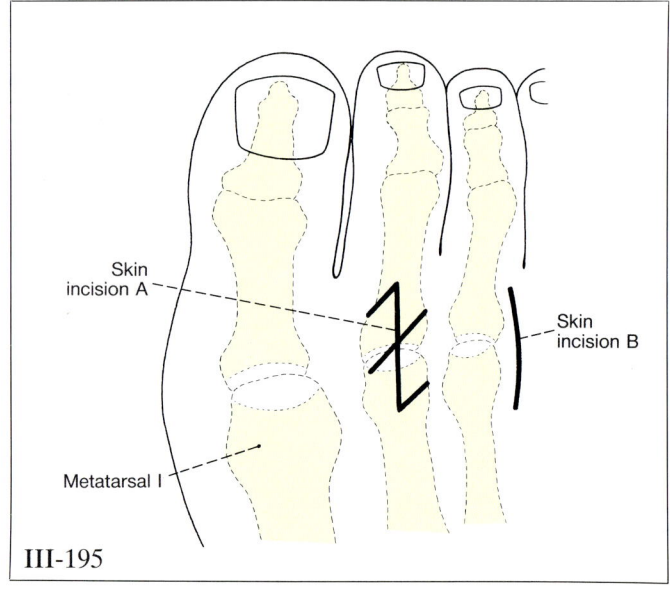

III-195

Metatarsophalangeal Joints II–V

Plantar Exposure of *Gocht*

Indication

Hammer toe operation with removal of bases of proximal phalanges

Operative Steps

1. Make a plantar, distally convex curved incision over the bases of the proximal phalanges across the width of the anterior part of the sole of the foot (Fig. III-196).
2. Develop the exposure by cutting through the subcutaneous fat longitudinally down to the flexor tendons, avoiding the laterally situated neurovascular bundles (Fig. III-197).
3. Split the aponeurosis and the annular ligaments of the tendons, and retract the tendons to either side (Fig. III-197).
4. Split the joint capsule and expose the metatarsophalangeal joint.

Note

For a better view of the operative field, elevate digits II–V with a gauze sling.

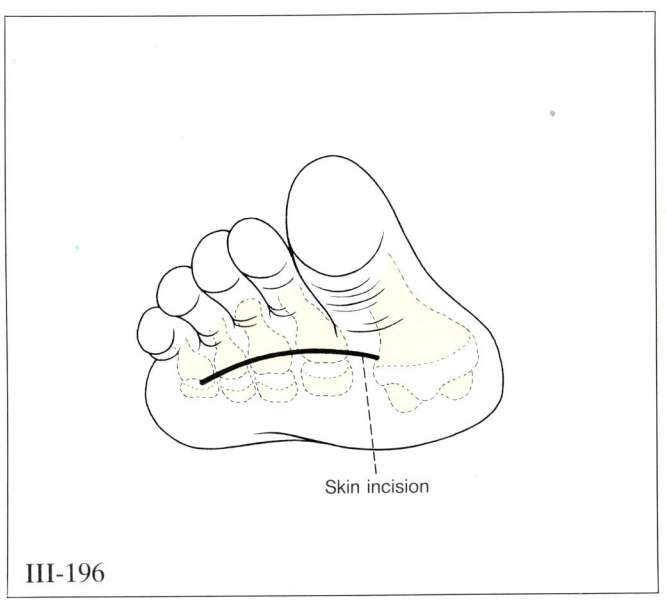

III-196

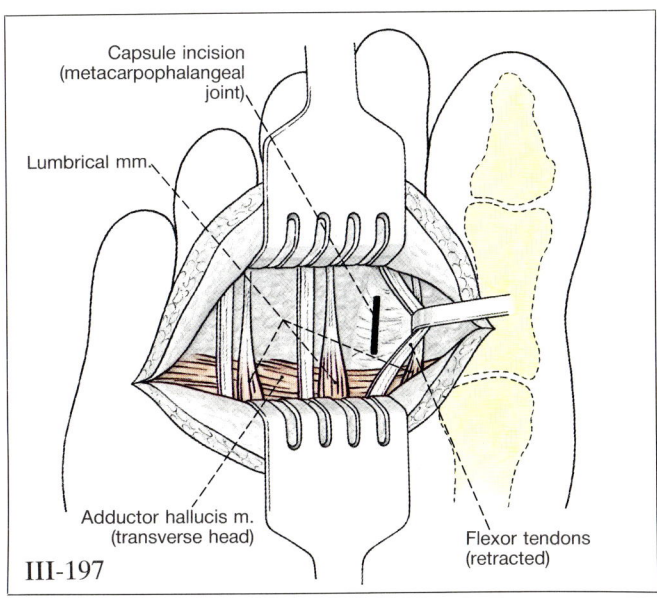

III-197

Alternative

The plantar exposure (Fig. III-198) can also begin with an elliptical skin incision. Removal of the piece of skin will cause a plantar pull on the toes during subsequent reapproximation of the skin edges.

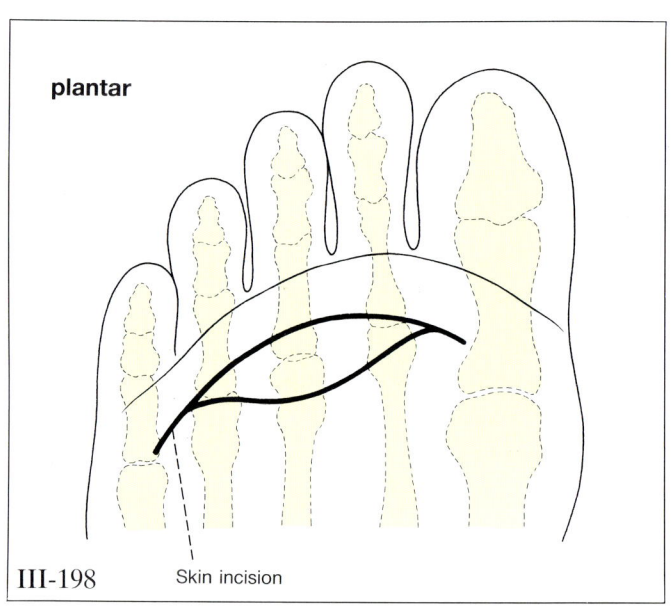

III-198 Skin incision

Proximal Interphalangeal Joint

Anterior Exposure

Indication

Hammer toe operation of *Hohmann*

Operative Steps

1. Make an approximately 2-cm-long longitudinal incision (Fig. III-199, skin incision A) over the proximal interphalangeal joint; alternatively, encircle a corn (Fig. III-199, skin incision B).
2. A bayonet-shaped incision over the proximal interphalangeal joint (Fig. III-200) gives the option of transverse removal of a corn (Fig. III-200, skin incision B).

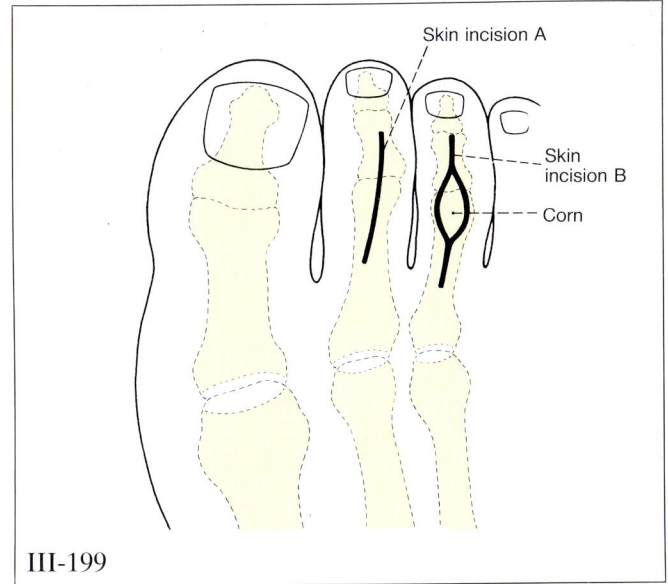

III-199

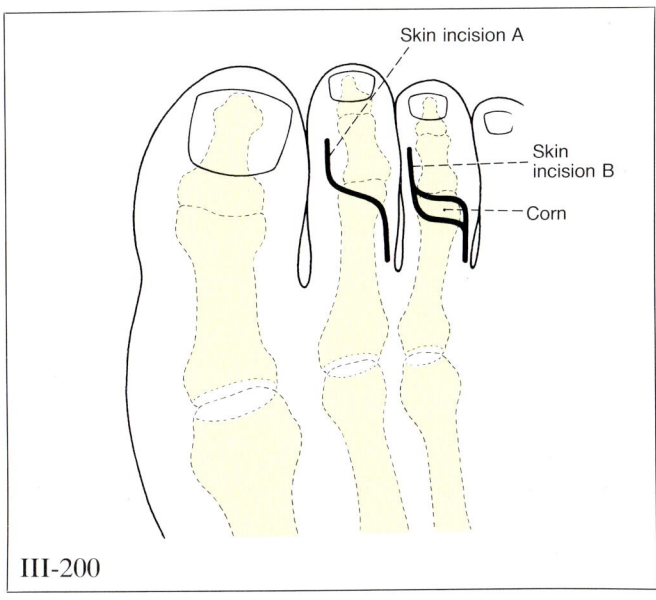

III-200

Proximal Interphalangeal Joint — Anterior Exposure

3. After exposing the extensor tendon, split it longitudinally and reflect the parts medially and laterally (Fig. III-201).
4. Split the joint capsule longitudinally and the proximal interphalangeal joint is exposed (Fig. III-202).
5. For an augmented exposure of the joint, use a scalpel to detach the capsule from the head of the proximal phalanx and the base of the middle phalanx.

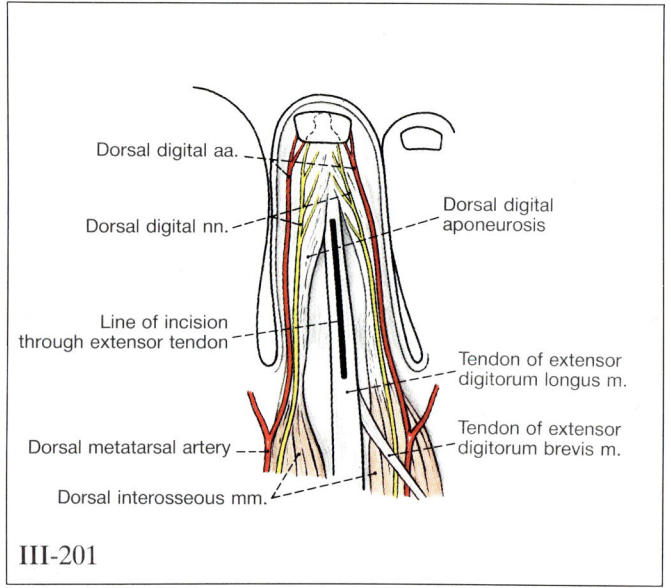

III-201

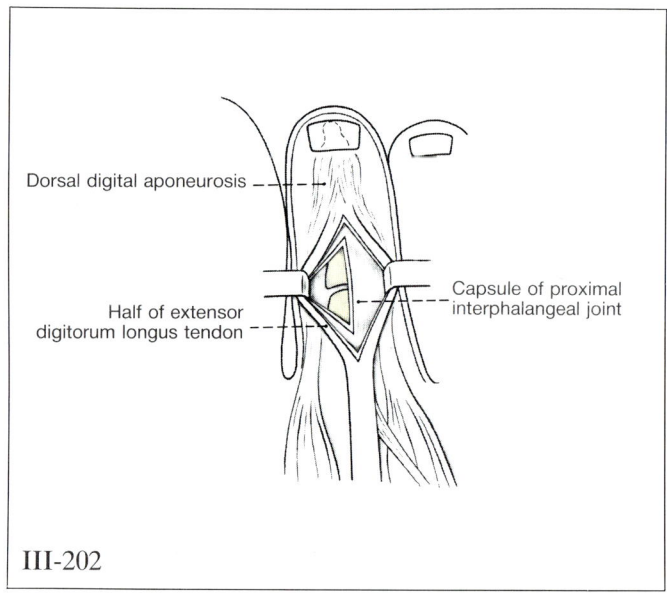

III-202

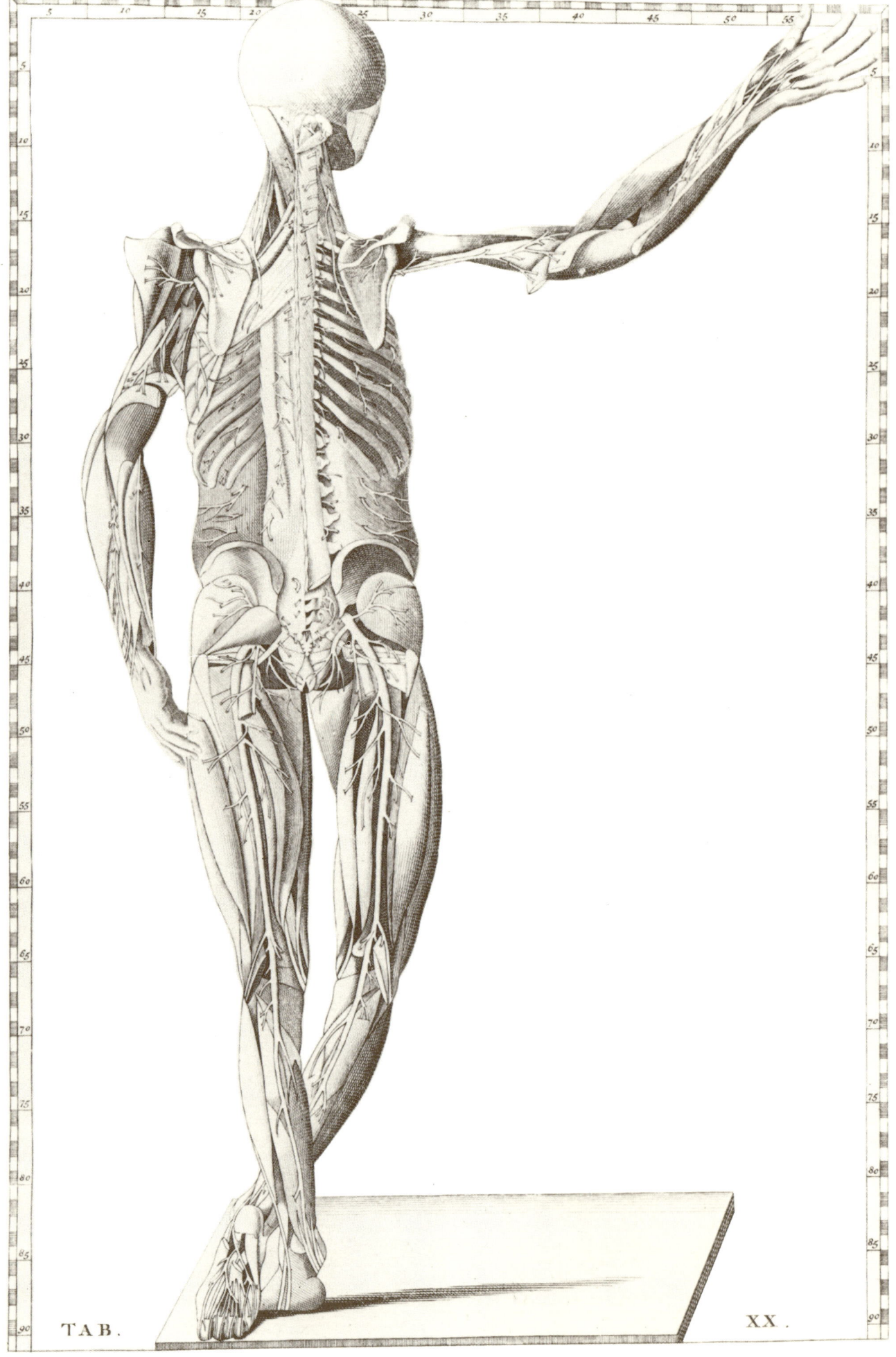

TAB. XX.